Peter J. Polverini
Editor

# Personalized Oral Health Care

## From Concept Design to Clinical Practice

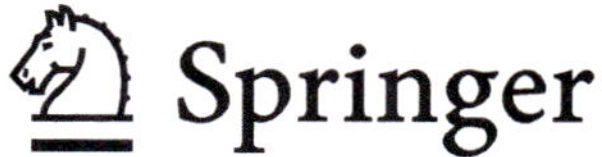

*Editor*
Peter J. Polverini
School of Dentistry
The University of Michigan
Ann Arbor, Michigan
USA

ISBN 978-3-319-23296-6 ISBN 978-3-319-23297-3 (eBook)
DOI 10.1007/978-3-319-23297-3

Library of Congress Control Number: 2015960763

Springer Cham Heidelberg New York Dordrecht London


Printed on acid-free paper

Springer International Publishing AG Switzerland is part of Springer Science+Business Media (www.springer.com)

# Preface

Personalized health care is an emerging concept that has gained considerable momentum in recent years. It is a system of care that proposes shifting the focus of care from disease management to disease prevention and health management, with a greater emphasis on prevention, risk assessment, and preemptive intervention. The future dental practice environment will no doubt place much more emphasis on disease prevention and on assessing disease risk. New technologies will provide dentists with greater capabilities to predict early disease onset and minimize disease progression and thus initiate treatment earlier that it is more cost-effective. This concept of personalized health care will have a transformative effect on the oral health-care system. If dentistry is to be part of this new health-care environment, future practitioners must be able to utilize the most up-to-date technologies that will enable risk assessment and facilitate the creation of a personalized health plan for their patients.

Many of these new technologies designed to aid in point-of-care decisions about disease risk or early diagnoses are evolving rapidly and reflect technological and knowledge-driven advances in genomics, proteomics, and metabolomics. It will no longer be necessary for dentists to rely solely on clinical biomarkers to assess disease onset and progression. Rather, the identification of patient-specific molecular profiles that reveal disease susceptibility or predict early disease onset will be among the principal tools used by the new practitioner. Genomic medicine will be a major catalyst in the implementation of personal oral health assessment and, along with new technologies such as salivary diagnostics, will reveal new biomarkers that will accelerate the evolution of personalized oral health care.

The driving force behind the movement to interprofessional education and collaborative practice is the acknowledged need to implement a holistic approach to health care to improve the overall quality of care. It is widely acknowledged that optimal patient care can only be achieved through the application of evidence-based practice, with a focus on quality improvement and through the participation of health professionals working in interdisciplinary teams that utilize the most up-to-date technology. The impetus for changing the culture of health professional education and care delivery is multifactorial, including not only safety issues but also fragmentation of health-care delivery, rising health-care costs, inadequate technological infrastructure for sharing information electronically, the movement to patient-centered health-care homes, and impending health reform.

With this background we have attempted to provide the reader with an overview of this emerging field of personalized oral health care. The topics chosen begin with a description by Dr. Harold Slavkin of what personalized health care will look like in a contemporary health-care environment. It continues with a description by Dr. Alex Vieira of how genomic technology will be applied to disease diagnosis and prevention, and Dr. Lynn Johnson describes how information technology will provide a platform for integrating patient information across the health disciplines. Dr. Nisha D'Silva discusses how discovery science has revealed important new biomarkers for oral cancer diagnosis and therapy. Dr. Will Giannobile describes the potential use of companion diagnostics and genetic testing in the dental office. Dr. Yvonne Kapila discusses how the field of metabolomics is being used as a "physiological fingerprint" of patients and thus is used to reveal important insights into a variety of diseases and patient responses to therapy. The application of genetic testing to risk assessment of two of the most common chronic oral diseases, dental caries and periodontal disease, is discussed by Dr. Tim Wright and Dr. Carlos Garaicoa-Pazmino et al., respectively. As we gain more insight into the genetic basis of chronic orofacial pain, Dr. Alex DaSilva provides a concise overview of how this information is being used to develop new strategies to diagnose and treat chronic orofacial pain. The last three chapters address the curricular changes that need to occur in dental education to prepare future practitioners for a personalized oral health-care environment (Dr. Peter Polverini), how personalized oral health care will impact health-care policy (Dr. Burton Edelstein), and what some of the opportunities and challenges are that will shape the future personalized oral health-care environment (Dr. Peter Polverini).

We hope this book stimulates broad discussion of this topic and stimulates additional research into the biological, social, and economic implications of this emerging approach to health care.

Ann Arbor, MI, USA Peter J. Polverini

# Contents

# Contributors

**Nisha J. D'Silva, BDS, MSD, PhD** Division of Oral Medicine, Pathology and Radiology, Department of Periodontics and Oral Medicine, University of Michigan School of Dentistry, Ann Arbor, MI, USA

**Alexandre F. DaSilva, DDS, DMedSc** Biologic and Material Sciences Department, University of Michigan School of Dentistry, Ann Arbor, MI, USA

**Ann M. Decker, DMD** Department of Periodontics and Oral Medicine, University of Michigan School of Dentistry, Ann Arbor, MI, USA

**Burton L. Edelstein, DDS, MPH** Section of Population Oral Health, Columbia University College of Dental Medicine, New York, NY, USA

Children's Dental Health Project, Washington, DC, USA

**Carlos Garaicoa-Pazmino, DDS** Department of Periodontics and Oral Medicine, University of Michigan School of Dentistry, Ann Arbor, MI, USA

**William V. Giannobile, DDS, DMedSc** Department of Periodontics and Oral Medicine, University of Michigan School of Dentistry, Ann Arbor, MI, USA

Department of Biomedical Engineering, College of Engineering, Ann Arbor, MI, USA

**Lynn A. Johnson, PhD** Periodontics and Oral Medicine, University of Michigan, School of Dentistry, Ann Arbor, MI, USA

**Yvonne L. Kapila, DDS, PhD** Department of Periodontics and Oral Medicine, University of Michigan, School of Dentistry, Ann Arbor, MI, USA

**Alexandra B. Plonka, DDS** Department of Periodontics and Oral Medicine, University of Michigan School of Dentistry, Ann Arbor, MI, USA

**Peter J. Polverini, DDS, DMSc** Department of Periodontics and Oral Medicine, University of Michigan School of Dentistry, Ann Arbor, MI, USA

Department of Pathology, University of Michigan Medical School, Ann Arbor, MI, USA

**Eileen Quintero, MSI** Division of Dental Informatics, University of Michigan School of Dentistry, Ann Arbor, MI, USA

**Harold C. Slavkin** Division of Biomedical Sciences, University of Southern California, Los Angeles, CA, USA

**Alexandre R. Vieira, DDS, MS, PhD** Department of Oral Biology, University of Pittsburgh School of Dental Medicine, Pittsburgh, PA, USA

**J. Tim Wright, DDS, MS** Department of Pediatric Dentistry, University of North Carolina School of Dentistry, Chapel Hill, NC, USA

# Abbreviations

| | |
|---|---|
| ACOs | Accountable care organizations |
| AGEs | Advanced glycation end products |
| AJCC | American Joint Committee on Cancer |
| aMCC | Anterior mid-cingulate cortices |
| ATM | Ataxia telangiectasia |
| BAA | Business associate agreement |
| Bcl2 | B-cell lymphoma 2 |
| CDC | Centers for Disease Control and Prevention |
| CGES | Clinical genome and exome sequencing |
| CGM | Continuous glucose monitoring [system] |
| CHF | Congestive heart failure |
| CHRT | Center for Health Research and Transformation |
| CMMI | Center for Medicare and Medicaid Innovation |
| CTSC | Cathepsin C gene |
| DLPFC | Dorsolateral prefrontal cortex |
| DMFS | Decayed, missing, and filled surfaces |
| DMFT | Decayed, missing, and filled teeth |
| DNA | Deoxyribonucleic acid |
| EGF | Epidermal growth factor |
| EHR | Electronic health record |
| ELISA | Enzyme-linked immunosorbent assays |
| ENCODE | Encyclopedia of DNA Elements |
| ePHI | Electronic protected health information |
| FDA | Food and Drug Administration |
| FE | Finite element |
| fNIRS | Functional near-infrared spectroscopy |
| GAgP | Generalized aggressive periodontitis |
| GCF | Gingival crevicular fluid |
| GPS | Global positioning systems |
| GWAS | Genome-wide association studies |
| HGP | Human Genome Project |
| HHS | Health and Human Services |
| HIF | Hereditary fructose intolerance |
| HIPAA | Health Insurance Portability and Accountability Act |
| HITECH | Health Information Technology for Economic and Clinical Health [Act] |
| HPV | Human papillomavirus |

HR-MAS High-resolution magic angle spinning
HRSA Health Resources and Services Administration
ICDAS International Caries Detection and Assessment System
IL Interleukin
IOM Institute of Medicine
IT Information technology
LAgP Localized aggressive periodontitis
LHS Learning Health System
LN-Met Lymph node metastatic tissues
LOC Lab-on-a-chip
MCPM Membrane choline phospholipid metabolism
MetS Metabolic syndrome [diseases]
MMPs Matrix metalloproteinases
NAT Normal adjacent tissue
NCCN National Comprehensive Cancer Network
NCI National Cancer Institute
NHGRI National Human Genome Research Institute
NHI National Heart Institute
NHOK Normal human oral keratinocytes
NIDCR National Institute of Dental and Craniofacial Research
NIDR National Institute for Dental Research
NIH National Institutes of Health
NSF National Science Foundation
OMIM Online Mendelian Inheritance in Man®
ONC Office of the National Coordinator
OPG Osteoprotegerin
OSCC Oral squamous cell carcinoma
PBRNs Practice-Based Research Networks
PCMHs Patient-centered medical homes
PCORI Patient-Centered Outcomes Research Institute
PCR(s) Polymerase chain reaction(s)
PLS Papillon-Lefevre syndrome
POC Point-of-care
PPA Personalized physiology analytics
RANKL Receptor activator of nuclear kappa B ligand
ROS Reactive oxygen species
RSFC Resting state functional connectivity
SaaS Software as a Service
SCC(s) Squamous cell carcinoma(s)
SNPs Single nucleotide polymorphisms
tDCS Transcranial direct current stimulation
TGFa Transforming growth factor alpha
TIMPs Tissue inhibitors of MMPs
TLRs Toll-like receptors
TMD Temporomandibular disorder(s)
TMS Transcranial magnetic stimulation

| | |
|---|---|
| TNM | Tumor size, nodal involvement, and metastases |
| TNP | Trigeminal neuropathic pain |
| TP | Trigger point |
| USDA | US Department of Agriculture |
| VEGF | Vascular endothelial growth factor |
| WHO | World Health Organization |

# Personalized Oral Medicine and the Contemporary Health Care Environment

1

Harold C. Slavkin

**Abstract**

There are major drivers required to realize the "tipping point" for personalized oral medicine—the scientific foundation, proof of principle to precede implementation, and a cultural and economic environment that celebrates innovation and emphasizes quality and cost-effective health prevention. In Malcolm Gladwell's acclaimed book *The Tipping Point*, he argues that success, such as emergence of Social Security legislation in the mid-1930s, Medicare and Civil Rights legislation in the 1960s, the recently enacted Affordable Health Care Act, and even personalized oral medicine, is dependent on people with social gifts at a specific time and place in history. We are about to reach the "tipping point" when society, patients, health policy and governments, industry, and health professionals embrace personalized diagnosis, treatment plans, therapeutics, and procedures that optimize comprehensive and cost-effective health care with predictable outcomes for all people. The completion of the Human Genome Project (HGP), recent cost-effective and rapid whole genome-wide sequencing methods, and instrumentation, along with bioinformatics to handle and annotate data collections, enable clinicians to formulate decisions based upon the patient's genotype and phenotype. Despite challenges, now is the time for health professionals to prepare for personalized oral medicine through pre- and postgraduate education programs.

## Introduction

What's missing in primary health care? Among all of the complex issues required to optimize health care in the United States, we need to align and integrate mental, vision, and oral care into primary health care for all people at all stages of the lifespan—from conception through hospice

H.C. Slavkin
Division of Biomedical Sciences, Center for Craniofacial Molecular Biology, Herman Ostrow School of Dentistry, University of Southern California, Los Angeles, CA, USA
e-mail: Slavkin@usc.edu; hslavk@gmail.com





P.J. Polverini (ed.), *Personalized Oral Health Care: From Concept Design to Clinical Practice*,
DOI 10.1007/978-3-319-23297-3_1

care. First, we must coordinate understanding of our patients' phenotype with their unique genotype [1]. Enter personalized oral medicine. Three significant steps must be recognized and completed to establish personalized oral medicine. First, complete the Human Genome Project (HGP) costing 1–2 % of the National Institutes of Health (NIH) budget from 1988 to October 2004. Second, accelerate scientific discoveries, informatics, and their translation to clinical practice in the post-genomic era (2004 through 2014 and beyond). Third, analyze and diffuse information, knowledge, and technology to educate health care policy makers, to recruit health professionals (medicine, dentistry, pharmacy, nursing and allied health professions) into personalized oral medicine, and to educate the larger society as to the value of their personal and unique medical and dental history, family history, human and microbial genomics, pharmacogenomics, and the cost-effective benefits derived from prospective health care. The first two steps have been completed!

Let's revisit the first point. Just 15 years ago, June 26, 2000, President Bill Clinton and UK Prime Minister Tony Blair received the "95 % working draft" of the human genome from the publically funded, international HGP led by Francis Collins of the NIH, and the private, for-profit company Celera Genomics led by Chief Scientist Craig Venter [2–4]. "Without a doubt, this is the most important and most wondrous map ever produced by mankind," announced President Clinton as he began his remarks [2]. In attendance were the teams of scientists and the scientific leadership of various federal agencies at the East Room of the White House (this author was in attendance as Director, National Institute of Dental and Craniofacial Research–NIDCR). The US federal consortium for the HGP led by Francis Collins included National Institutes of Health (NIH); Centers for Disease Control and Prevention (CDC); the Department of Energy; the Food and Drug Administration (FDA); Health and Human Services (HHS) Secretary's Advisory Committee on Genetics, Health, and Society; Health Resources and Services Administration (HRSA); National Science Foundation (NSF); and the US Department of Agriculture (USDA). The US federal program-sponsored sequencing was performed in 20 universities and research centers in the US, United Kingdom, Japan, France, Germany, and China. The cost from 1988 to 2003 was $3 billion appropriated by the US Congress. The competing Craig Venter private Celera Genomics venture was initiated in 1998 and cost $300 million.

The HGP is the most ambitious biological research program ever undertaken by either governments or the private sector. The mission is to map all the genes in the entire three-billion-letter genetic code embodied within DNA in each of the ten trillion of human somatic cells in one person. The six feet in length of DNA within each cell nucleus contains 23 pairs of chromosomes containing functional genes (genes that encode enzymes, regulation of cell processes, and structural genes such as collagens, keratins, and beyond) and (nonfunctioning) pseudo-genes. In addition, we possess additional functional genes in the maternally inherited mitochondrial DNA and, of course, the unique DNA found within each of the 100 trillions of microorganisms that comprise the human microbiome (oral cavity included). Conceptually, the nuclear, mitochondrial, and microbial sources of DNA have become "the human genome."

Thereafter, the complete human nuclear genome sequence, including 21,000 functional and 19,000 nonfunctional or pseudo-genes, was published in April 2003 and finalized in 2004 [5]. This treasure trove of information was rapidly used to identify countless genes involved in health and disease in humans, primates, mice, chickens, fish, roundworms, and fruit flies. In tandem, numerous studies explored the biological function(s) of genes and investigated chromatin (histone and non-histone chromosomal proteins) and epigenetics, and small RNAs as regulatory elements. These and related studies were launched and catalogued by the National Human Genome Research Institute (NHGRI) as Encyclopedia of DNA Elements (ENCODE) [6]. This remarkable effort focused on how genes are regulated vis-à-vis alternative splicing (one gene generates multiple and different mRNA transcripts), gene–gene interactions, epigenetics (e.g., acetylation, methylation), as well as an array of gene mutations operant during embryonic development as well as postnatal life.

The year 2000 was also the year in which Malcolm Gladwell published his first book *The Tipping Point* [7]. According to Gladwell, "Specific types of people are responsible for bringing about large levels of change" [7]. Arguably, "the biological revolution," in the words of Sir Francis Crick, offers personalized health care as a tipping point for this time in history—from the discovery of the structure and suggested functions of DNA and the clinical applications from genomics and pharmacogenomics to the realization of tissue and organ regeneration.

We now live in an era of molecular dentistry and medicine, an era that is delivering innovative ways to prevent, diagnose, treat, and even cure the diseases and disorders that inflict mortality and morbidity upon the human condition [8–30]. As we ponder the near future, we need to recognize that complex human diseases or multifactorial genetic diseases are the most common forms of human genetic disease (e.g., non-Mendelian craniofacial birth defects, tooth decay, periodontal diseases, head and neck cancers, chronic craniofacial–oral–dental pain conditions); these do not present well-delineated Mendelian patterns of inheritance but tend to be expressed within families. Meanwhile, the emerging opportunity for prospective health care will shift the emphasis from disease treatment and management to prevention and wellness management [29].

The second point needs some clarification. In the decade following the completion of the HGP in 2004 (2004–2014), standing upon the shoulders of the previous 60 years of accomplishments derived from "the biological revolution", is termed the post-genomic decade. This decade contained spectacular advances in science—notably the International HapMap Project, ENCODE, numerous advances in nucleic acid sequencing technology, bioinformatics for large and complex genetic data, the completion with annotation of two dozen published individual human genomes including that of James Watson and the complete sequence of Craig Venter [30–33], and instrumentation and associated technologies that significantly reduced costs, increased accuracy, and increased speed for complete individual human genome-wide sequencing [33–36]. Today a complete human genome can be sequenced within 12 h for a cost of $1000 per patient [35, 36].

Finally, the third remaining point needs some explanation. Using Gladwell's terms, numerous connectors, mavens, and salesmen lectured and wrote peer-reviewed journal articles about the expanding foundation for personalized oral medicine with enormous implications, opportunities, and challenges for health professionals. These efforts continue, and many recommendations are now found in the most recent NIDCR Strategic Plan (2014–2019) [37]. Included within this strategic plan is a call to expand the foundation for personalized or precision oral medicine [38].

In Gladwell's definition, "a tipping point is the moment of critical mass, the threshold, the boiling point" [7]. In his analysis, the tipping point is reached as a result of "The law of the few"; the men and women cited above would be considered "connectors" or people in a community who know large numbers of people and who are used to making introductions; they facilitate change through large social networks [7]. In addition, and often not heralded, are another group of people who function as "information specialists" or "mavens"; they propagate "word-of-mouth epidemics." Finally, again based on Gladwell's model, there are "salesmen" or persuaders who are often charismatic people with highly effective negotiation skills such as news anchors Walter Cronkite (CBS) and Peter Jennings (ABC). Of course, for the social or cultural epidemic to flourish, it requires the nexus formed by Gladwell's "The Law of the Few" (connectors, mavens, and salesmen), "The Stickiness Factor" (based on the specific content of a message), and always "The Power of Context," meaning within a specific time and place in human history [7].

## Purpose of This Chapter

This chapter provides background, challenges, and opportunities to enable the reader to celebrate and champion personalized oral medicine as an integral to primary health care [1, 8–14, 16, 17, 25–27, 29, 37, 38]. Arguably, *the* grand challenge remaining of the post-genomic era is to gain a detailed understanding of the heritable variation within the human genome [19, 20, 23–27, 33–36]. Characterization of this genetic variation among individuals, and within families, communities, and populations will illuminate the essential clinical understanding of differential susceptibility to disease, differential response to therapeutics (pharmacogenomics), and the complex interaction of genetic and environmental factors that result in specific phenotypes [30–36].

As we approach the tipping point, transformational changes in health care are clearly in view, driven by advances in science and technology, with convergence of information and knowledge spanning diverse fields of inquiry. One formidable factor is that national health care spending reached $2.5 trillion in 2009. The economic recession and rising unemployment in many sectors, plus the changing demographics and baby boomers aging into Medicare, predict significant influences on health care spending from 2009 to 2019 to reach $4.5 trillion [39]. As a result, federal and state government spending will account for more than half of all US health care spending by 2019 [39].

In part, the tipping point will materialize from social pressures and the economics of health care. In tandem, we will gain a deeper understanding of signaling pathways, molecular interactions, and increasing numbers of novel biomarkers that indicate health and wellness as well as the diagnosis and progression of disease [6, 15, 17, 19–28, 34, 38]. Further, the craniofacial–oral–dental complex provides many opportunities to assess risk, stratify patients as to relative risk or susceptibility, prevent and diagnose diseases and disorders, and inform and guide therapeutics (pharmacogenomics) and other treatments [37, 40].

Health professionals know that the craniofacial–oral–dental complex can be readily accessed and repeatedly sampled for tooth decay (dental caries) development and progression; periodontal diseases; saliva as an informative body fluid; biofilm-associated microorganisms on tooth, prostheses, and mucosal surfaces; and oral mucosal tissue lesions, with minimal difficulty or patient discomfort [1, 10, 40–46]. We are on the threshold of interprofessional primary health care that includes mental, vision, and oral health professionals. Now is the time for health professionals to prepare for the arrival of personalized oral medicine [1, 8–14, 16, 17, 23, 25, 27, 29, 37, 38].

## Agents of Change (Connectors, Mavens, and Salesmen): The Essential Scientific Foundation and Proof of Principle

Prior to, during, and following World War II, a series of "little things" can easily be identified that make a big difference. The realization and organization of these "little things" can eventually reach a critical mass, the threshold, the boiling point, and be named "The Tipping Point" [7]. In no small measure, progress in the biological and related health sciences has been and continues to be the result of people with unique talents as described as "connectors, mavens, and salesmen" using the terms of Gladwell [7]. What follows here are a few examples that eventually will result in the tipping point for personalized oral health.

## Phenotype vs. Genotype

Although the study of genetics began before Johann Gregor Mendel, his innovations using phenotypic characteristics of pea plants (e.g., color, shape, texture) in the 1860s resulted in a theory of inheritance based upon three profound principles: (1) an organism's phenotype (what it looks like, how it functions, how it behaves) cannot be used as a basis for determining the organism's genotype (the organism's genomics); (2) the law of segregation states that genes retain their individuality and do not combine to form a new blended trait; and (3) the law of independent assortment states that every gene has both dominant and recessive forms, which explains in part why traits can skip generations. Mendel's work was not initially recognized and remained obscure until the twentieth century when it was recognized in the "fly room" at Columbia University in New York [47, 48].

## The First Pieces of the DNA Puzzle

The year 1869 was the landmark year in genetic research when Friedrich Miescher first identified what he called "nuclein" within the nucleus of white blood cells (the term "nuclein") soon became "nucleic acid" and then "deoxyribonucleic acid" (DNA) [49]. Thereafter, discrete studies by Phoebus Levene and Erwin Chargaff independently contributed critical details of the DNA molecule [50].

### Chromosomes Carry Genes

Walter Sutton and Theodor Boveri demonstrated in 1902 that chromosomes carry genetic material as critically analyzed by Victor McKusick [51]. Thomas Hunt Morgan and colleagues deduced that the gene for color blindness must lie on the X chromosome because of its distinctive pattern of inheritance—fathers did not pass it on to sons, and it was rare among women. Morgan's team, working at Columbia University, conducted a series of additional experiments on the fruit fly to determine how a mutation would be inherited. From these studies, they concluded that specific mutated genes are carried on specific chromosomes. This series of discoveries and the elegant analyses of the evidence formed the foundation for their classic treatise *The Mechanism of Mendelian Heredity* published in 1915 [52].

### DNA Causes Bacterial Transformation

Oswald Avery and his colleagues suggested in 1944 that DNA, rather than a protein as widely believed at that time, may be the actual hereditary material of bacteria, transferred between bacteria, and could be analogous to genes found in viruses, yeast, plants, and animals [53].

*A dentist isolates and purifies the first DNA samples used for X-ray diffraction studies by Rosalind Franklin that provided the essential evidence from adenoviral DNA used by James Watson and Francis Crick.* It was Norman Simmons, a dental graduate of 1939 from the Harvard School of Dental Medicine in Boston and PhD in Experimental Pathology from Rochester University in 1950, who isolated and purified the DNA used by Rosalind Franklin in the early 1950s [54–56]. It was Irwin Chargaff who discovered that A (adenosine) hybridizes to T (thymidine) and C (cytosine) hybridizes to G (guanosine) [50]—combined with the critical observations from X-ray crystallography work by Rosalind Franklin, Norman Simmons, and Maurice Wilkins—that contributed to Watson and Crick's derivation of the three-dimensional, double-helical model for the DNA structure [57].

## Post-World War II Progress in Many Areas

Political leadership and the dreadful legacy from the war motivated international and domestic economic, educational, and social changes of great magnitude. The creation of the United Nations with the World Health Organization (WHO), the GI Bill in the USA, the legislation for building land grant universities and interstate highways, the Marshall Plan to rebuild Europe, the rebuilding of Japan, and significant immigration of outstanding scientists to the USA (prior to and following WW II), each served as discrete yet synergistic advances that increased support for biomedical, physical, chemical, and behavioral sciences [58–60]. Vannevar Bush, director of the Office of Science and Technology in Roosevelt's administration, had a plan for the NIH that was eventually realized in 1948 with the National Institute for Dental Research (NIDR), the National Cancer Institute (NCI), and the National Heart Institute (NHI) [59, 60].

In tandem, physics, engineering, computations, and communications were each accelerated through major investments from industry, government (Departments of Defense, Energy, and Agriculture as well as the National Science Foundation), and a number of not-for-profit foundations. These significant investments rapidly translated into increased numbers of engineers, scientists, health care professionals, and associated health care support industries (manufacturing, distribution, insurance, technology support).

*A dentist, Robert Ledley, was one of the first to envision using computers to create a mathematized biology that would enhance computerized medical (and dental) diagnosis.* Professor Robert Stevens Ledley (a dental graduate of the New York University School of Dentistry of 1948 and MS in Physics from Columbia University in 1950) recruited childhood friend Margaret Oakley Dayhoff to join him at the National Biomedical Research Foundation at Georgetown University Medical Center in 1960. Dayhoff was the first person to establish a computer-based biological database. By 1962, these two highly gifted individuals worked together to cooperate, collaborate, and develop the field of informatics with computer programs to aid in the experimental determination of proteins based upon the genetic code for each amino acid as found in messenger as well as unique transfer RNAs [61–63]. Thereafter, hundreds of discrete discoveries with computer programs, instrumentation, and high-throughput gene and protein sequencing resulted in biology experiencing many of the same changes that revolutionized physics and chemistry in the twentieth century [61–63]. Imagine biology, before computers, polymerase chain reactions (PCR) [64], rapid sequencing of DNA and RNA, genomics, pharmacogenomics, bioinformatics, and the enormous opportunities for government and venture capital funding with unlimited applications for improving the human condition [1, 5, 6, 18–20, 22–27, 34–36, 61, 65].

## Return on Investments in Oral Medicine

On June 26, 1948, President Harry Truman signed into law the creation of the National Institute for Dental Research (NIDR) [60, 66, 67]. Along with the institutes for cancer and heart diseases and disorders, NIDR invested federal funds to address the societal needs to understand, treat, manage, and eventually prevent craniofacial–oral–dental diseases and disorders [60, 66]. Investments were required for building a scientific research workforce through training grants and fellowships. Investments were required to build facilities and infrastructure within the intramural as well as extramural communities [60, 66, 67]. The first major accomplishment was derived from chemistry and demonstrated in clinical trials that fluoride in drinking water produced a significant reduction in tooth decay and, thereafter, became a major public health tool to improve public health [59, 60, 66].

Numerous investments followed, such as the creation of the very first Intramural Genetics Branch within the NIH Campus in 1957 to address genetic diseases of the craniofacial–oral–dental complex, led by Carl Witkop [60, 66, 67]. Witkop received his DDS from the University of Michigan in 1949 and MS in Oral Pathology in 1950. His interests focused primarily on hereditary abnormalities of the teeth, pigment metabolism abnormalities, and oral manifestations of hereditary dermatological conditions. In tandem, federal funding also supported research, translational and clinical, related to periodontal disease, congenital and acquired craniofacial malformations, autoimmune diseases, tooth and bone diseases, infectious diseases and disorders, acute and chronic pain, and human behavior, as well as basic research investigations of neoplastic diseases, cell migrations, extracellular matrix molecules, mechanisms of invertebrate as well as vertebrate biomineralization, genetic mechanisms that control growth and development, oral mucosal immunology, oral microbiology (viruses, bacteria, yeast), genomics of specific pathogens, the oral microbiome, FaceBase, and much more [58–60, 66–74].

More recently, investments were made in gene therapy associated with the production of saliva [10], biomimetics studies for tooth and root regeneration, and much more. Collectively, the return on investments has profoundly improved the oral health of the American people (and beyond), and there is much yet to be accomplished looking to the future [1, 8–14, 16, 17, 25–27, 29, 34, 37–39, 46,

67]. In particular, current efforts are focused to reduce or eliminate craniofacial–oral–dental health disparities; to reduce or eliminate tooth decay, oral cancers, periodontal diseases, temporomandibular joint diseases, Sjogren's diseases, and neurological diseases and disorders (e.g., Bell's palsy, trigeminal neuralgia, chronic facial neuropathies); and to improve the management of chronic facial pain (Table 1.1)

**Table 1.1** Discrete step toward "tipping point" for personalized oral medicine

| Date | Accomplishment |
|---|---|
| 1861 | Principles of Inheritance (JG Mendel) |
| 1944 | DNA and Bacterial Transformation (Avery) |
| 1950s | Preparation of DNA for crystallography (Simmons/Franklin) |
| 1953 | Structure/Function DNA (Watson and Crick) |
| 1964 | Genetic Code, mRNA, tRNAs, transcription (Nirenberg team and others) |
| 1970s | Recombinant DNA technology (Boyer, Rutter, and others) |
| 1988–2004 | Human Genome Project (HGP) (Collins' team and Venter's team) |
| 1980s–Present | Candidate genes for diseases and gene therapy translational medicine/dentistry |
| 1990s–Present | Head and Neck Cancer Genome (NIDCR and NCI, Hosts) |
| 2000–Present | Single nucleotide polymorphisms (SNPs) |
| 2000–Present | Mendelian versus complex human diseases and disorders, gene–gene and gene–environment interactions, epigenetics, and major chronic diseases |
| 2008–Present | Genome-wide association scans (GWAS) for craniofacial–oral–dental diseases and disorders (e.g., tooth decay, periodontal diseases, craniofacial pain, head and neck cancers) |
| 2010–Present | Personalized oral medicine |
| 2011 | Exome sequencing of solid tumors from head and neck squamous cell carcinoma |
| 2013 | FDA approval for rapid genome sequencing from Illumina ($1000 genome in 12 h) |
| 2014 | Toward the "tipping point" for personalized health care |
| 2015 | U.S. Federal support for precision or personalized medicine and dentistry |

## Examples from Genomic Applications for Congenital and Acquired Craniofacial–Oral–Dental Diseases and Disorders

The following highlights a few selected examples from applications derived from the HGP in the post-genomic era (2004–2014). Genetic factors are at the root cause of numerous diseases and disorders, including congenital non-syndromic (e.g., cleft lip and cleft palate) and syndromic craniofacial anomalies (e.g., craniosynostosis, ectodermal dysplasia), dental anomalies (e.g., number, shape, timing of eruption and tooth replacement, amelogenesis imperfecta, and molecular biology of enamel gene products), periodontal diseases (i.e., inherited Mendelian as well as complex human multigene, gene–environment, diseases), tooth decay (dental caries), and oropharyngeal cancer [1, 8–14, 16, 17, 25–27, 29, 37, 38, 47, 52, 60–81]. Genome-derived information has been shown to enable a more comprehensive understanding of disease etiology and permits earlier diagnosis, allowing for preventive measures prior to disease onset and progression [1, 8, 9, 13, 14, 81–84]. As a generality, genetic mutations in polarizing signals (e.g., Shh, BMPs, Wnt5a, Smad2-4), growth factors and their cognate receptors (Egf and Egfr, Fgfs and Fgfrs), transcriptional factors (Dlx, Hox, Pitx2, Tbx22), cell cycle regulation factors (e.g., p53), cell adhesion molecules (E-cadherin, connexin43), and extracellular matrix molecules (e.g., Col2A1, Mmp2, Timp1-3, laminins, fibronectins) are implicated in the genetic variances that cause diseases and disorders. These examples provide "proof of principle" for personalized oral medicine and provide rapid determination of risk and precise personal diagnostics [1, 9, 11, 21, 22, 24, 28, 30, 33, 83].

*The most common diseases affecting the US population are complex disorders that result from defects in multiple genetically controlled systems in response to environmental challenges.* Human diseases such as childhood obesity, periodontal diseases, tooth decay, head and neck cancers, cardiovascular diseases, cerebrovascular diseases, type 2 diabetes, chronic obstructive pulmonary disorders, schizophrenia, and dementias (including Alzheimer's disease) each demonstrate complex genetic inheritance that will require sophisticated analysis. For example, metabolic syndrome diseases (MetS) are a global pandemic of enormous health, economic, and social concern that affects a significant portion of the world's population [83]. MetS includes abdominal obesity, hyperglycemia, hypertriglyceridemia, low high-density lipoprotein cholesterol, hypertension, periodontal disease, and type 2 diabetes mellitus, based upon European studies [84]. However, geography and ethnicity provide further variations within African, Hispanic, and/or Asian populations. For example, type 2 diabetes has a unique gene mutation found in Hispanic people [85].

## Exploring the Genomics of Periodontal Diseases

Periodontal diseases represent complex human diseases of the oral cavity. They are characterized by inflammatory responses associated with hard as well as soft tissues within the periodontium in response to commensal and pathogenic oral microorganisms (oral microbiome). These conditions are associated with a number of systemic associations along with macro- and micro-environmental factors (e.g., age, gender, ethnicity, family health history, obesity, cardiovascular disease, type 2 diabetes, pregnancy, smoking, diet, hygiene habits) [66, 69, 83–91]. In addition to the cardinal signs of inflammation, periodontal diseases present other phenotypes including gingival pocket formation, clinical attachment loss (measured in millimeters), bleeding upon probing examination, and loss of tooth-supporting alveolar bone as assessed by radiographic examination and tooth mobility [86–88]. As the disease progresses, tooth mobility and chronic destruction of soft and hard tissue are readily apparent. Periodontal diseases are presented in 40 % of the adult US population and are considered to be the primary cause of tooth loss among adults [86, 87].

The author is using "diseases" advisedly and offers that critical observations, documentations, and assessments of clinical phenotypes are profoundly important toward correlation of phenotype with genotype (e.g., phenomics) [1, 92]. This is particularly important when considering periodontal disease(s) as related to age, gender, ethnicity, composition of biofilms, and systemic diseases (e.g., type 2 diabetes, insulin levels, gonadotrophic hormone levels, puberty, pregnancy, obesity) [11, 12, 69, 83–91]. For example, epidemiologic studies indicate that biofilm-induced gingival inflammation is universal in children and adolescents without any evidence of gingival tissue or alveolar bone destruction. This condition is typically called gingivitis (without periodontal disease). However, children and adolescents can present the signs and symptoms of chronic destructive periodontal disease with soft tissue and bone loss. These children and adolescents present with rapid, destructive bone loss localized to permanent incisors and first molar teeth. This is termed localized aggressive periodontitis (LAgP). Another observation is found in children and adolescents with more teeth associated with destructive bone loss, and this is termed generalized aggressive periodontitis (GAgP).

Each example demonstrates an association with age, gender, and ethnicity, as well as with systemic disease associations and hormonal levels associated with puberty. Each would be considered non-Mendelian inheritance (single gene mutation) but rather as a complex human disease (multiple gene variances with gene–environment interactions). A number of significant research opportunities arise with respect to genome-wide association studies (GWAS) to identify multiple gene variances correlated with specific clinical phenotypes [82–91].

Meanwhile, Papillon–Lefevre syndrome (PLS) is an autosomal recessive disorder characterized by palmoplantar hyperkeratosis and severe early onset generalized aggressive periodontitis that results in premature loss of the primary and secondary dentitions. A major gene locus for PLS is mapped to a 2.8-centaMorgan interval on chromosome 11q14. This region contains six known genes including the lysosomal protease cathepsin C gene (CTSC) [14, 82]. A number of significant research opportunities arise related to understanding the functions of CTSC as related to periodontal disease susceptibility within complex diseases. What regulates tissue-specific gene expression of cathepsin C [82]? In addition to the cardinal features of PLS, PLS patients are reported to present increased susceptibility to infection, and this may reflect additional effects of specific cathepsin C mutations or the epigenetic effects from other gene loci. Further complications arise in that all PLS patients do not show CTSC mutations, yet their phenotype aligns well with ectodermal dysplasias.

In these examples the reader should appreciate that genotyping is critically dependent upon astute clinical observations that enable understanding of how gene variance results correlate with phenotype in health or disease. The reader should realize that genome GWAS identify hundreds of genetic variants associated with complex human diseases and traits. However, most genetic variants so far confer small increments in risk and explain a small portion of familial clustering. This inevitably leads questions as to how to explain "missing" heritability [91–93].

A number of recent studies demonstrate that 45 % of genetic variance can be explained by considering all SNPs simultaneously [19, 23–25, 92–94]. The emerging approach to complex human diseases is to consider incomplete linkage disequilibrium between causal variants and genotyped SNPs and to employ stringent significance tests to large data sets. This was employed to demonstrate that common SNPs explain a large proportion of the heritability for human height [92].

## Exploring the Genomics of Tooth Decay

The number one chronic disease of children and adults is tooth decay or "dental caries." Available information demonstrates that tooth decay is a chronic disease that is caused by discrete bacteria found within the oral microbiome, excessive carbohydrates derived from the diet, host genomics as well as microbial genomics, and environmental factors. The heritability of dental caries has been estimates to be from 30 to 60 % [95–97]. This condition is a classical example of a complex human disease reflecting gene–gene and gene–environment interactions. Genome-wide association scans (GWAS) identified a number of genes associated with risk for tooth decay in children as well as adults [97].

## Exploring the Genomics of Head and Neck Cancers

Relatively common head and neck cancer phenotypes include melanoma, basal cell carcinoma, and squamous cell carcinoma. Oral squamous cell carcinoma (OSCC) is a major cause of morbidity and mortality worldwide, with presentation of more than 275,000 new cases reported each year and over 120,000 deaths every year [98]. OSCC is the sixth most common neoplastic disease in the developed world. OSCC-associated morbidity and mortality remain high and have not improved in over four decades [25, 40, 46, 58, 59]. One explanation for the lack of improvement indicates that tumor size and lymph node involvement and stage (I to IV) do not provide guidance for clinical outcome. Apart from tobacco, alcohol, and direct sunlight, human papillomavirus (HPV) infection is another known risk factor for OSCC.

OSCC results from progressive genetic changes leading to malignancy in a multistep process. Current progress in the discovery of genetic biomarkers is rapidly advancing. At this point in the journey, it is clear that one biomarker for head and neck cancers will not materialize. Rather, multiple gene-based markers associated with specific causes within specific ethnic groups will eventually become the foundation for diagnosis and therapeutics, as shown in the list here:

## Progress in Genomics of Head and Neck Squamous Cell Carcinoma (HNSCC) Tumors Using Whole-Exome Sequencing[1, 2] [99]

- TP53 is the most common gene in HNSCC, a gene that encodes p53 protein known to regulate the cell cycle, programmed cell death, DNA repair, and transcriptional control.
- NOTCH1 is the second most common gene mutation in HNSCC and also functions in blood cancer acute lymphoblastic leukemia.
- CDKN2A, PIK3CA, HRAS, and FBXW7 are other gene mutations found in HNSCC tumors and represent part of the neoplastic signature.

## Exploring the Genomics of Chronic Craniofacial–Oral–Dental Pain

Migraine headaches and temporomandibular joint and muscle disorders are the most common causes of chronic craniofacial–oral–dental pain. In 2011, the Institute of Medicine (IOM) of the National Academies of Science published a report on the public impact of chronic pain entitled "Relieving Pain in America" [99]. This study highlighted that 25 % of adult Americans experience chronic pain and that women experience pain much more often than men, and yet their accounts of pain are often dismissed by male health care professionals [99–103]. A number of genes have been discovered that are associated with chronic facial pain (e.g., orofacial myalgia), and additional genes have been discovered to influence or modulate nociception—the neuronal process of encoding and processing noxious mechanical, thermal, and chemical stimuli vis-à-vis nerve endings called nociceptors located in the skin, periodontium, periosteum, joint surfaces, and muscles of mastication and facial expression [25, 100–103]. These advances enable improved correlations between phenotype and genotype and improved and more precise diagnostics and selection of therapeutics based upon genomics (Table 1.2) [103].

**Table 1.2** Genomic variant types associated with examples of phenotypes possibly associated with comparable DNA variants in craniofacial–oral–dental diseases and disorders

| Variant type | Associated phenotype(s) |
|---|---|
| Repetitive DNA, including trinucleotide repeats | Fragile X syndrome, Huntington's disease |
| Copy-number variants | DiGeorge syndrome (22q11.2 deletion syndrome), Charcot–Marie–Tooth disease type 1A |
| Long insertion–deletion variants | Resistance to HIV viral infection |
| Structural variants | Chromosomal translocations as in adult leukemia and spontaneous abortions |
| Aneuploidy | Down's syndrome, Turner's syndrome |
| Epigenetic alterations | Prader–Willi syndrome, Beckwith–Wiedemann syndrome, methylation of CpG islands in E-cadherin and COX-2 genes in periodontal disease |

Personalized oral medicine offers risk assessment, stratification of patients, diagnosis, treatment vs. treatment-nonresponsive individuals, individual responses to therapeutics (i.e., pharmacogenomics) based upon individual mechanism-specific genotype coupled with critical phenotypes (phenomics). The multiple genetic variance basis of many oral diseases and disorders defines the inflammatory response of individuals, regulation of the cell cycle, and DNA replication in specific cell types, epigenetics, and a host of other biological mechanisms that define an individual's threshold for resistance or susceptibility to specific diseases

## A "Situation Audit" of the Contemporary Health Care Environment: Does the Environment Celebrate Innovation, Comprehensive Primary Health Care for all People, and with an Emphasis on Wellness and Health Prevention?

At the time of writing this chapter, US health care is, candidly, a *work in progress* and replete with

[1] Exome is the complete set of exons, or protein-encoding sequences, found within the human nuclear genome and which represent about 1 % of the total DNA.

[2] These studies by Agrawal and colleagues (2011) focused on tumors from patients with history of tobacco consumption and also tested negative for human papillomavirus (HPV).

contradictions in no small measure due to a lack of alignment, cooperation, and coordination between the federal and state governments around health care. The scope of practice, provisions of patient benefits within Medicaid, reimbursements for health care providers, and health insurance regulations are often disparate between the federal and the various state governments. There are also enormous differences around health care progression such as prevention, prospective health care, a health home, home self-care, virtual health care, and wellness. Prospective health care means predictive, preventive, personalized, and participatory health care and wellness programs. Further, significant conceptual disconnects are most exaggerated around mental, vision, and oral health care around our nation. These have each been amplified and intensified during the legislative processes to initiate the Affordable Health Care Act.

Demographers and health policy experts suggest that the number of adults 50 and over will reach 132 million by 2030, an increase from 2000 of more than 70 %. In 2030, one out of five citizens will be 65 or older. Between 2012 and 2060, the number of individuals age 65 years and older will increase from 43.1 to 92 million in the United States [39]. Further, it is now well documented that as adults age, risk for developing chronic diseases and disorders increases.

Today, seven out of ten deaths result from chronic diseases and disorders, each with oral complications. Of the ten most commonly prescribed medications, six are used to treat chronic diseases with oral complications. The seven most common chronic diseases faced by older adults include oral systemic connections or associations including the following: (1) arthritis (associated with TMJ, xerostomia, and bleeding), (2) cancers (chemotherapy, radiation therapy associated with oral mucositis, candidiasis, and xerostomia), (3) chronic obstructive pulmonary disorders (associated with oral leukoplakia, erythroplakia, squamous cell carcinoma, xerostomia, and candidiasis), (4) type 2 diabetes (associated with periodontal disease, candidiasis, neuropathy, oral mucosal ulcerations, "poor" healing, compromised inflammatory response, and xerostomia resulting from medications), (5) heart diseases (possible hematoma, excessive bleeding, taste changes, and xerostomia), (6) hypertension (associated with lichenoid drug reactions, gingival overgrowth, xerostomia, and taste changes), and (7) mental health diseases and disorders (associated with excessive biofilm formations, lichenoid reactions, tooth decay, gingivitis, periodontal disease, and xerostomia).

According to Truffer and colleagues [39], oral health care expenses in 2009 reached $101 billion for the treatment of two-thirds of the US population, using only 7 % from public funds. That same year, oral health conditions treated in the so-called medical care system (head and neck birth defects, oropharyngeal cancers, and trauma) were $95.9 billion. Total health care that year reached $2.5 trillion. It is projected that health care expenses will reach $4.5 trillion by 2019 or 19.3 % of GDP. Succinctly, the US spends more than all of the major industrial nations combined on health care yet receives much less as measured by morbidity and mortality across the lifespan.

In tandem, a number of studies have highlighted that there are gaps or disconnects between societal needs and formal health professional education (medicine, dentistry, pharmacy, nursing, and the allied health professions) [104]. Over the last five decades, there has been a call to include human genetic education into the curriculum of North American dental education [105–111]. Despite these efforts, little has been accomplished. In the twenty-first century, there continues to be a call for human genomics to be integrated into oral health professional education [1, 8–14, 16, 17, 25–27, 29, 37, 38, 58, 59, 67, 73, 74, 89–91, 95–97, 99, 105–111, 126]. Throughout the industrial nations, the mantra offered is "smarter, faster, and cheaper" health care services with an emphasis upon prevention of chronic diseases and disorders. Such collective thinking as articulated in the United States argues that major revisions in the "health care system" must increase translational and clinical research, reduce costs, increase performance outcomes, and be based upon prevention services that meet the societal needs and requirements for health and wellness [112–115].

### Examples of Online Databases That Assist Clinicians in Differential Diagnosis or Candidate Gene Identification for Syndromic Disorders Before CGES[3] Is Performed

**Free Access**

- Genetic Testing Registry (www.ncbi.nlm.nih.gov/gtr)
- HuGE Navigator (http://hugenavigator.net/HuGENavigator)
- Human Gene Mutation Database (www.biobase-international.com/product/hgmd)
- Online Mendelian Inheritance in Man (www.omim.org)
- Phenomizer (http://compbio.charite.de/phenomizer)
- SimulConsult (www.simulconsult.com)
- Entrez (National Center for Biotechnology Information) (http://www.ncbi.nlm.nih.gov/gquery/gquery.fcgi)

**Subscription or Fee Required for Access**

- Isabel (www.isabelhealthcare.com/home/default)
- London Medical Databases (http://lmdatabases.com)
- POSSUM (www.possum.net.au)

## Future Directions for Personalized Oral Medicine: Next Steps

The emergence of genomic information, knowledge, and technology continues to illuminate our understanding of craniofacial–oral–dental diseases and disorders. Increasingly, these scientific discoveries are informing clinical practice [1, 9, 10, 16, 17, 25–27, 29, 34, 37, 38, 41–46, 58–60, 66–83, 87–91, 95–103, 112–115, 126]. It is becoming increasingly evident that the knowledge from genomics will yield predictive genetic tests for dozens, if not hundreds, of conditions, reduce risk through various interventions routinely used for preimplantation genetic diagnosis, provide guidelines for translating pharmacogenomics knowledge to bedside and chairside (especially related to drugs used for oncology), utilized by primary care health professionals, and likely be inequitable especially in the developing world [116–125].

### The Major Challenge: Chronic Diseases

Technologies for genome-wide sequence interrogation profoundly advances identification of informative gene loci associated with complex diseases [116–125]. One enormous challenge is the gap between correlations and causality. We have a limited theoretical framework derived from Mendelian genetics for complex human diseases and disorders and an incomplete molecular understanding of chronic diseases and their individual pathophysiology [125].

### The Second Dimension to the Human Genome: The Epigenome

Mapping the epigenome will provide significant information for each cell type during embryogenesis and subsequent postnatal growth and development in health and disease. Specifically when, where, and how do epigenetic factors such as acetylation and methylation regulate gene expression and function [117–119]?

*Within oral medicine and related health professions, we must provide high school, college, and preclinical education in human and microbial genetics, genomics, and genetic counseling.* For many decades, clinical scholars have been advocates for human and microbial genetics, and more recently genomics, to be an integral component of the preclinical and clinical education and training of oral health professionals [13, 16, 17, 25–27, 29, 67, 105–111, 126]. Despite formal

[3] CGES means clinical genome and exome sequencing. There is presently a spectrum of genomic variants, from nucleotide insertions and deletions of at least 8–10 base pairs (e.g., ACTGATTGCT) through copy-number variants that are less effectively assayed by current CGES technology.

recommendations, very modest progress has been accomplished [111, 112].

**Conclusions**

In concert, the standards in virtually every state in the United States have failed to keep pace with changes in the biological sciences, especially genomics, omitting concepts related to genetic complexity, the importance of environment to phenotype variation, differential gene expression, and the differences between inherited and somatic genetic diseases. A multidisciplinary analysis of primary health care recommends that medical, dental, pharmacy, and nursing professional education must be revised to address the diseases and disorders found in the greater society [111, 112]. In addition, in order to make significant improvements in the public's craniofacial–oral–dental health requires major revisions in oral health professional education [1, 13, 16, 110–112].

To address these issues as related to modern human genetics and genomics, the recent Macy report provides a detailed curriculum for genomics that will enable oral health professionals to use the knowledge and practical applications for risk assessment, stratification of patients, selection of therapeutics based on pharmacogenomics, and diagnostics [1, 8–14, 25, 27, 29, 67–70, 111, 112, 117]. Recent progress toward interprofessional health care supports the adoption of the Macy Report and a new laboratory manual entitled "Genetics of Complex Human Disease" [116–122]. In tandem, we must create practical CE courses that enable practitioners to gain access to the content and applications related to personalized oral medicine (e.g., "Genomics and Clinical Dentistry"). Further, we must provide essential knowledge for health care policy experts as well as insurance, manufacturing, and distribution industries. In tandem, we will continue to experience a next-generation sequencing revolution that will impact upon personalized oral medicine [32, 34, 36, 116–126].

Finally, enabling the future of personalized oral medicine requires a few significant lessons based upon the experiences from the last few decades. First, free and open access to human genome and microbiome data is critical for the rapid progress of the biomedical sciences. Second, accelerating innovations for technology and informatics clinical research and development with an emphasis upon multidisciplinary health professional teams will continue to be a key to success. Third, phenomics or the accurate identification and alignment of genetic and phenotypic, as well as environmental, risk factors are a major driver to success. Applying genome-wide sequencing and SNPs technology to classical Mendelian disorders has revealed fascinating variance within the phenotype as well as genotype [126–128]. These efforts must also coordinate with human behaviors to achieve optimal benefits. Fourth, support for public–private partnerships is critical to advance drug development coupled with pharmacogenomics. One example is to enhance the relationship between the FDA, NIH, and big and small pharmaceutical companies. Finally, we must ensure individual privacy and effective and continuous education for health care providers and the larger society about genomic health care and ensure an appropriate health care system reimbursement for the cost of evidence-based, cost-effective preventive services.

## References


1. Slavkin HC. From phenotype to genotype: enter genomics and transformation of primary health care around the world. J Dent Res. 2014;93(7 supp 1): 3s–6.
2. President Clinton's speech of 26th June 2000 at 10:19 am (EDT). Avaialable at: http://www.genome.gov/pfv.cfm?pageID=10001356.
3. International Human Genome Sequencing Consortium. Initial sequencing and analysis of the human genome. Nature (London). 2001;409: 860–921.
4. Venter JC, Adams MD, Myers EW, Li PW, Mural RJ, Sutton GG, et al. The sequence of the human genome. Science. 2001;291:1304–51.
5. International Human Genome Sequencing Consortium (IHGSC). Finishing the euchromatic

sequence of the human genome. Nature. 2004;431:931–45.
6. Encyclopedia of DNA Elements (ENCODE). Available at: http://www.encodeproject.org. Accessed 3 Oct 2014.
7. Gladwell M. The tipping point: how little things can make a difference. New York: Little, Brown and Company; 2000.
8. Collins FS, Tabak LA. A call for increased education in genetics for dental health professionals. J Dent Educ. 2004;68:807–8.
9. Garcia I, Tabak LA. A view of the future: dentistry and oral health in America. J Am Dent Assoc. 2009;140:44s–8.
10. Wong DTW. Salivaomics. J Am Dent Assoc. 2012;143(10 suppl):19s–24.
11. Giannobile WV, Braun TM, Caplis AK, Doucette-Stamm L, Duff GW, Kornman KS. Patient stratification for preventive care in dentistry. J Dent Res. 2013;92:694–701.
12. Giannobile WV, Kornman KS, Williams RC. Personalized medicine enters dentistry: what might this mean for clinical practice? J Am Dent Assoc. 2013;144:874–6.
13. Glick M. Expanding the dentist's role in health care delivery: is it time to discard the Procrustean bed? J Am Dent Assoc. 2009;140:1340–2.
14. Hart TC, Hart PS, Bowden DW, Michalec MD, Callison SA, Walker SJ, et al. Mutations of the cathepsin C gene are responsible for Papillon-Lefevre syndrome. J Med Genet. 1999;36:881–7.
15. Hornstein RB, Shuldiner AR. Genetics of diabetes. Rev Endocr Metab Disord. 2004;5:25–36.
16. Johnson L, Genco RJ, Damsky C, Haden NK, Hart S, Hart TC, et al. Genetics and its implications for clinical dental practice and education: report of panel 3 of the Macy Study. J Dent Educ. 2004;72(2 Suppl):86–94.
17. Kornman KS, Duff GW. Personalized medicine: will dentistry ride the wave or watch from the beach? J Dent Res. 2012;91(7 Suppl):8S–11.
18. Cook-Deegan R. The gene wars: science, politics, and the human genome. New York: WW Norton & Co.; 1994.
19. Feero WG, Guttmacher AE, Collins FS. Genomic medicine – an updated primer. N Engl J Med. 2010;362(21):2001–11.
20. McDermott U, Downing JR, Stratton MR. Genomics and the continuum of cancer care. N Engl J Med. 2010;364:340–50.
21. Farzadegan H, Vlahov D, Solomon L, Muñoz A, Astemborski J, Taylor E, et al. Detection of human immunodeficiency virus type 1 infection by polymerase chain reaction in a cohort of seronegative intravenous drug users. J Infect Dis. 1993;168(2):327–31.
22. Epstein CJ, Erickson RP, Wynshaw-Boris A, editors. Inborn errors of development. 2nd ed. New York: Oxford University Press; 2008.
23. Boccia S, Brand A, Brand H, Ricciardi G. The integration of genome-based information for common diseases into health policy and healthcare as a major challenge for public health genomics: the example of the methylenetetrahydrofolate reductase gene in non-cancer diseases. Mutat Res. 2009;667(1–2):27–34.
24. Frank-Raue K, Frank-Raue RS. Molecular genetics and phenomics of RET mutations: impact on prognosis of MTC. Mol Cell Endocrinol. 2010;322:2–7.
25. Slavkin HC, Navazesh M, Patel P. Basic principles of human genetics: a primer for oral medicine. In: Greenberg M, Glick M, Ship J, editors. Burket's oral medicine. 11th ed. Ontario: BC Decker Inc.; 2008. p. 549–68.
26. Slavkin HC. The future of research in craniofacial biology and what this will mean for oral health professional education and clinical practice. Aust Dent J. 2014;59(1 Suppl):1S–5.
27. Slavkin HC, Santa Fe Group. Revising the scope of practice for oral health professionals. J Am Dent Assoc. 2014;145:228–30.
28. Williams AL, Jacobs SB, Moreno-Macías H, Huerta-Chagoya A, Churchhouse C, Márquez-Luna C, the SIGMA Type 2 Diabetes Consortium, et al. Sequence variants in SLC16A11 are a common risk factor for type 2 diabetes in Mexico. Nature. 2013;506:97–103.
29. Polverini PJ. A curriculum for the new dental practitioner: preparing dentists for a prospective oral health care environment. Am J Pubic Health. 2012;102(2):e1–3. doi:10.2105/AJPH.2011.300505.
30. Watson J. Living with my personal genome. Pers Med. 2009;6:607–10.
31. Venter CJ. A life decoded: my genome, my life. New York: Viking Press; 2009.
32. Venter CJ. Multiple personal genomes await. Nature. 2014;464:676–7.
33. Collins FS. The language of life: DNA and the revolution in personalized medicine. New York: HarperCollins Publishers; 2010.
34. Collins FS. Has the revolution arrived? Nature. 2014;464:674–5.
35. Davies K. The $1,000 genome: the revolution in DNA sequencing and the new era of personalized medicine. New York: Free Press; 2010.
36. Collins FS, Hamburg MA. First FDA authorization for next-generation sequencer. N Engl J Med. 2013;369:2369–71.
37. NIDCR Strategic Plan 2014–2019. Available at: http://www.nidcr.nih.gov. Accessed 10 Oct 2014.
38. Garcia I, Kuska R, Somerman MJ. Expanding the foundation for personalized medicine: implications and challenges for dentistry. J Dent Res. 2013;92 suppl 1:3–10s.
39. Truffer CJ, Keehan S, Smith S, Cylus J, Sisko A, Poisal JA, et al. Health spending projections through 2019: the recession's impact continues. Health Aff. 2010;29(3):522–9.

40. U.S. Department of Health and Human Services. Oral health in America: a report of the Surgeon General. Rockville: US Department of Health and Human Services/National Institute of Dental and Craniofacial Research/National Institutes of Health; 2000.
41. Slavkin HC. The Surgeon General's report and special needs patients: a framework for action for children and their caregivers. Spec Care Dentist. 2001;21(3):88–94.
42. Slavkin HC. Expanding the boundaries: enhancing dentistry's contribution to overall health and well being of children. J Dent Educ. 2001;65(12): 1323–34.
43. Kleinman DV. The future of the dental profession: perspectives from Oral Health in America: a report of the Surgeon General. J Am Coll Dent. 2002;69(3):6–10.
44. Crall JJ. Oral health policy development since the Surgeon General's Report on Oral Health. Acad Pediatr. 2009;9(6):476–82.
45. Lewis CW. Dental care and children with special needs: a population perspective. Acad Pediatr. 2009;9(6):420–6.
46. Petersen PE. Global policy for improvement of oral health in the 21st century – implications to oral health research of World Health Assembly 2007, World Health Organization. Community Dent Oral Epidemiol. 2009;37(1):1–8.
47. Mendel GJ. Experiments concerning plan hybrids. Proc Nat Hist Soc Brunn IV. 1865;3–47.
48. Andrei A. Experiments in plant hybridization (1866), by Johann Gregor Mendel. In: Embryo project encyclopedia (04 Sept 2013). ISSN: 1940–5030. Available at: http://embryo.asu.edu/handle/10776/6240.
49. Miescher F. Ueber die chemische Zusammensetzung der Eiterzellen. Medicinisch-chemische Untersuchungen. 1871;4:441–60.
50. Chargaff E, Zamenhof S, Green C. Composition of human desoxypentose nucleic acid. Nature. 1950;165(4202):756–7.
51. McKusick VA. Walter Sutton and the physical basis of Mendelism. Bull Hist Med. 1960;34:487–97.
52. Morgan TH, Sturtevant AH, Muller HJ. The mechanism of Mendelian heredity. New York: Kessinger Publishing; 1915.
53. Avery OT, MacLeod CM, McCarty M. Studies on the chemical nature of the substance inducing transformation of pneumococcal types: induction of transformation by a deoxyribonucleic acid fraction isolated from pneumococcus type III. J Exp Med. 1944;79(2):137–58.
54. Simmons NS, Blout ER. The structure of tobacco mosaic virus and its components: ultraviolet optical rotary dispersion. Biophys J. 1960;1(1):55–62.
55. Wilkins MHF. The molecular configuration of nucleic acids. Nobel lecture, 11 Dec 1962. Available at: (http://cmbi.bjmu.edu.cn/news/report/2003/DNA50/source/wilkinslecture.pdf). Accessed 29 Sept 2014.
56. Chambers DA, editor. DNA the double helix: perspective and prospective at forty years. New York: The New York Academy of Sciences; 1995.
57. Watson JD, Crick FH. Molecular structure of nucleic acids: a structure for deoxyribose nucleic acid. Nature. 1953;171:737–8.
58. Snead ML, Slavkin HC. Science is the fuel for the engine of technology and clinical practice. J Am Dent Assoc. 2009;140:17s–24.
59. Slavkin HC. The evolution of the scientific basis for dentistry: 1936 to now and its impact on dental education. J Dent Educ. 2012;76:28–35.
60. Guttman JL. The evolution of America's scientific advancements in dentistry in the past 150 years. J Am Dent Assoc. 2009;140:8s–15.
61. Stevens H. Life out of sequence: a data-driven history of bioinformatics. Chicago: The University of Chicago Press; 2013.
62. Ledley RS. Digital electronic computers in biomedical science. Science. 1959;130:1232.
63. Waterman MS. Introduction to computational biology: maps, sequences, and genomes. London: Chapman & Hill; 1995.
64. Mullis K. Dancing naked in the mind field. New York: Vintage Books; 1998.
65. Crick F. What a mad pursuit: a personal view of scientific discovery. New York: Basic Books; 1988.
66. Harris RR. Dental science in a new age: a history of the National Institute of Dental Research. Rockville: Montrose Press; 1989.
67. Slavkin HC. Birth of a discipline: craniofacial biology. Newtown: Aegis Communications; 2012.
68. Zero DT, Fontana M, Martinez-Miler EA, Ferreira-Zandona A, Ando M, Gonzalez-Cabezas C, et al. The biology, prevention, diagnosis and treatment of dental caries. J Am Dent Assoc. 2009;140:25s–35.
69. Armitage GC, Robertson PB. The biology, prevention, diagnosis and treatment of periodontal diseases: scientific advances in the United States. J Am Dent Assoc. 2009;140 Suppl 1:36s–44.
70. Cohen Jr MM, MacLean RE, editors. Craniosynostosis: diagnosis, evaluation, and management. New York: Oxford University Press; 2000.
71. Gorlin RJ, Slavkin HC. Embryology of the face. In: Tewfik TL, Der Kaloustian VM, editors. Congenital anomalies of the ear, nose, and throat. Oxford: Oxford University Press; 1997. p. 287–96.
72. Der Kaloustian VM. Introduction to medical genetics and dysmorphology. In: Tewfik TL, Der Kaloustian VM, editors. Congenital anomalies of the ear, nose, and throat. Oxford: Oxford University Press; 1997. p. 3–28.
73. Slavkin HC. What the future holds for ectodermal dysplasias: future research and treatment directions. Am J Med Genet. 2009;149A:2071–4.
74. Dixon MJ, Marazita ML, Beaty TH, Murray JC. Cleft lip and palate: understanding genetic and environmental influences. Nat Rev Genet. 2011;12: 167–78.

75. Snead ML, Zeichner-David M, Chandra T, Robson KJH, Woo SLC. Construction and identification of mouse amelogenin cDNA clones. Proc Natl Acad Sci U S A. 1983;80:7254–8.
76. Snead ML, Lau EC, Zeichner-David M, Fincham AG, Woo SLC, Slavkin HC. DNA sequence for cloned cDNA for mouse amelogenin reveal the amino acid sequence for enamel-specific protein. Biochem Biophys Res Commun. 1985;129:812–8.
77. Lau EC, Mohandas TK, Shapiro LJ, Slavkin HC, Snead ML. Human and mouse amelogenin gene loci are on the sex chromosomes. Genomics. 1989;4: 162–8.
78. Lau EC, Simmer JP, Bringas Jr P, Hsu DD-J, Hu CC, Zeichner-David M, et al. Alternative splicing of the mouse amelogenin primary RNA transcript contributes to amelogenin heterogeneity. Biochem Biophys Res Commun. 1992;188(3):1253–60.
79. Pugach MK, Gibson CW. Amelogenin gene regulation. In: Goldberg M, editor. Amelogenins: multifaceted proteins for dental and bone formation and repair (frontiers between science and clinic in odontology), vol. 1. Paris: Bentham Books; 2010. p. 19–24.
80. Chun YHP, Hu JCC, Simmer JP. The non-amelogenins ameloblastin and enamelin. In: Goldberg M, editor. Amelogenins: multifaceted proteins for dental and bone formation and repair (frontiers between science and clinic in odontology), vol. 1. Paris: Bentham Books; 2010. p. 42–55.
81. Wright JT. Consequences of amelogenin mutations in amelogenesis imperfect. In: Goldberg M, editor. Amelogenins: multifaceted proteins for dental and bone formation and repair (frontiers between science and clinic in odontology), vol. 1. Paris: Bentham Books; 2010. p. 88–98.
82. Hart TC, Hart PS, Michalec MD, Zhang Y, Firatli E, Van Dyke TE, et al. Haim-Munk syndrome and Papillon-Lefevre syndrome are allelic mutations in cathepsin C. J Med Genet. 2000;37:88–9.
83. Shimazaki Y, Saito T, Yonemoto K, Kiyohara Y, Lida M, Yamashita Y. Relationship of metabolic syndrome to periodontal disease in Japanese women: the Hisayama Study. J Dent Res. 2007;86(3):271–5.
84. Kassi E, Pervanidou P, Kaltsas G, Chrousos G. Metabolic syndrome: definitions and controversies. BMC Med. 2011;9:48–62.
85. The SIGMA Type 2 Diabetes Genetics Consortium. A low frequency variant in HNF1A has a large effect on type 2 diabetes risk in a Latino population. JAMA. 2014. doi:10.1001/jama.2014.6511.
86. Loe H, Brown LJ. Early onset periodontitis in the United States of America. J Periodontol. 1991;62:608–16.
87. Pihlstrom BL, Michalowicz BS, Johnson NW. Periodontal diseases. Lancet. 2005;366:1809–20.
88. Van Dyke TE, Serhan CN. Resolution of inflammation: a new paradigm for the pathogenesis of periodontal diseases. J Dent Res. 2003;82(2):82–90.
89. Vaithilingam RD, Safii SH, Baharuddin NA, Ng CC, Cheong SC, Bartold PM, et al. Moving into a new era of periodontal genetic studies: relevance of large case–control samples using severe phenotypes for genome-wide association studies. J Periodontal Res. 2014. doi:10.1111/jre.12167.
90. Rhodin K, Divartis K, North KE, Barros SP, Moss K, Beck JD, et al. Chronic periodontitis genome-wide association studies. J Dent Res. 2014;93(9):882–90.
91. Divaris K, Monda KL, North KE, Olshan AF, Reynolds LM, Hsueh WC, et al. Exploring the genetic basis of chronic periodontitis: a genome-wide association study. Hum Mol Genet. 2013;22(11):2312–24.
92. Houle D, Govindaraju DR, Omholt S. Phenomics: the next challenge. Nat Rev Genet. 2010;11:855–63.
93. Yang J, Benyamin B, McEvoy BP, Gordon S, Henders AK, Nyholt DR, et al. Common SNPs explain a large proportion of the heritability for human height. Nat Genet. 2010;42:565–9.
94. Manolio TA, Collins FS, Cox NJ, Goldstein DB, Hindorff LA, Hunter DJ, et al. Finding the missing heritability of complex diseases. Nature. 2009. doi:10.1038/nature08494.
95. Shuler CF. Inherited risks for susceptibility to dental caries. J Dent Educ. 2001;65(10):1038–45.
96. Wang X, Willing MC, Marazita ML, Wendell S, Warren JJ, Broffitt B, et al. Genetics and environmental factors associated with dental caries in children: the Iowa Fluoride Study. Caries Res. 2012;46(3):177–84.
97. Shaffer JR, Feingold FE, Wang X, Tcuenco KT, Weeks DE, De Sensi RS, et al. Heritable patterns of tooth decay in the permanent dentition: principal components and factor analyses. BMC Oral Health. 2012. doi:10.1186/1472-6831-12-7.
98. Warnakulasuriya KAAS, Harris CK, Scarrott DM, Watt R, Gelbier S, Peters TJ, et al. An alarming lack of public awareness towards oral cancer. Br Dent J. 1999;187(6):319–22.
99. Agrawal N, Fredrick MJ, Pickering CR, Bettegowda C, Chang K, Li RJ, Fakhry C, Xie TX et al. Exome sequencing of head and neck squamous cell carcinoma reveals inactivating mutations in NOTCH1. Science 2011;333:1154–7.
100. Cohen RL, Settleman J. From cancer genomics to precision oncology—tissue's still an issue. Cell. 2014;157:1509–13.
101. Osazuwa-Peters N. Human papillomavirus (HPV), HPV-associated oropharyngeal cancer, HPV vaccine in the United States—do we need a broader vaccine policy? Vaccine. 2013;31(47):5500–5.
102. Institute of Medicine United States Committee on Advancing Pain Research, Care and Education. Relieving pain in America: a blueprint for transforming prevention, care, education, and research. Washington, DC: National Academies Press; 2011.
103. Dao TT, LeResche L. Gender differences in pain. J Orofac Pain. 2000;14:169–84.

104. Sato H, Droney J, Ross J, Olesen AE, Staahl C, Andresen T, et al. Gender, variation in opioid receptor genes and sensitivity to experimental pain. Mol Pain. 2013;9:48–57.
105. James S. Human pain and genetics: some basics. Br J Pain. 2013;7(4):171–8.
106. Slavkin HC. Distinguishing Mars from Venus: emergence of gender biology in health and disease. J Am Dent Assoc. 1998;129:357–61.
107. Frenk J, Chen L, Bhutta ZA, Cohen J, Crisp N, Evans T, et al. Health professionals for a new century: transforming education to strengthen health systems in an interdependent world. Lancet. 2010;376:1923–58.
108. Kopel H, editor. The teaching of human genetics in dental education. Los Angeles: University of Southern California Press; 1979.
109. Sanger R, editor. Guidelines for the teaching of human genetics in dental education. Denver: University of Colorado Press; 1979.
110. Salinas CF, Jorgenson RJ, editors. Dentistry in the interdisciplinary treatment of genetic diseases. New York: Alan R. Liss, Inc.; 1980.
111. Fields M, editor. Dental education at the crossroads. Washington, DC: Institute of Medicine, National Academy of Sciences; 1995.
112. Kohn LT, editor. Academic health centers: leading change in the 21st century. Washington, DC: Institute of Medicine, National Academy of Sciences; 2003.
113. DePaola D, Slavkin HC. Reforming dental health professions education: a white paper. J Dent Educ. 2004;48(11):1139–50.
114. Hendricson WD, Cohen PA. Oral health care in the 21st century: implications for dental and medical education. Acad Med. 2001;76(12):1181–206.
115. Sung N, Crowley W, Genel M, Salber P, Sandy L, Sherwood L, et al. Central challenges facing the national clinical research enterprise. J Am Med Assoc. 2003;289:1278–87.
116. Crowley Jr WF, Sherwood L, Salber P, Scheinberg D, Slavkin HC, Tilson H, et al. Clinical research in the United States at a crossroads: proposal for a novel public-private partnership to establish a national clinical research enterprise. J Am Med Assoc. 2004;291(9):1120–6.
117. Kupersmith J, Sung N, Myron G, Slavkin HC, Califf R, Bonow R, et al. Creating a new structure for research on healthcare effectiveness. J Investig Med. 2005;53(2):67–72.
118. Slavkin HC, Sanchez-Lara P, Chai Y, Urata M. A model for interprofessional health care: lessons learned from craniofacial teams. J Calif Dent Assoc. 2014;42(9):637–44.
119. Agundez JAG, Esguevillas G, Amo G, Garcia-Martin E. Clinical practice guidelines for translating pharmacogenomics knowledge to bedside: focus on anticancer drugs. Front Pharmacol. 2014; 5(188):1–4.
120. Chakravarti A, Clark AG, Mootha VK. Distilling pathophysiology from complex disease genetics. Cell. 2013;155:21–6.
121. Rivera CM, Ren B. Mapping human epigenomes. Cell. 2013;155:39–55.
122. Dougherty MJ, Pleasants C, Solow L, Wong A, Zhang H. A comprehensive analysis of high school genetics standards: are states keeping pace with modern genetics? CBE Life Sci Educ. 2011;10:318–27.
123. Wang L, McLeod HL, Weinshilboum RM. Genomics and drug response. N Engl J Med. 2011;364(12): 1144–53.
124. Al-Chalabi A. Genetics of complex human disease: a laboratory manual. New York: Cold Spring Harbor Laboratory Press; 2014.
125. Biesecker LG, Green RC. Diagnostic clinical genome and exome sequencing. N Engl J Med. 2014;370(25):2418–25.
126. Slavkin HC, Navazesh M, Patel P. Basic principles of human genetics: a primer for oral medicine. In: Gliok M, editor. Burket's oral medicine 12th edition. Shelton, Connecticut: People's Medical Publishing House-USA 2015. p. 625–52.
127. Koboldt DC, Steinberg KM, Larson DE, Wilson RK, Mardis ER. The next-generation sequencing revolution and its impact on genomics. Cell. 2013;155:27–38.
128. Driss A, Asare KO, Hibbert JM, Gee BE, Adamkiewicz TV, Stiles JK. Sickle cell disease in the post genomic era: a monogenic disease with a polygenic phenotype. Genomics Insights. 2009;2: 23–48.

# 2 Genomic Approaches to Disease Diagnosis and Prevention

Alexandre R. Vieira

**Abstract**
Genomic approaches are the basis for proposing personalization of medicine, a philosophy that customizes healthcare using molecular analysis to guide medical decisions tailoring them to individual patients. Specific treatments will be prescribed only to patients who will positively respond to them, avoiding additional suffering and costs and focusing on therapies that better suit each particular case. This chapter briefly revisits the current state of the art of genomics, transcriptomics, proteomics, and pharmacogenomics and proposes that greater emphasis on phenomics will possibly accelerate discovery and implementation of a healthcare system that utilizes molecular information for bedside care.

## Introduction

The genetics field came a long way in regard to utilizing genetic variation to identify linkage between specific loci and phenotypes. From the first suggestion that linkage could be used to physically locate genes in chromosomes in 1911 to genome-wide genotyping scans utilizing array-base devices with more than one million single nucleotide polymorphisms (Fig. 2.1), fulfilling the promise to utilize genomic approaches to clinically manage patients is on the horizon [1–5].

A.R. Vieira, DDS, MS, PhD
Department of Oral Biology, University of Pittsburgh School of Dental Medicine, Pittsburgh, PA, USA
e-mail: ARV11@pitt.edu

## Gene Mapping

Physically locating chromosomal regions and genes that are linked or associated with disease phenotypes was the initial focus of much of the effort to unveil genetic causes of common diseases. The technology quickly advanced from a few markers to more than one million markers that can be efficiently interrogated, as seen in Fig. 2.1. After more than a decade of work, it is clear that those methods are powerful enough to detect causes of conditions that are rare and influenced by strong gene effects (Fig. 2.2). For typically more common diseases, in which more than one gene contributes to the condition and each gene has a small effect, the detection of associations does not translate into any relevant information worth utilizing in the management of



P.J. Polverini (ed.), *Personalized Oral Health Care: From Concept Design to Clinical Practice*,
DOI 10.1007/978-3-319-23297-3_2

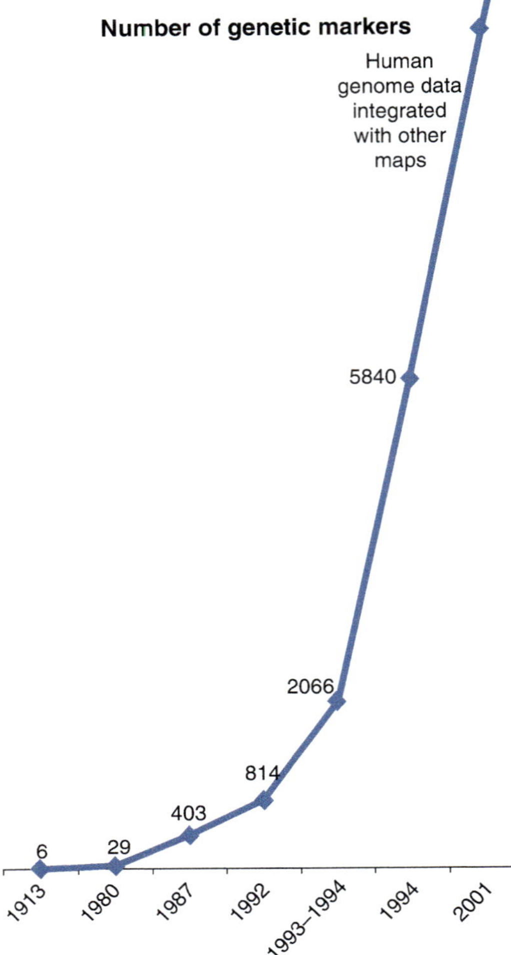


**Fig. 2.1** Timeline and evolution of the number of genetic markers available for genomic analysis. From the first publication in 1913 to the integration of data from the human genome project with other physical maps of the genome, there are a few million genetic variants identified that can be potentially interrogated in genomic analyses

patients. Again, the exception is for families with "private" and rare mutations. "Private" in this context means the mutation is so rare it is unlikely it will even be seen again in another case outside the family. This scenario becomes of interest just for the family and the identification of the mutation in all affected family members will help with genetic counseling explaining the mode of inheritance and risks for new offspring (Fig. 2.3). Due to the low frequency, it is very unlikely a mutation like this will attract the interest of private corporations to develop a product for genetic testing.

## Direct Sequencing

One of the consequences of the human genome project was the rapid development of technologies that made it more efficient to obtain DNA sequence reads. Machines today can obtain reads of millions of base pairs in the same time that just a few base pairs were obtained 30 years ago. This evolution permits a whole genome to be sequenced (or a whole exome or the sequencing of the portion of DNA that codes for protein). Those methods have been used to unveil the genetic variants that cause disease in cases where expected mutations cannot be identified [6]. One good example is an analysis of a family segregating KGB syndrome (KGB stands for the initials of the affected patients in the original report and includes distinct craniofacial anomalies, macrodontia of the maxillary central incisors, short stature, mental retardation, and skeletal anomalies), in which a mutation in *ANKRD11* (ankyrin repeat-containing cofactor 1 or ankyrin repeat domain 11) was identified [7]. This work demonstrated that mutations in *ANKRD11* cause KGB syndrome, outlining a fundamental role of the gene in craniofacial, dental, skeletal, and nervous system development and function and providing a tool for genetic screening of suspected cases.

## Transcriptomics

Gene expression profiling (which includes mRNA transcripts that reflect the genes that are being actively expressed at any given time) is seen as a precursor for the proteome. For diagnostic purposes, assessing profiles in saliva was of great interest due to the noninvasive nature of saliva collection. Array technology generated even more interest, but closer evaluation of the origins of expression microarray and reverse transcription-PCR (RT-PCR) signals in human saliva revealed discouraging results [8]. RNA-specific RT-PCR strategies cannot eliminate

**Fig. 2.2** Most diseases are influenced by more than one gene, with relatively small to moderate effects. Genetic variants in these genes that lead to disease tend to have relatively small to moderate allele frequencies as well. Association studies are excellent for detecting diseases that are common with highly frequent disease-causing genetic variants. Conversely, linkage approaches are excellent for detecting rare diseases that have uncommon alleles with very strong effects. Most diseases, however, are polygenic in nature, can be modulated by environmental factors, may have epigenetics influences, and cannot be fully assessed by linkage or association approaches

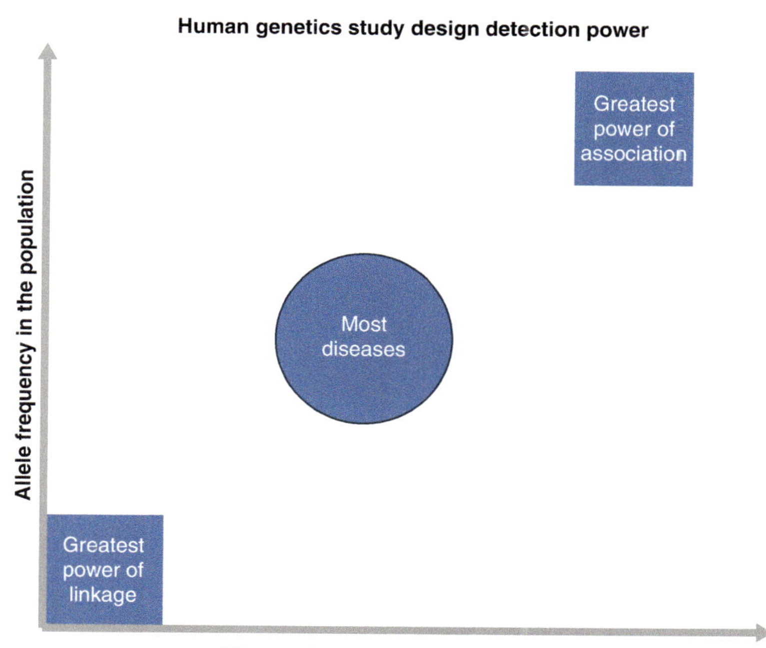


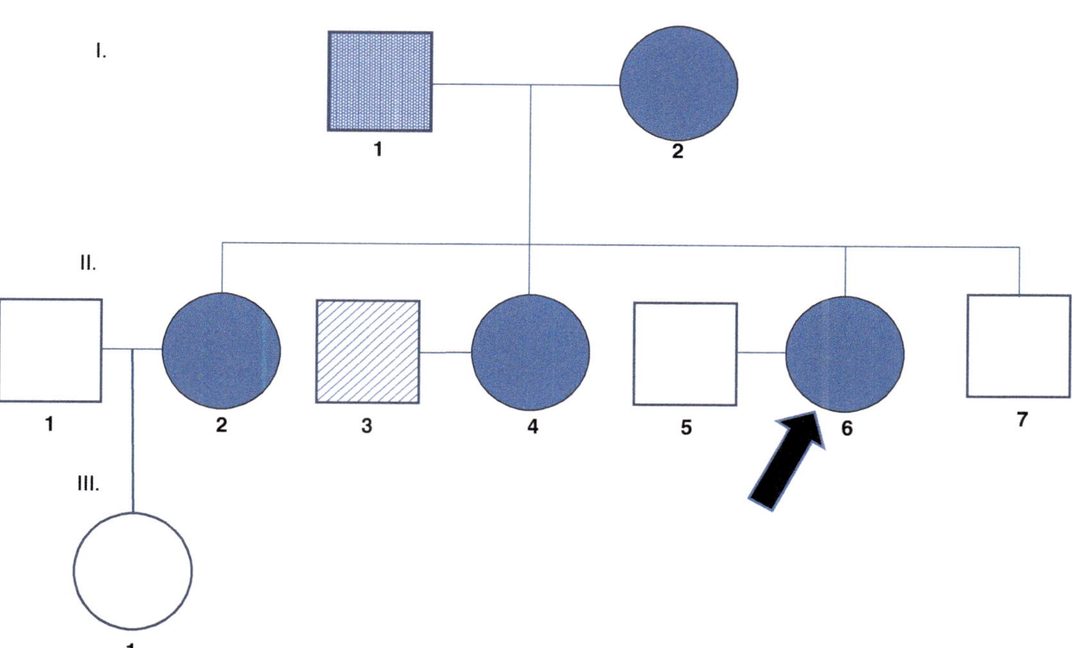


**Fig. 2.3** Family-segregating oligodontia. Squares indicate males, circles females. Blue indicates affected individuals (details of affection status below). Individuals I.2, II.2, II.4, and II.6 have severe forms of oligodontia. Individual I.1 has only five teeth missing (hypodontia indicated by a shade under the blue color) and individual II.3 hypodontia of three teeth (*stripped blue marked*). All individuals with blue color are heterozygous for the *WNT10A* mutation F228I. The individual II.3 does not carry a *WNT10A* mutation, indicating his hypodontia has a different etiology. Individual II.6, marked with the black arrow, requested genetic counseling and was advised her chance of having a child with oligodontia was 50 %

confounding signals from contaminating genomic DNA, suggesting that saliva extracts do not support mRNA expression studies.

## Proteomics

Since genomics did not immediately translate into curing diseases, the direct identification of the products of the genes, the proteins, gained increased interest. Proteomics has been the focus of several initiatives hoping to explore the function of genomes by providing insight on the overall level of intracellular protein composition, structure, and activity. Mass spectrometry, chips, and reversed-phase microarrays are some of the current technologies implemented in proteomic studies. Virtually, proteomics has been explored in every possible source of substrate from the oral cavity: enamel and acquired pellicle cells, dentin, skin fibroblasts, saliva, root canal and periapical sources, pulp cells, periodontal cells, gingival fluid and cells, teeth, clinical isolates from caries and biofilm, epithelial cells, and squamous cell carcinomas cells and serum [9].

## Pharmacogenomics

There is great interest in studying the role of genetics in drug response. Genetic variation influences drug absorption, distribution, metabolism, elimination, and receptor target effects. This approach will permit the personalization of treatments by selecting individuals who will respond and/or benefit from certain drugs and, conversely, avoiding certain therapies in individuals who will not respond to certain medications. Individuals carrying genetic variants in *CYP2D6* (cytochrome P450 2D6) and *OPRM1* (mu-type opioid receptor) have distinct responses to halothane, isoflurane, and fentanyl [10]. Head and neck squamous cell carcinomas displaying a *PIK3CA* (phosphatidylinositol 4,5-bisphospate 3-kinase catalytic alpha isoform) mutation may be more resistant to erlotinib (EGFR tyrosine kinase inhibitor, EGFR stands for epidermal growth factor receptor), indicating that the mutational status of *PIK3CA* may be used to select preclinical models for response to erlotinib. A *GSTT1*-lacking fetus (GSTT1 stands for glutathione S-transferase theta 1) from a mother who smokes 15 cigarettes or more per day will have a nearly 20-fold increase of developing cleft lip and palate [11].

These examples are relevant because the identification of the above gene mutations in patient subpopulations that exhibit more effective responses and/or an improved benefit/risk upon treatment will become a central part of care management. This scenario is even more relevant when one realizes that drug development appears to be at an impasse, with delivery of new products being at an all-time low [12]. Genetic variant prevalence in the population, the cost of genetic variant testing, and the cost of choosing the wrong treatment are key parameters in the evaluation of the economic viability of personalized medicine. Mathematical models suggest that upfront testing costs are likely offset by avoided nonresponse treatment costs [13].

## Phenomics

The challenges, however, of incorporating molecular information for supporting clinical decisions (both diagnosis and treatment) are still abundant, from skepticism of the usefulness of these approaches and their underlying costs to the difficulties in translating results that suggest an increased risk at the population level without providing a clear meaning for the individual. There is still much to be learned about the interplay between genetics background and disease onset and prognosis.

To accelerate this process, a refocus on the measurement of the physical and biochemical traits—phenomes—has been proposed. There are two strong reasons to justify this effort. Genome-wide association studies for complex traits and diseases require a large number of observations to overcome the multiple testing issues and to permit that relatively small individual contribution from genes to be detected. If we assume a multiplicative mode of inheritance, sample size of cases identical to that of controls, depending on the disease frequency, thousands of samples are potentially required (Table 2.1).

Cases or affected individuals are typically defined by having a particular disease or condition (i.e., been born with cleft lip and palate, having a diagnosis of periodontitis, having had caries experience). In the case of cleft lip and palate, scientists have demonstrated that a more sophisticated clinical description, for example, one that includes the status of the dentition, provides new opportunities for identifying association with genes (Fig. 2.4). Subtypes of oral clefts based on dental abnormalities have been proposed [15]:

### Cleft Lip With or Without Cleft Palate (CL/P)

Unilateral right
- With/without tooth agenesis outside the cleft area

Unilateral left
- With/without tooth agenesis outside the cleft area
- With/without microdontia or supernumerary teeth on the noncleft side
- With/without multiple dental anomalies

Bilateral
- With/without tooth agenesis outside the cleft area
- With/without supernumerary teeth
- With/without malposition of lower canines
- With/without multiple dental anomalies

"Unsuccessful" bilateral (unilateral CL/P with agenesis of the lateral incisor on the noncleft side)
- With/without multiple dental anomalies

### Cleft Palate Only (CPO)

Complete
- With/without tooth impaction
- With/without multiple dental anomalies

Incomplete
- With/without tooth malposition

Binary definitions can be redefined by utilizing multiple parameters (i.e., affected teeth,

**Table 2.1** Number of individuals necessary to obtain 80 % power in genome-wide association studies

| Study design | Linkage disequilibrium between genetic marker and disease-causing mutation | Case-control | — | Family-based (transmission disequilibrium test, TDT) |
|---|---|---|---|---|
| Frequency of rare allele in the population | — | Relative risk of disease-causing genotype = 0.1 | Relative risk of disease-causing genotype = 0.01 | — |
| 0.01 | 1 | 6312 | 7712 | 16,520 |
| — | 0.75 | 11.084 | 13.526 | 26,975 |
| — | 0.5 | 24,616 | 30,002 | 55,304 |
| Corresponding disease prevalence | — | 10.2 % | 1.0 % | — |
| 0.1 | 1 | 776 | 986 | 1972 |
| — | 0.75 | 1368 | 1736 | 3.278 |
| — | 0.5 | 3052 | 3866 | 6856 |
| Corresponding disease prevalence | | 12.1 % | 1.2 % | — |
| 0.5 | 1 | 386 | 616 | 964 |
| — | 0.75 | 688 | 1096 | 1720 |
| — | 0.5 | 1554 | 2472 | 3880 |
| Corresponding disease prevalence | — | 22.5 % | 2.3 % | — |

Estimates from: Ohashi and Tokunaga [14]

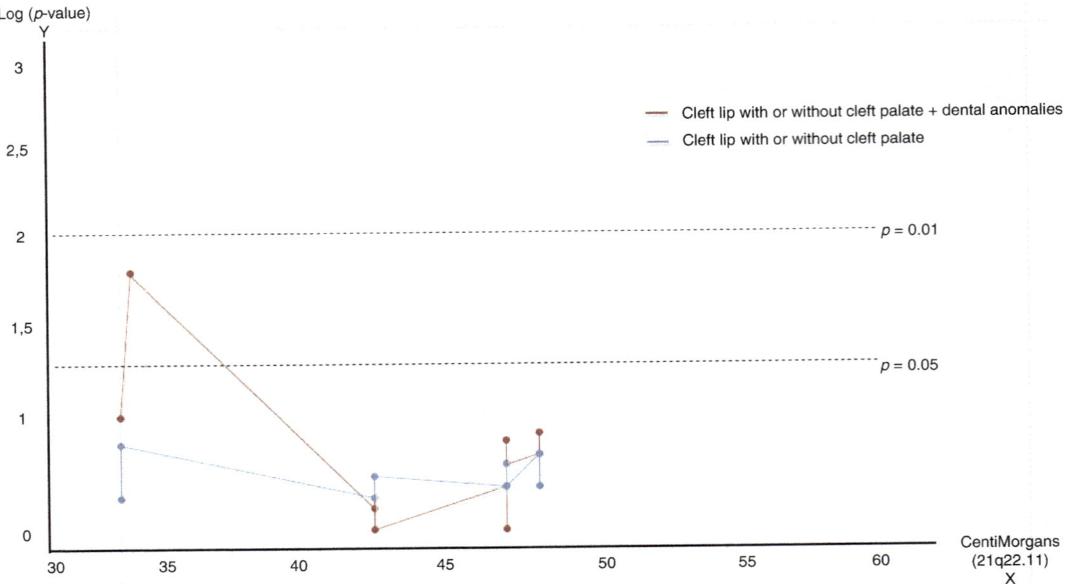


**Fig. 2.4** When association data for chromosome 21q22.11 was analyzed with the definition of affection status as having been born with cleft lip and palate, no association was detected (*blue line*, which is below the threshold of $p = 0.05$). When the same data was analyzed by defining affected status by having been born with cleft lip and palate, with or without having dental anomalies (tooth agenesis, supernumerary teeth, microdontia), an association was detected in the locus of *GART* (phosphoribosylglycinamide formyltransferase; pink line picking around 34 centMorgans, cM) (From: Vieira et al. [16])

presence of certain microorganisms, severity), which will likely lead to groups of affected individuals that have much closer case presentations. This will decrease heterogeneity and likely enrich for common genetic contributions, either from the same gene or from genes in the same pathway. The downside of this approach is the need for identifying larger amounts of affected individuals to obtain the desirable minimal number of cases for analysis.

## Conclusions

It is recommended that scientists interested in all disciplines of dentistry start to rethink case definitions and to utilize more complex case definitions for their studies.

If one takes the cariology field as an example, DMFS/dmfs scores are more indicative of disease severity than DMFT/dmft scores. However, for decayed teeth, the D1–D4 scale will provide an even more precise definition of severity, similar to the 0–6 scale of the International Caries Detection and Assessment System. However, those scales only indicate individual caries experience and do not necessarily convey information about the pathogenesis. The addition of other caries etiology variables will enhance these clinical definitions by discriminating individuals who perform suboptimal oral hygiene, have specific diet preferences, present specific bacterial colonization, or a combination of these. It is unlikely that genomic approaches will be useful to all fields of dentistry unless more sophisticated clinical descriptions are incorporated in the analyses of disease-causing factors, both genetic and nongenetic.

## References

1. Botstein D, White RL, Skolnick M, Favis RW. Construction of a genetic linkage map in man using restriction fragment length polymorphisms. Am J Hum Genet. 1980;32:314–31.

2. Donis-Keller H, Green P, Helms C, Cartinhour S, Weiffenbach B, Stephens K, et al. A genetic linkage map of the human genome. Cell. 1987;51:319–37.
3. Gyapay G, Morissette J, Vignal A, Dib C, Fizames C, Millasseau P, et al. The 1993–94 Généthon human genetic linkage map. Nat Genet. 1994;7:246–339.
4. Murray JC, Buetow KH, Weber JL, Ludwigsen S, Scherpbier-Heddema T, Manion F, et al. A comprehensive human linkage map with centimorgan density. Cooperative Human Linkage Center (CHLC). Science. 1994;265:2049–54.
5. The International Human Genome Mapping Consortium. A physical map of the human genome. Nature. 2001;409:934–41.
6. Choi M, Scholl UI, Ji W, Liu T, Tikhonova IR, Zumbo P, et al. Genetic diagnosis by whole exome capture and massively parallel DNA sequencing. Proc Natl Acad Sci U S A. 2009;106:19096–101.
7. Sirmaci A, Spiliopoulos M, Brancati F, Powell E, Duman D, Abrams A, et al. Mutations in ANKRD11 cause KBG syndrome, characterized by intellectual disability, skeletal malformations, and macrodontia. Am J Hum Genet. 2011;89:289–94.
8. Kumar SV, Hurteau GJ, Spivack SD. Validity of messenger RNA expression analysis of human sliva. Clin Cancer Res. 2006;12:5033–9.
9. Rezende TMB, Lima SMF, Petriz BA, Silva ON, Freire MS, Franco OL. Dentistry proteomics: from laboratory development to clinical practice. J Cell Physiol. 2013;228:2271–84.
10. Eng G, Chen A, Vess T, Ginsburg GS. Genome technologies and personalized dental medicine. Oral Dis. 2012;18:223–35.
11. Shi M, Christensen K, Weinberg CR, Romitti P, Bathem L, Lozada A, et al. Orofacial cleft risk is increased with maternal smoking and specific detoxification-gene variants. Am J Hum Genet. 2007;80:76–90.
12. Dere WH, Suto TS. The role of pharmacogenomics and pharmacogenomics in improving translational medicine. Clin Cases Miner Bone Metab. 2009;6:13–6.
13. Stallings SC, Huse D, Finkelstein SN, Crown WH, Witt WP, Maguire J, et al. A framework to evaluate the economic impact of pharmacogenomics. Pharmacogenomics. 2006;7:853–62.
14. Ohashi J, Tokunaga K. The power of genome-wide association studies of complex disease genes; statistical limitations of indirect approaches using SNP markers. J Hum Genet. 2001;46:478–82.
15. Letra A, Menezes R, Granjeiro JM, Vieira AR. Defining cleft subphenotypes based on dental development. J Dent Res. 2007;86:986–91.
16. Vieira AR, McHenry TG, Daack-Hirsch S, Murray JC, Marazita ML. Candidate gene/loci studies in cleft lip/palate and dental anomalies finds novel susceptibility genes for clefts. Genet Med. 2008;10:668–74.

# 3 Health Information Technology (Health IT): The Future of Personal Medicine

Lynn A. Johnson and Eileen Quintero

**Abstract**

Health IT is changing the focus of healthcare providers from curing illness to empowering the individual to improve their personal health. Cloud computing stores big data for safe and easy access by individuals, mobile devices are used to enter data during a health event, wearable sensors detect changes in our bodies' physical changes, and social media permits sharing our health information to support communities. These four health IT trends combine to generate the big data that personalizes healthcare and feeds the electronic systems of the learning health system (LHS). The learning health system continuously analyzes this data as well as the data from hospital electronic health records and other healthcare entities. The continuous data aggregation and analysis allows the "learning" of the learning health system to occur. Subsequently, each of us, as well as our healthcare providers, uses health IT to access this "learned" knowledge to proactively improve our health. Health IT combined with the learning health system is anticipated to shorten the 17-year "bench-to-bedside" gap between knowledge discovery and its application in personal health to 17 months.

## Introduction

> According to an Arabian proverb, "He who has health, has hope. And he who has hope, has everything." [1]

The future of health and of healthcare depends upon health information technology. Health information technology, also known as health IT, is an overarching framework of health information that ensures the secure exchange of health information between patients, providers, insurers, hospitals,

L.A. Johnson, PhD (✉)
Periodontics and Oral Medicine,
University of Michigan, School of Dentistry,
Ann Arbor, MI, USA
e-mail: lynjohns@umich.edu

E. Quintero, MSI
Division of Dental Informatics,
University of Michigan School of Dentistry,
Ann Arbor, MI, USA



P.J. Polverini (ed.), *Personalized Oral Health Care: From Concept Design to Clinical Practice*,
DOI 10.1007/978-3-319-23297-3_3

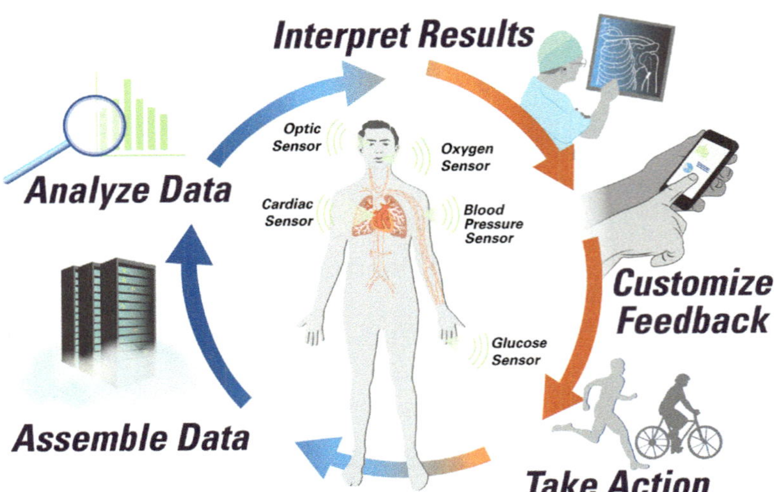


**Fig. 3.1** The learning health system cycle (assemble data, analyze data, interpret results, customize feedback, and take action) with the pillars of health IT (cloud, social media, sensors, mobile devices). The learning health system operates in the cloud; data are gathered using sensors, social media, and mobile devices; and practitioners and patients receive and act upon information provided on mobile devices

government agencies, and other healthcare entities [2]. Already providers are carrying tablets [3], and patients are wearing devices that track their vital signs, sleep patterns, pulse, and physical activity [4]. This information is beginning to join the electronic record systems in hospitals and health research databases to improve and personalize the information required to improve health. Whereas up to this point healthcare considerations have primarily focused solely on illness, health IT is shifting the healthcare community toward improving how we practice healthcare [5]. As such, health IT is becoming increasingly relevant for making better, faster, evidence-based decisions for treatment and patient care. We propose that the four pillars of health IT are the cloud, mobile devices, sensors, and social media. Most importantly, these four pillars generate the big data that could fuel a learning health system (LHS): a system that can continuously study and improve itself (Fig. 3.1). This chapter will first discuss the LHS and then the four technology pillars that support it.

## The Learning Health System: From Big Data to Knowledge to Use

In recent years there has been growing recognition that our current health systems have consistent problems that result in suboptimal practices, high costs, and concerns about patient safety [6].

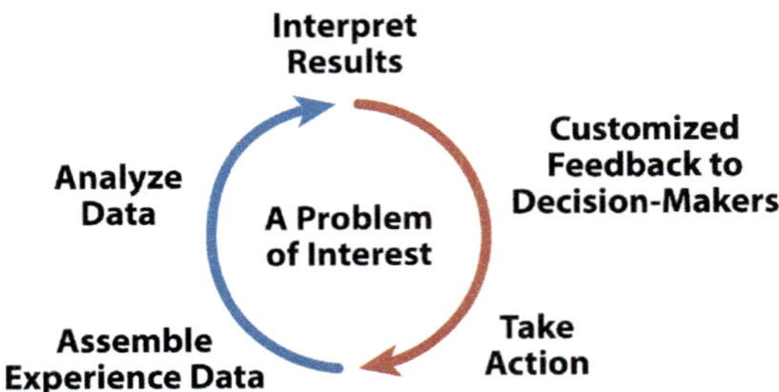


**Fig. 3.2** The virtuous cycle of the learning health system. A learning cycle (C. Friedman. Adapted with permission from "Toward Complete and Sustainable Learning Systems." Available at http://medicine.umich.edu/sites/default/files/2014_12_08-Friedman-IOM%20LHS.pdf)

From this realization has emerged the concept of a learning health system (LHS). The LHS concept, first expressed by the Institute of Medicine in 2007, is now being adopted across the country and around the world [7, 8]. The concept borrows advancements backing technological areas such as machine learning, self-learning code, recommender systems, and artificial intelligence.

The LHS consists of a series of "virtuous cycles" of continuous learning to address specific health problems. The cycle begins with collection and analysis of big data to generate new knowledge (see Fig. 3.2 left/blue side of the cycle). Stakeholders can interact with that new knowledge to provide only the relevant information required at that time to solve a case (see Fig. 3.2 right/red

side of the cycle). Stakeholders might be clinicians, patients, or even researchers. Once a decision is made, the decision and results are fed back into the system as data and influence the outcomes of the next analysis of big data. Thus, the system "learns" by taking the results of the last patient-care decision into account when generating the results of the next stakeholder request. A set of learning cycles forms the LHS. The LHS enables continuous access to relevant health data from entities across the nation, conduct of analyses that convert the data to useful knowledge, and transmission of that knowledge to all stakeholders in formats that promote positive action and health-promoting behavioral change [9]. The overall goal is to more rapidly change stakeholder behavior toward evidence-based treatment decisions in order to improve health, as well as to transform our healthcare organization by creating more instantaneously collaborative environments for comparing treatment results.

Gathering "big data" is currently a hot topic. The emphasis on aggregating and analyzing big data ("blue side" of Fig. 3.2) creates only half of a learning system, because the cycle terminates at "12 o'clock" (see Fig. 3.2) and cannot complete itself. Absent a mechanism to deliver what is learned into actual practice and document the practice changes that result, these limited efforts will continue to propagate the frequently cited 17-year "bench-to-bedside" gap between knowledge discovery and its general application in practice [10]. This latency is likely to increase as the rate of new knowledge generation increases, in absence of an accompanying mechanism to promote the uptake of this new knowledge [11]. In order to make continuous learning and improvement possible, attention needs to shift to also being able to continuously learn from big data in order to drive meaningful improvement ("red side" of Fig. 3.2). We challenge the community to reduce the "bench-to-bedside" gap from 17 years to 17 months or 17 weeks.

The LHS has the potential to reduce the time between discovery and application of health research findings not only by providing automated identification of cases to which new findings apply but also by identifying clinical patterns of positive outcomes in real time. Our current methods for clinical research and clinical trials of new procedures or medical innovations require time for setup of the experiment and completion with a defined number of participants. Performed by one or a few doctors, significant "n" requires significant time. The LHS could facilitate faster research through identification of "n" through natural practice. In dentistry the realization that research can be significantly sped by inclusion of outcomes data collected in private practice rather than limiting data collection to specific studies has prompted a movement to include, educate, and standardize data collection for private practice. In 2005 the National Institute of Dental and Craniofacial Research (NIDCR) awarded three separate grants for a total of $75 million over 7 years to foster participation for evidence-based data collection and research on the part of all dentists in private practice settings [12]. The establishment of these practice-based research networks (PBRNs) allows practicing dentists to contribute to research and also apply current findings to their patient care [13]. The positive influence of direct application of research to clinical decision-making can be viewed in this quote:

> As my career developed, I began to seriously wonder at the end of the day if I actually improved the health of my patients. When I reviewed the research I realized that in fact some of my most basic questions related to caring for patients could not satisfactorily be answered. Involvement in practice-based research has allowed me to ask and begin to answer clinical questions that actually matter to me and my patients. Additionally, conducting research in my own practice has helped me implement change in my practice at a much quicker rate. The results that I have been involved in producing just mean so much more to me now! [14]

Still, submission of data and searching for clinical answers require additional time and effort. In an environment where even Amazon automatically recommends books based on the books you have purchased before, it raises the question of whether health information systems could include such recommendations.

In Michigan, the Center for Health Research and Transformation (CHRT) has initiated "Learning Health for Michigan," an initiative targeted at achieving a statewide LHS [15]. At the national level, the Office of the National Coordinator (ONC) for health IT has specifically articulated the LHS as a 10-year goal and the pinnacle achievement of health information technology [16]. At the global level, efforts based in the European Union [17] have advanced the LHS agenda, and interest in the concept is appearing in Japan, Australia, and Argentina [18], as well as other countries around the world.

Implementation plans for the LHS make the case for a system that both allows access to diverse data without interfering with security and ownership of that data, bypassing any territorial concerns, and provides a systematic and operationalized method for creating personalized health information that is current and relevant to an individual case. It has the potential to decrease the time required for new research knowledge and treatment outcomes data to be applied in practice and thereby improve health for all of the world's population.

## LHS Technology Pillar #1: Cloud

### Case Study

On October 29, 2012, Hurricane Sandy deposited 4 feet of contaminated water in the Sea Bright, NJ, dental practice of Drs. Michele Brucker and Kevin Colleir. Very few of their paper charts were salvaged and none of the radiographs. Drs. Brucker and Colleir were grateful for the support offered by the dental community, from guidance on legal issues to dentists who opened their offices to Brucker and Colleir to provide care to their patients. However, without their records, contacting and caring for patients was a challenge. Now electronic records are a priority for them [19]. Compare this to the story of periodontists Dr. Saljae Aurora and Christopher Chung from Vancouver, British Columbia [20], who had lost all of their computers, monitors, and printers in a burglary. Because they use a cloud electronic health record (EHR), they used their home laptops to access their patients' information. They were able to see all scheduled patients, schedule new appointments, document all procedures, bill for treatments, and in all ways conduct their normal dental practice.

## How Cloud Computing Works

Cloud computing is a term that avoids all sensibilities. You cannot see, touch, smell, hear, or taste a computing cloud, but most of us use it. The basic concept behind the cloud is that all of your data, and sometimes your software programs, are stored via the Internet and that you can access them from any device, anywhere and at any time. This is such a significant change in how we use technology that we will describe how cloud computing works and how it is encouraging the transformation of healthcare.

Computers communicate over wireless networks, and clinicians now use handheld devices such as phones and tablets to enter and access patient information over these wireless networks. Storing information in the cloud means that you are saving information somewhere other than on a portable storage device or the device you are currently using, and that you will be able to access that information, and mostly likely previous versions of that information, from a different device at any time. Often the computer servers that make this possible are owned and operated by another company.

Cloud software means that the software files are installed somewhere else, but that it is possible to use the software via a web browser or other interface from your device. In this case, each action, such as recording a health history, calculating a bill, or communicating with a patient, is an operation that is executed on a server that is located somewhere unknown to yourself, and you see the results. That server might be in the next town or even halfway around the world. The video *Cloud Computing Explained* [21] has an easy-to-understand explanation of cloud computing.

### Software as a Service (SaaS)

If there is one technical term associated with cloud computing that everyone needs to know, it is software as a service, also known as SaaS (pronounced sah-ss, rhymes with glass). Cloud computing provides storage as a service and software as a service by which software service providers can enjoy the virtually infinite and elastic storage and computing resources [22]. It is subscription-based utilization of computer hardware and software over the Internet, similar to the way utility companies supply gas and electricity [23]. With SaaS you do not purchase software that you own and install; instead, you buy a subscription to the cloud software or cloud storage and the rights to use it for the duration of your subscription. Because it is cloud based, the service runs on a server in an unknown location. You do not need to install, update, back up, or perform any of the myriad tasks associated with software on a day-to-day basis. Instead those operations occur behind the scenes.

Subscriptions are now sold for both storage and software, with the "as a service" signifying that you pay to use but not to own, maintain, or upgrade. Business has used cloud computing because it allows capacity and functionality to increase on the fly without a major investment in infrastructure, personnel, or licensing fees. Also, when a computer, laptop, tablet, etc. fails, businesses can use a different device and still be able to access their information. Cloud architecture can potentially be superior to traditional electronic health record (EHR) infrastructure in terms of security, economy, efficiency, and utility [24].

## Cloud in Healthcare

Using EHRs to share information between patients and providers helps to improve diagnosis, promote self care, and improve patients' knowledge of their health. The use of cloud electronic EHRs is increasing steadily in North America and Europe [25] in both dentistry [26–28] and medicine [29–31]. They allow clinicians to access their patients' records on a variety of devices, i.e., computers, as well as on tablets and smartphones, as long as there is an Internet connection. It is anticipated that cloud EHRs will improve individual patient care, but it will also bring many public health benefits, including:

- Early detection of infectious disease outbreaks around the country [32]
- Improve tracking of chronic disease management [33]
- Collect de-identified cost and service quality information for analysis to discover how to minimize healthcare costs while increasing quality of care [2]

### Security

Federal legislation intended to safeguard the privacy and security of electronic protected health information (ePHI) has evolved since the 1996 Health Insurance Portability and Accountability Act (HIPAA) [34]. The Health Information Technology for Economic and Clinical Health (HITECH) Act, part of the American Recovery and Reinvestment Act of 2009, is also relevant because it has several provisions that strengthen the civil and criminal enforcement of the HIPAA rules, mainly by defining levels of culpability and corresponding penalties [35]. Of special relevance to cloud-based EHRs is the January 2013 HIPAA Omnibus Rule [36] which expanded the HIPAA requirements to include business associates (vendors or service providers that maintain and store ePHI), where previously only covered entities (hospitals, clinics, and insurers) had originally been held to uphold the HIPAA regulations. Now cloud EHR providers are as liable for noncompliance as are covered entities. As a result, covered entities are required to put a business associate agreement (BAA) into place with any service provider who has access to ePHI, thereby guaranteeing the service provider's compliance with HIPAA [37].

HIPAA requires anyone who stores ePHI to fulfill numerous physical and technical requirements. The IT security requirements can distract clinicians from patient-care activities. For example, a practice needs to detail when backups are performed, where off-site backups are stored, and how media is destroyed. In addition, the practice must document that the procedures described in the policy are performed. By using a cloud service, the practice is relieved from the responsibility of writing and documenting many of the HIPAA requirements. Instead, the cloud EHR provider shoulders those obligations. It is anticipated that clinicians will not want to be burdened with the IT security requirements of HIPAA and instead will pay to have that security provided for them [38].

## Cloud: Impact on Patient Care

The LHS requires personal health information from numerous and varied patients in a myriad of EHR systems to be joined with existing and new knowledge generated through research. The connecting of health and research information would not be possible without this information first being located in the cloud. The siloed nature of traditional in-house EHRs hampers movement toward the LHS through old incompatible architectures and a focus on operating servers, backups, and other non-health-related activities. By moving the EHR software and storage of its associated PHI to the cloud, the focus of resources can instead be on improved data exchange and enhancing patient and clinician access to relevant health and research information that will improve health decisions at the time they are required. The LHS makes the case for a system that allows access to diverse data without interfering with security and ownership of that data and that provides a systematic and operationalized method for creating personalized health information that is both current and relevant to an individual case.

## LHS Technology Pillar #2: Mobile Devices

### Case Study

Jennifer is preparing for tomorrow's research presentation when the right side of her head begins to throb and she feels nauseous. She needs to turn off the lights in her office, place a cool cloth over her eyes, and rest for about 1 h before she can work again. She describes the pain as though her brain is exploding. It feels like someone took a baseball bat and beat the side of her skull with it and jabbed an ice pick into her right eye.

### Discussion

Medical entrepreneurs have taken advantage of public obsession with apps to leverage a new model for data collection. Frustrated with the loss of data inherent in after-the-fact pain reporting, Dr. Alex DaSilva and his partners create the application *PainTrek* [39, 40], which allows patients to report pain as it's occurring. This iOS application provides a 3D head and facial map based on a squared grid system, with vertical and horizontal coordinates, using anatomical landmarks. Each quadrangle, measuring approximately 1.6 cm × 1.6 cm, frames well-detailed craniofacial and cervical areas for the patient to "paint" to express his/her exact pain location, quality, and intensity (Fig. 3.3). Additional survey questions offer more details. Using a scrolling timeline, patients and their clinicians can now graphically compare pain levels for various incidents and understand the impact of different treatments or external influences.

Any information the patient reports while the migraine is occurring is instantly accessible by the healthcare team for improved pain diagnosis and management. *PainTrek* statistically measures the change in the area of pain and its intensity after a specific treatment, as well as the impact on the patients' lives. Patient and clinicians can now track pain levels as they change over time for conditions such as migraines or fibromyalgia.

The value of an application such as *PainTrek* goes beyond its use to document and improve the health of a single patient and into the research realm to create new knowledge that can lead to the improved health of numerous patients. *PainTrek* has been used by researchers to verify the efficacy of a temporomandibular disorder (TMD) treatment. In a study, 24 TMD patients used *PainTrek* to systematically record their pain as well as complete an associated pain-related questionnaire. One-half of the patients received an electrical stimulation treatment and the other half received a placebo treatment. Those patients who received the stimulation treatment reported 50 % pain relief after 1 month as recorded by *PainTrek* [41].

Previously, TMD or pain research studies required patients to complete pain rating scales

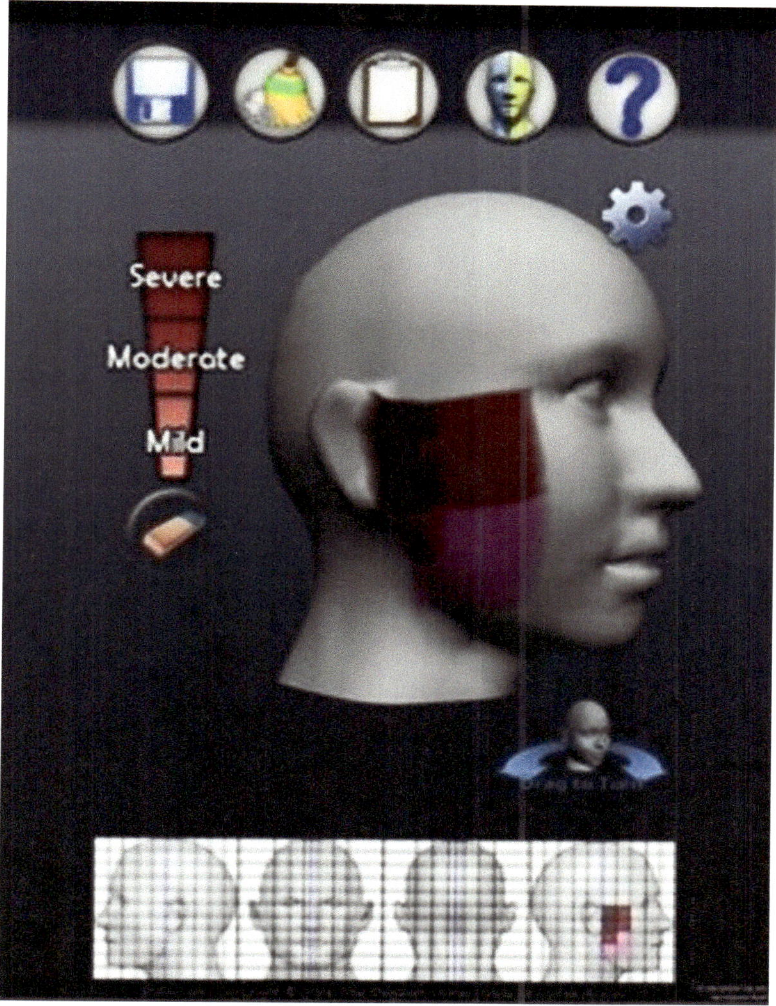


**Fig. 3.3** The patient used *PainTrek* to "paint" the location and severity of the pain they experienced (Image provided by Alex DaSilva)

(0 = no pain to 10 = worst pain) for analysis. The results were usually presented in a table or chart intended for researchers only. *PainTrek* provides a more nuanced and detailed analysis for researchers as well as an easily understood visual analysis for non-researchers such as patients. The summative visual results of the active group (treatment group receiving the stimulation) are displayed in Fig. 3.4. While a scan of these results clearly demonstrates improvement (green indicates decreased pain; red indicates increased pain), behind each image is detailed pain intensity and location data which can be downloaded for additional complex analyses. This research study illustrates how a single mobile application can provide information that is easily understood by patients and researchers alike. Patients can now make more informed treatment decisions; concurrently, researchers can discover new knowledge to help numerous and varied patients.

## Mobile Devices: Impact on Patient Care

*PainTrek* is an example of a mobile application that has the potential to improve the life of a migraine sufferer such as Jennifer (see earlier case study) by personalizing how information related to her headaches is gathered. Before

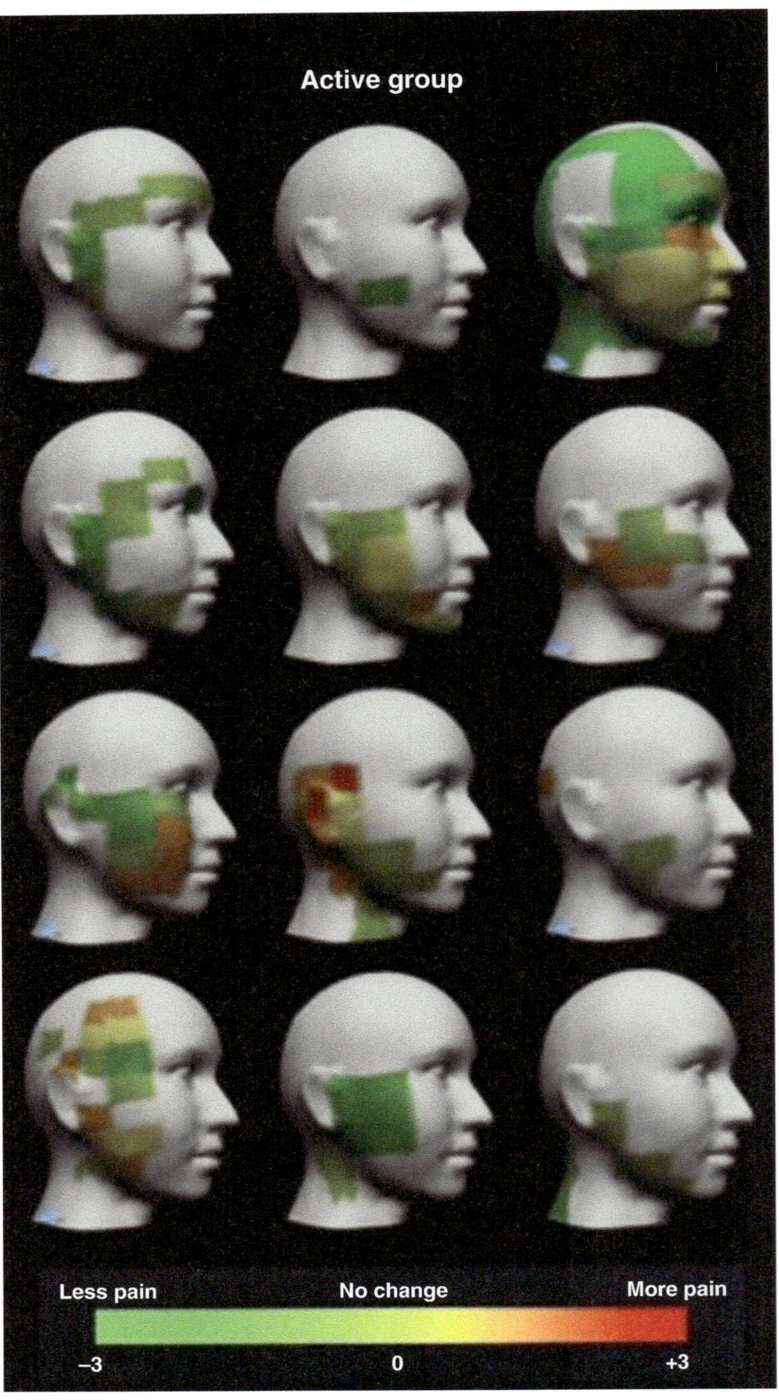


**Fig. 3.4** Summation of patient reported pain intensity and location in the TMD treatment study (Image provided by Alex DaSilva)

*PainTrek*, a patient would retrospectively write notes to be shared with the clinician at a later time. Alternatively, the patient would try to accurately recall characteristics of the pain incident, frequently with great difficulty. *PainTrek* is being used to study head and neck pain [42, 43] that will subsequently lead to the improvements in the health of pain patients [44]. In essence,

*PainTrek* decreases recall bias from the care of patients with pain.

Mobile devices enable real-time data collection that, when combined with software, creates the potential to reduce errors and accelerate diagnosis and treatment selection. Error reduction and expedited diagnostic and treatment decision can, in turn, decrease healthcare costs. This data can be combined with other data in the LHS in order for the LHS disease cycle to continue to learn and thus provide ongoing and improved health information that will improve the health of other patients.

## LHS Technology Pillar #3: Sensors

### Case Study

James, a 54-year-old male, is an avid bicyclist. He was diagnosed with type 1 diabetes 9 years ago. In the last 2 years James has developed additional problems with neuropathy in his feet and face. For most of his diabetic life, he used needle sticks to test his blood glucose level, followed by an insulin injection seven to ten times each day. This greatly impacted his daily routine, and the neuropathy made him give up the sport he loved—bicycling. Recently James started using an OmniPod [45] with a continuous glucose monitoring (CGM) system. The CGM continuously checks his glucose levels 24 h each day. Based on the glucose level, the OmniPod delivers the insulin without a tube, like most insulin pumps. James is now cycling again and is not in fear of tangling tubes in his equipment. Like other pumps, the OmniPod significantly reduces highs and lows, thereby decreasing the risk of diabetic complications [46]. James now goes about his life with less worry about hypoglycemia than he did when using injections [47]. He now has control over his life with diabetes.

## Discussion

Diabetes mellitus affects approximately 9.3 % of the US population, or 29.1 million people [48], and approximately 450,000 of these people use CGMs and insulin pumps to manage their diabetes [49]. Sensors have changed the way type 1 diabetics live with diabetes. CGMs and other sensor technologies can more accurately and continuously take measurements of the human body. A sensor with a tiny electrode inserted under the skin measures blood glucose levels. This information can then be wirelessly transmitted via Bluetooth to a display device which notifies the patient if their glucose reaches a high or low limit. This information is stored for uploading so that the patient understands the long-term trends of their glucose levels. Thus, the patient is now alerted before reaching their glucose limit. Diabetics now have early notifications, alerts for low or highs even when sleeping, and insight into how food, exercise, medication, and illnesses impact their diabetes [50].

When insulin pump technology such as the OmniPod is combined with a continuous blood glucose monitoring system, the technology seems promising for real-time control of blood sugar levels. With the size of the last insulin injection, combined with the elapsed time and a programmable metabolic rate, the insulin pumps estimate the insulin remaining in the bloodstream and report it to the patient. This supports the injection of a new insulin bolus before the effects of the last bolus are complete and thus prevents the patient from overcompensating for high blood sugar [51].

Sensor technology for diabetes cannot be discussed without a parallel dialog about the accompanying algorithms. These algorithms are now sophisticated enough to automatically control the insulin delivery based on feedback of the blood glucose level. When the loop is closed, the system functions like an artificial pancreas [52].

Diabetes patients are not the only patients for whom sensors are changing their lives and improving their health. Wearable devices with sensors are now readily available to patients and are revolutionizing information gathering. A key element to this shift is remote monitoring. The convergence of pervasive wireless networks, cloud technology, miniaturization, and noninvasive biosensors is rapidly making the concept of monitoring patients as they go about their daily lives a reality. Skin patches detect temperature, heart rate, perspiration, and movement. These sensors are now starting to detect ailments such as heart disease through cardiac monitoring. PhysIQ [53] has demonstrated the power of sensor technology and just how deeply individual health can be impacted. PhysIQ daily monitors patients with chronic diseases and provides early notification of any changes directly to clinicians. All of this will lead to increased knowledge, cost reductions, and overall improvements in individualized care. PhysIQ is considered the first personalized physiology analytics platform.

Congestive heart failure (CHF) results in over 1,000,000 hospitalizations annually. Physicians at the University of Chicago are assessing if sensors, combined with the cloud-based predictive analytics of PhysIQ, can reliably identify CHF earlier than current methods [54]. They predict that by using a secure website, physicians will be warned of a negative change in a patient's physiology and will be able to proactively intervene and prevent a hospitalization. The physicians anticipate that quality of care will improve and healthcare costs will decrease.

The US Department of Veterans Affairs Center for Innovation is using PhysIQ's proprietary personalized physiology analytics (PPA) technology to investigate the unique interplay between continuous physiological signals such as heart rate, respiration rate, oximetry, blood pressure, and any number of other signals, creating a dynamic multivariate baseline for each patient [55]. No variable is viewed in isolation, and the PhysIQ algorithms identify meaningful deviations and interactions from an individual's baseline that often cannot be otherwise ascertained.

## Sensors: Impact on Patient Care

Sensors provide better knowledge of individual health through monitoring and can increase mobile health and telehealth capabilities. It is anticipated that the ability to extend the geography of care through sensors may drive down health costs through early detection and even treatment. For example, signs of an oncoming heart attack may alert a patient so that they can be at a care facility during the critical early minutes following the heart attack.

It is important to understand that sensors, combined with mobile technology and bioinformatics, create a new type of physiological analytics that is based on an individual's personalized baseline. They are not based upon population data—that is, they do not use "big data." Systems like the PhysIQ platform are changing chronic disease management into a proactive health delivery model. The next step is to integrate the information gathered by these devices with other systems to allow these systems to "learn" and then to answer questions about health at the time it is needed.

## LHS Technology Pillar #4: Social Media

### Case Study

"What are you doing right now?" One response to this question was "Just bit into a chocolate biscuit and a tooth fell out. Just had to take a 2 paracetamol to kill the pain. Visit to the dentist tomorrow." This was one of the tweets (a microblog of 140 characters or fewer) included in a social media research study about dental pain. The researchers discovered that Twitter users shared health information related to their dental pain, including the impact of the pain on their day and what they did to relieve the pain. Some of the tweets even inquired about advice from other Twitter users [56].

### Discussion

Twitter and other social media sites are changing how individuals approach their personal health. The case study above reinforces other studies that demonstrate that people experiencing pain are likely to engage at social media sites to share their disease, its symptoms and treatment, and more online [57]. Health information openly shared on social media sites is changing the face of population health.

*The New York Times* reported on a February 2011 outbreak of legionellosis in San Francisco that alerted the local health authorities and the Centers for Disease Control and Prevention (CDC) through Facebook [58] and Wikipedia [59] entries. A CDC officer read the symptoms posted on Facebook, recommended diagnostic tests, and referred the victims to the CDC's online questionnaire.

*Healthmap* [60], a website that tracks global outbreaks in real time, uses data mining strategies from news aggregators, blogs, and Twitter, as well as official reports to describe human and animal disease outbreaks. The mobile app *Outbreaks Near Me* [61] uses global positioning systems (GPS) so that you can stay clear of disease locations when traveling overseas or even track flu outbreaks in your community.

Social media sites help you track your workouts, including the time and distance, and determine the number of calories burned. Online support groups are formed and "followers" discuss training goals such as weight loss. Fitocracy [62], an award-winning app, allows you to track your workouts and daily habits. You get your own trainer starting at $1/day to keep you motivated and on track. The coach will assess your needs and create a personal training program, including workouts and a nutrition plan. Finally, wearable fitness trackers such as Jawbone [63] and Fitbit [64] track your activity and sleep and provide the option of sharing this information on social media sites with your "followers."

Research has proven that peers have a significant impact on health behavior. When people are losing weight around you, you are more likely to lose weight, and when they are quitting smoking, you are more likely to cease smoking. Social media is a modern community that can also impact our health behavior. A few examples of the power of social media on health behavior follow.

Researchers' compiled data from 12 studies, involving 1,884 participants, spread across the USA, Europe, east Asia, and Australia, which examined social networking services for weight loss. The amalgamated results showed that people who used these services achieved a collective modest, but significant, decrease in body mass index (BMI) by a value of 0.64.

PatientsLikeMe [65] is an online platform for patients with life-changing illnesses. These patients share their experience, find other patients like them matched on demographic and clinical characteristics, and learn from the aggregated data reports of others to improve their health. The goal of the website is to help patients answer the question: "Given my status, what is the best outcome I can hope to achieve, and how do I get there?"

Research demonstrated that a substantial proportion of members of PatientsLikeMe experience benefits from participating in the community. Much of the benefit comes from peer-to-peer interaction to aid decision-making [66]. Patients reported making more informed treatment decisions as a result of using the site, particularly around managing side effects. Members felt that they improved management of their symptoms and were better able to communicate with peers experiencing the same problems [67].

## Social Media: Impact on Patient Care

Health policy researcher and surgeon Dr. Hutan Ashrafian, from the Department of Surgery and Cancer, Imperial College London, succinctly summarizes the power of social media on health behavior: "One advantage of using social media over other methods is that it offers the potential to be much more cost-effective and practical for day-to-day use when compared to traditional approaches. The feeling of being part of a community allows patients to draw on the support of their peers as well as clinicians. They can get advice from their doctor without the inconvenience or cost of having to travel, and clinicians can provide advice to many patients simultaneously" [68]. In addition, information about successful health behavior can be shared with the specific disease LHS cycle in order for the system to continue to learn so that others with similar conditions can improve their health.

## The Learning Health System: A Case Study

This chapter began with a discussion of health IT and how the four pillars of health IT (cloud, mobile devices, sensors, and social media) generate the big data that can potentially fuel the learning health system (LHS). To date the LHS does not exist; however, a few dental schools have started work on the cloud and mobile pillars that will lay the foundation for an LHS. These dental schools have started to explore the use of cloud EHRs delivered on tablets and other mobile devices in order to reduce the up-front capital costs of purchasing and installing software, servers, backups, and other infrastructure. Since cloud EHR companies are new to the market, they tend to be designed with the user in mind and are more intuitive to use [69]. Students expect modern capabilities from the dental school EHR, such as patient records, including radiographs and other images, to be accessible anywhere they have an Internet connection, including on mobile devices. Students ask to collaborate with faculty via secure e-mail or web conference on their phones about a patient they encountered at an outreach rotation [70]. Dental school administrators expect that all records will be available at all times, even immediately after a disaster; that security will continually meet all school, state, and federal regulations; [71] and that the increasing costs of EHR systems will diminish [72]. The cloud EHR that operates on mobile devices meets these requirements.

Eventually these dental schools expect that the data generated by the dental school EHRs will be combined with data from the two additional pillars—sensors and social media. Data from the EHRs merged with data gathered by oral [73] and medical sensors as well as social media information about successful dental behavior can be combined into an LHS cycle in order for the LHS to continue to learn about oral health conditions and consequently provide patients and care providers answers to specific oral and general health questions.

Consequently, the University of Michigan, University of Pittsburgh, and University of North Carolina are partnering with Internet2 to seek a cloud EHR solution that meets the needs of dental education. The result is an innovative collaboration between the cloud EHR service provider ICE Health Systems, the three dentals schools, and Internet2 [74, 75]. This is the first time a service provider has agreed to work with dental schools to develop an EHR that would meet their needs. This collaboration is focused on supporting the patient care, education, and research missions of academic dentistry with the long-term goal of improving patient outcomes, first in oral health and then in all of health, through a learning health system.

### Conclusions

Movements in technology impact patient care in all settings, from hospital to private practice. Private practices already juggle system advancements in digital radiology, prescriptions, referrals, or in collaboration with laboratories. The motivations for changing to electronic systems can be myriad, from peer pressure to legislation. Sometimes technology might be adopted solely for patient comfort. In Whitmore Lake, Michigan, the offices of Gentle Dental promise that the patient experience will be positive because their offices are "equipped with state-of-the-art technology that enables us to provide superior care for you and your family," including digital X-rays, TV watching, heated blankets, and games for the kids [76].

Health IT has evolved from computers that took an entire room to process a few numbers to current mobile or wearable computers with processors, connectivity, and software. This chapter has discussed four current health IT trends that are impacting personal health: (1) the growth of computer farms that create a "cloud" for storing and processing data; (2) the movement toward smaller, more mobile devices used by patients; (3) the development of sensors that detect physiologic and chemical changes in the human body; and (4) the evolution of sharing personal health information to inform support communities. The amalgamation of sensors monitoring our physical health with personalized mobile devices and sharing of health information, when combined with cloud computing, makes data collection, access, and distribution feel inseparable from our personal life. In short, health IT is creating new ways for each of us to proactively monitor and proactively improve our health.

Currently health IT is trending toward empowering the individual. Health IT also has the potential to combine the big data used for personalizing health and combine it with research findings and data from cloud-based EHR systems in hospitals and other healthcare entities to power the learning health system (LHS). Once a LHS disease cycle is developed, it will continuously access relevant health information from entities across the nation, conduct analyses that convert the data to useful knowledge, and transmit that knowledge to individuals and health stakeholders in ways that accelerate health-enhancing behavioral change. The dream of the health IT combined with the LHS is anticipated to shorten the 17-year "bench-to-bedside" gap between knowledge discovery and its application in personal health to 17 months. That may be the biggest transformation to ever occur in healthcare.

## References

1. Akesson J. Arabic proverbs and wise sayings (English and Arabic edition). Lund: Pallas Athena Distribution; 2011. Available at: http://www.quotes.net/quote/16548.
2. Chaudhry B, Wang J, Wu S, Maglione M, Mojica W, Roth E, et al. Systematic review: impact of health information technology on quality, efficiency, and costs of medical care. Ann Intern Med. 2006; 144(10):742–52.
3. Healthcare IT News. The usage of tablets in the healthcare industry. 2012. Available at: http://www.healthcareitnews.com/blog/usage-tablets-healthcare-industry. Accessed Jan 2015.
4. Schrum J. Fitness trackers: motivating you to move. Consumer Electron Assoc. Available at: http://www.ce.org/CorporateSite/media/CEA-Consumer-Info/health%20and%20fitness/FitnessTrackers.pdf. Accessed Jan 2015.
5. Kholsa V. Technology will replace 80% of what doctors do. Fortune. 2012. Available at: http://tech.fortune.cnn.com/2012/12/04/technology-doctors-khosla/.
6. Institute of Medicine. Best care at lower cost: the path to continuously learning health care in America. A consensus report from the Institute of Medicine. 2012. Available at: http://www.iom.edu/Reports/2012/Best-Care-at-Lower-Cost-The-Path-to-Continuously-Learning-Health-Care-in-America.aspx. Accessed Jan 2015.
7. Olsen L, Aisner D, McGinnis JM. The learning healthcare system. Washington: National Academies Press; 2007.
8. Law N, Yuen A, Fox R. Educational innovations beyond technology: nurturing leadership and establishing learning organizations. New York: Springer; 2011.
9. Friedman C, Rubin J, Brown J, Buntin M, Corn M, Etheredge L, et al. Toward a science of learning systems: a research agenda for the high-functioning Learning Health System. J Am Med Inform Assoc. 2015;22(1):43–50.
10. Morris Z, Wooding S, Grant J. The answer is 17 years, what is the question: understanding time lags in translational research. J Royal Soc Med. 2011;104(12):510–20.
11. Friedman C, Rigby M. Conceptualising and creating a global learning health system. Int J Med Inform. 2013;82(4):e63–71.
12. NIH National Institute of Dental and Craniofacial Research. Dental practice-based research to improve oral health and to support the adoption of evidence-based clinical practice. Available at: http://www.nidcr.nih.gov/grantsandfunding/See_Funding_Opportunities_Sorted_By/ConceptClearance/CurrentCC/PracticeBasedResearch.htm?_ga=1.186430441.1990314821.1416494358.
13. NIH National Institute of Dental and Craniofacial Research. Strategic plan 2014–2019. Available at: http://www.nidcr.nih.gov/research/ResearchPriorities/StrategicPlan/Documents/nidcr-strategic-plan-2014-2019.pdf?_ga=1.186430441.1990314821.1416494358.
14. NIH National Institute of Dental and Craniofacial Research. The role of practitioners in the new National Dental Practice-Based Research Network. Available at: http://www.nidcr.nih.gov/Research/DER/ClinicalResearch/Archive/?_ga=1.186430441.1990314821.1416494358.
15. Center for Healthcare Research & Transformation. A learning health state for Michigan. Available at: http://www.chrt.org/events/a-learning-health-state-for-michigan/. Accessed Oct 2014.
16. Office of the National Coordinator for Health Information technology (ONC). Federal Health Information Technology Strategic Plan 2011–2015. Available at: http://www.healthit.gov/sites/default/files/utility/final-federal-health-it-strategic--plan-0911.pdf. Accessed Nov 2014.
17. Delaney B. TRANSFoRm: Translational research and patient safety in Europe. Available at: https://joinup.ec.europa.eu/node/134978. Accessed Nov 2014.
18. Rubin JC, Friedman CP. Weaving together a healthcare improvement tapestry: learning health system

brings together health data stakeholders to share knowledge and improve health. J AHIMA. 2014;85(5):38–43.

19. Fox K. New Jersey dentists lose office, gain hope after hurricane. ADA News. 2013. Available at: http://www.ada.org/en/publications/ada-news/2013-archive/february/new-jersey-dentists-lose-office--gain-hope-after-hurricane. Accessed Nov 2014.
20. Inspire Periodontics & Implants. Available at: http://inspirevancouver.com/home.htm. Accessed Nov 2014.
21. Sheehan M, Wayne T. Cloud computing explained [video]. Uploaded by HighT3chDad on Sep 29, 2008. Available at: http://www.youtube.com/watch?v=QJncFirhjPg. Accessed 15 Mar 2011.
22. Armbrust M, Fox A, Griffith R, Joseph AD, Katz R, Konwinski A, et al. Above the clouds: a Berkeley view of cloud computing. 2009. Technical Report No. UCB/EECS-2009-28. Available at: http://www.eecs.berkeley.edu/Pubs/TechRpts/2009/EECS-2009-28.html.
23. Katzan Jr H. On an ontological view of cloud computing. Commun Assoc Comput Machinery. 2010;3:1.
24. Schweitzer EH. Reconciliation of the cloud computing model with US federal electronic health record regulations. J Am Med Inform Assoc. 2012;19:161–5. doi:10.1136/amiajnl-2011-000162.
25. Perera G, Holbrook A, Thabane L, Foster G, Willison DJ. Views on health information sharing and privacy from primary care practices using electronic medical records. Int J Med Inform. 2011;80(2):94–101. doi:10.1016/j.ijmedinf.2010.11.005.
26. ICE Health Systems. Available at: http://icehealthsystems.com/. Accessed Oct 2014.
27. Dovetail. Available at: http://dovetail.co/. Accessed Oct 2014.
28. Dentisoft Technologies. Dentisoft Office Cloud Pro Software. Available at: http://www.dentisoft.com/. Accessed Oct 2014.
29. Practice Fusion. Available at: http://www.practicefusion.com. Accessed Oct 2014.
30. GE Healthcare. Centricity EMR. Available at: http://www3.gehealthcare.com/en/Products/Categories/Healthcare_IT/Electronic_Medical_Records/Centricity_EMR. Accessed Oct 2014.
31. Scriptnetics. Inc. MedScribbler. Available at: http://www.medscribbler.com/. Accessed Oct 2014.
32. Brownstein JS, Freifeld CC, Madoff LC. Digital disease detection—harnessing the web for public health surveillance. N Engl J Med. 2009;360:2153–7.
33. Hillestad R, Bigelow J, Bower A, Girosi F, Meili R, Scoville R, et al. Can electronic medical record systems transform health care? Potential health benefits, savings, and costs. Health Aff. 2005;24(5):1103–17.
34. Wu SS, editor. Guide to HIPAA security and the law. Chicago: ABA Section of Science & Technology Law; 2007.
35. U.S. Department of Health & Human Services. Health Information Technology for Economic and Clinical Health (HITECH) Act. Fed Reg 160: Health Insurance Reform: Security Standards; Final Rule. 2009. Available at: http://www.gpo.gov/fdsys/pkg/FR-2013-01-25/pdf/2013-01073.pdf.
36. U.S. Department of Health & Human Services. Health Information Privacy: Omnibus HIPAA Rulemaking. Available at: http://www.hhs.gov/ocr/privacy/hipaa/administrative/omnibus/index.html. Accessed Nov 2014.
37. Li M, Yu S, Ren K, Lou W. Securing personal health records in cloud computing: patient-centric and fine-grained data access control in multi-owner settings. Security and privacy in communication networks. Lecture Notes of the Institute for Computer Sciences. Soc Informat Telecommun Eng. 2010;50:89–106.
38. Kuo AM. Opportunities and challenges of cloud computing to improve health care services. J Med Internet Res. 2011;13(3):e67.
39. Dasilva A, Maslowski E, Sheehan S. PainTrek. Available at: http://um3d.dc.umich.edu/portfolio/paintrek/. Accessed Dec 2014.
40. UM3DLab. PainTrek-Mobile Pain Tracking and Analysis (Beta-v0.9). Available at: https://www.youtube.com/watch?v=CP8tvz2nmpY. Accessed Dec 2014.
41. Donnell A, Nascimento T, Lawrence M, Gupta V, Zieba T, Truong D, et al. High-definition and non-invasive brain modulation of sensorimotor dysfunction in chronic TMD. Brain Stimulation. 2015. (In press).
42. DaSilva AF, Nascimento T, DosSantos M, Lucas S, Van Holsbeeck H, DeBoer M, et al. μ-opioid activation in the prefrontal cortex in migraine attacks – brief report I. Ann Clin Transl Neurol. 2014;1(6):439–44.
43. DaSilva AF, Nascimento TD, Love T, DosSantos MF, Martikainen IK, Cummiford CM, et al. 3D-neuronavigation in vivo through a patient's brain during a spontaneous migraine headache. J Vis Exp. 2014;88:50682.
44. Nascimento T, DosSantos M, Lucas S, Van Holsbeeck H, DeBoer M, Maslowski E, et al. μ-opioid activation in the midbrain during migraine allodynia – brief report II. Ann Clin Transl Neurol. 2014;1(6):445–50.
45. OmniPod. OmniPod Insulin Management System. Available at: http://www.myomnipod.com/2013. Accessed Dec 2014.
46. National Diabetes Information Clearinghouse. DCCT and EDIC: the diabetes control and complications trial and follow-up study. Available at: http://diabetes.niddk.nih.gov/dm/pubs/control/index.aspx. Accessed Nov 2014.
47. Maione A. OP 27 psychological aspects of diabetes. Presented at the 43rd Annual Meeting of the European Association for the Study of Diabetes. Amsterdam. 2007.
48. National Center for Chronic Disease prevention and Health Promotion, Center for Disease Control and Prevention. National Diabetes Statistics Report 2014. Available at: http://www.cdc.gov/diabetes/pubs/statsreport14/national-diabetes-report-web.pdf. Accessed 20 Nov 2014.

49. Schaffer N. The role of human factors in the design and development of an insulin pump. J Diabetes Sci Technol. 2012;6(2):260–4.
50. Grunberger G, Bailey TS, Cohen AJ, Flood TM, Handelsman Y, Hellman R, et al. Statement by the American Association of Clinical Endocrinologists Consensus Panel on insulin pump management. Endocr Pract. 2010;16(4):746–62.
51. Schmeken H. Insulin on board: pumps and their bolus wizard. Diabetes Hands Foundation. Available at: http://www.tudiabetes.org/forum/topics/insulin-on-board-pumps-and-their-bolus-wizard. Accessed Nov 2014.
52. Joseph TA, Solanki J, Choudhary OP, Chouksey S, Malvia N, Chaturvedi P et al. Towards a wearable non-invasive blood glucose monitoring device. International Conference on Recent Trends in Physics (ICRTP 2012). J Phys. Conference Series 365 (2012); 012004:1–5.
53. PhysIQ. Available at: http://www.physiq.com/. Accessed Nov 2014.
54. Burke M. PhysIQ (formerly VGBio). Chicago Innovation Exchange at the University of Chicago. Available at: https://cie.uchicago.edu/innovation-fund/company/physiq-formerly-vgbio. Accessed Nov 2014.
55. Kappe B. VGBio's [PhysIQ] Vitalink: Predictive Analytics for Remote Patient Monitoring. [Hardware/software development blog.] Available at: http://blog.pathfindersoftware.com/blog/bid/279681/VGBio-s-Vitalink-Predictive-Analytics-for-Remote-Patient-Monitoring. Accessed Nov 2014.
56. Heaivilin N, Gerbert B, Page JE, Gibbs JL. Public surveillance of dental pain via Twitter. J Dent Res. 2011;90(9):1047–51.doi:10.1177/0022034511415273. Epub 18 Jul 2011.
57. Fox S. The engaged e-patient population: people turn to the Internet for health information when stakes are high and the connection fast. Washington: Pew Internet and American Life Project; 2008.
58. Garrity B. Social media join toolkit for hunters of disease. The New York Times. 2011. Available at: http://www.nytimes.com/2011/06/14/health/research/14social.html?pagewanted=all&_r=4&. Accessed Nov 2014.
59. Wikipedia. Legionnaires disease. Available at: http://en.wikipedia.org/wiki/Legionnaires%27_disease. Accessed Nov 2014.
60. Brownstein J, Freifed C. Healthmap. Harvard University. 2014. Available at: http://healthmap.org/en/. Accessed Nov 2014.
61. Freifeld C, Brownstein J. Outbreaks Near Me. 2007. Available at: http://healthmap.org/outbreaksnearme/. Accessed Nov 2014.
62. Fitocracy. 2014. Available at: https://www.fitocracy.com/. Accessed 2014.
63. Jawbone. 2014. Available at: https://jawbone.com/. Accessed Dec 2014.
64. Fitbit. 2014. Available at: http://www.fitbit.com/. Accessed Dec 2014.
65. PatientsLikeMe. 2014. Available at: https://www.patientslikeme.com/. Accessed Nov 2014.
66. Fox S, Jones S. The social life of health information: Americans' pursuit of health takes place within a widening network of both online and offline sources. Washington: Pew Internet & American Life Project; 2009. Available at: http://www.pewinternet.org/Reports/2009/8-The-Social-Life-of--HealthInformation.aspx.
67. Wicks P, Massagli M, Frost J, Brownstein C, Okun S, Vaughan T, et al. Sharing health data for better outcomes on PatientsLikeMe. J Med Internet Res. 2010;12(2), e19. doi:10.2196/jmir.1549. Epub 14 Jun 2010.
68. Ashrafian H, Toma T, Harling L, Kerr K, Athanasiou T, Darzi A. Social networking strategies that aim to reduce obesity have achieved significant although modest results. Health Aff. 2014;33(9):1641. doi:10.1377/hlthaff.2014.0370.
69. Mandl KD, Mandel JC, Murphy SN, Bernstam EV, Ramoni RL, Kreda DA, et al. The SMART Platform: early experience enabling substitutable applications for electronic health records. J Am Med Inform Assoc. 2012;19(4):597–603. doi:10.1136/amiajnl-2011-000622. Epub 17 Mar 2012.
70. Johnson L, Genuis M, Spallek H, Rankin D. The Electronic Health Record (R)evolution. An invited presentation at the Internet2 Global Summit. Denver; 2014.
71. Berd J. Forecasting the future of dental software—it's in the cloud! The Progressive Dentist Magazine. 2014. Available at: http://theprodentist.com/forecasting-the-future-of-dental-software-its-in-the-cloud/. Accessed Nov 2014.
72. Spallek H, Johnson L, Kerr J, Rankin D. Costs of health IT: beginning to understand the financial impact of a dental school EHR. J Dent Educ. 2014;78:1542–51.
73. Yirka B. Team develops tooth embedded sensor for oral activity recognition. Phys Org. 2013. Available at: http://www.Users/cranialfacial/Downloads/2013-09-team-tooth-embedded-sensor-oral.pdf. Accessed Jan 2015.
74. Creech M. The Universities of Michigan, North Carolina at Chapel Hill and Pittsburgh to spearhead Internet2 NET+ ICE-EHR Offering. Available at: http://www.internet2.edu/news/detail/6992/. Accessed Nov 2014.
75. Engel S. Dentistry in the cloud: molding electronic health records to research and education. Int Sci Grid This Week. 2014. Available at: http://www.isgtw.org/feature/dentistry-cloud-molding-electronic-health--records-research-and-education. Accessed Nov 2014.
76. Gentle Dental. Available at: http://www.smilelakeview.com/.

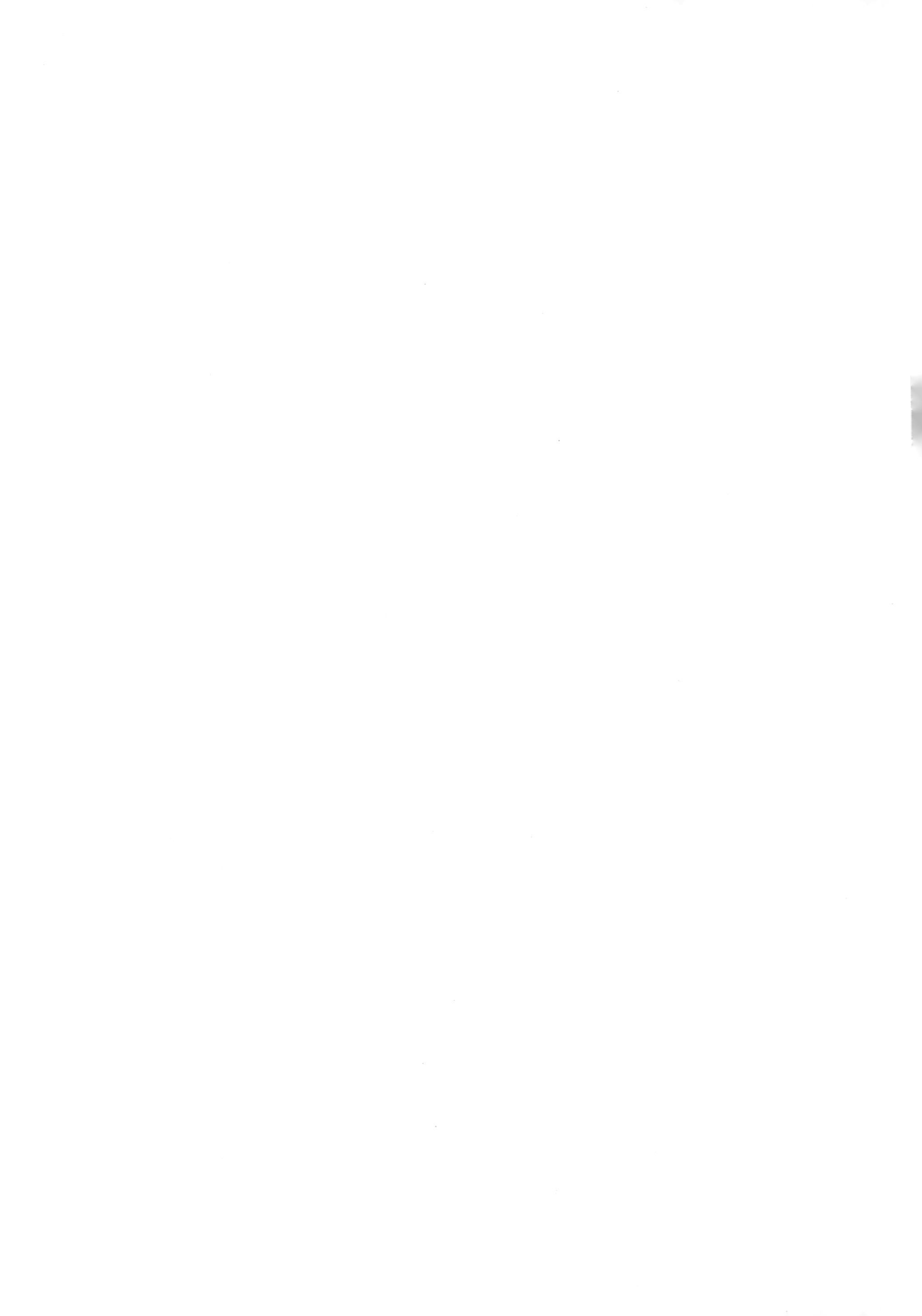

# 4 Biomarkers for Individualized Oral Cancer Therapy

Nisha J. D'Silva

**Abstract**
This chapter focuses on personalized medicine for oral cancer, with emphasis on selection of current and future therapies. Specifically, treatment selection of radiation, chemotherapy, and surgery and customized strategies for selection of targeted therapy are discussed. Worldwide, head and neck cancer is the sixth most common cancer by incidence and the fifth most common cause of cancer-related deaths. More than 90 % of oral cancers are squamous cell carcinomas (SCCs), which are the focus of this chapter. SCC arises from the oral cavity including lip, oropharynx/tonsil, larynx, and hypopharynx. The risk factors for SCC are tobacco, alcohol, and human papillomavirus 16 (HPV16). HPV-positive SCC usually occurs in the oropharynx, and HPV-negative SCC usually occurs in the oral cavity, larynx, and hypopharynx. Personalized medicine is customization of treatment to the individual patient. The goals of personalized medicine are to improve clinical outcome, reduce side effects, and decrease expenses. Currently personalized medicine in oral cancer is based on tumor stage and location, but not tumor biology. Unfortunately, two patients with similar tumor stage may respond differently to the same therapy. Identification at the time of diagnosis of an early-stage lesion that will behave aggressively will facilitate selection of appropriate aggressive treatment at the time of initial diagnosis. However, aggressive treatment is not appropriate for all early-stage lesions due to toxicity of treatment. Although targeted treatment has been developed for SCC, it is not used in a customized approach. This chapter discusses evolving approaches to customize therapy based on the biology of the individual tumor. Furthermore, targeted therapy and potential biomarkers to match therapy to patients are also discussed.

N.J. D'Silva, BDS, MSD, PhD
Division of Oral Medicine, Pathology and Radiology,
Department of Periodontics and Oral Medicine,
University of Michigan School of Dentistry,
Ann Arbor, MI, USA
e-mail: njdsilva@umich.edu



P.J. Polverini (ed.), *Personalized Oral Health Care: From Concept Design to Clinical Practice*,
DOI 10.1007/978-3-319-23297-3_4

## Introduction

Personalized, or precision, medicine matches therapy to individuals who will benefit from it [1]. Personalized medicine requires classification of individuals into subgroups based on susceptibility to a specific disease or response to a specific type of treatment [1]. The intent of the customized approach is to improve clinical outcome while reducing side effects and expenses [1]. Customization of patient management may be based on clinical parameters and/or genomic, proteomic, transcriptomic, and metabolomic signatures. This chapter will focus on personalized medicine for head and neck/oral cancer.

Worldwide, head and neck cancer is the sixth most common cancer by incidence, with about 600,000 new cases a year [2]. Globally, it is the fifth most common cause of cancer-related deaths [3]. The main tumors that comprise head and neck cancers are squamous cell carcinomas (SCCs), nasopharyngeal cancers, and malignant salivary gland tumors. More than 90 % of head and neck cancers are SCCs [4, 5], which are the focus of this chapter. SCCs arise from the oral cavity (~46 %), including the lip, oropharynx/tonsil (~12 %), larynx (~35 %), and hypopharynx (~8 %) [6]. The risk factors for SCC are tobacco, alcohol, and human papillomavirus 16 (HPV16), which is a risk factor primarily for oropharyngeal SCC [2].

Presently, personalized medicine for SCC is based on tumor stage and location but not tumor biology [6]. The American Joint Committee on Cancer (AJCC) staging system is based on tumor size, nodal involvement, and metastases (TNM), with early-stage (stage I or II) lesions having localized tumors <4 cm with no lymph node involvement or metastases. SCC usually presents at an advanced stage (stage III and IV), characterized by large primary tumors, possibly with nodal involvement and metastases. Early-stage SCC is usually treated with surgery or radiation, whereas late-stage disease is given multimodality treatment including chemotherapy/radiation or chemotherapy/radiation/surgery [4, 7, 8]. Patients with advanced SCC usually die from locoregional recurrence [9]. Due to minimal improvement in survival in four decades, the emphasis moved to dose escalation, but this is limited by toxic effects on patients. Complications of radiation include xerostomia, osteoradionecrosis, neck stiffness, and speech and swallowing difficulties [10]. Chemotherapeutic agents may include DNA-damaging agents and antimetabolites [7], which also have adverse side effects. The goals of treatment are to eliminate the cancer, preserve or restore function, and maintain/improve the quality of life [8]. The survival of patients with SCC has not improved dramatically in four to five decades. New treatment options are needed to improve survival and quality of life.

Tumor recurrence and spread decrease survival of SCC patients. Most SCC cases are advanced at diagnosis, and ~30 % of advanced cases recur within the first two years of treatment [11]. Recurrent tumor leads to failure of primary treatment and poor clinical outcome [4, 7, 12]. After failure of primary treatment, subsequent treatment options are not particularly effective [12]. The median survival time for patients with recurrent and/or metastatic SCC is less than a year [13]. Consequently, SCC patients are monitored by frequent clinical examinations and diagnostic imaging after treatment [14]. What is needed is an effective and comparatively inexpensive approach for monitoring tumor recurrence. Customized treatment selection and screening frequency are the goals of personalized medicine in SCC.

Targeted therapy, which is treatment against critical molecules that promote tumor progression, has been developed. However, except for cetuximab, a monoclonal antibody against EGFR, targeted therapy has been ineffective against SCC or is not used in the context of selected patients (personalized medicine). Given the emerging literature on genetic, proteomic, transcriptomic, and metabolomic signatures that predict responsiveness to therapy, personalized medicine based on tumor biology is a reasonable goal for SCC. The emphasis of this chapter will be biomarkers that facilitate selection of existing treatment and emerging targeted therapy.

## Prediction of Therapeutic Response (Treatment Selection)

Current treatment selection for SCC is based on tumor stage [15] rather than prediction of patient response to specific therapy [7]. Early-stage oral cavity SCC is treated with surgery alone, and 5-year survival is excellent. However, 3–37 % of patients with early-stage lesions will develop recurrent or second primary tumors and die of their disease in less than 5 years [16–18]. These individuals would likely benefit from aggressive treatment at the outset, but based on current knowledge, the group cannot be separated from those patients with early-stage SCC who respond well to therapy [19]. Aggressive treatment is not appropriate for all early-stage lesions due to physical and emotional challenges including facial disfiguration, feeding and speech impediments, dry mouth, taste abnormalities, and poor quality of life [20]. Treatment options for recurrent disease are sparse [21]. In a customized treatment approach, individuals with early-stage SCC that will behave aggressively would be identified at initial diagnosis and receive aggressive treatment. For example, a small study suggests that rap-1GAP is expressed in low N-stage SCC that respond well to therapy [22].

In understanding the discussion on personalized medicine in SCC, the following explanation of terms may be of value. Overall survival is the time that the patient survives, regardless of the cause of death. Cause-specific survival is the duration that a patient survives before dying from the disease itself, not an unrelated cause. Disease-free survival is the duration that the patient survives after treatment, without evidence of disease. In contrast, progression-free survival is the duration that a person survives after completion of treatment that stabilized the disease but did not eliminate it, i.e., the disease did not progress. A local recurrence is disease at the same site after removal of the primary tumor. A second primary cancer is a new tumor that is at a site distinct from the first tumor. For example, if a patient had a SCC on the tongue and later developed a SCC on the buccal mucosa, the buccal mucosa lesion would be a second primary tumor.

Etiologic factors, tumor histopathology, and other tumor biomarkers may predict response to existing therapy (surgery, radiation, chemotherapy), thereby informing treatment selection.

### Etiologic Factors

HPV16, tobacco, and alcohol are the major etiologic factors for SCC [23]. Tobacco and alcohol have a synergistic effect in the etiology of HPV-negative SCC [2, 24]. The synergistic impact, if any, of tobacco on HPV-positive SCC is unknown [25]. In the USA, the decrease in tobacco smoking correlated with a decrease in tobacco-related SCC [26, 27]. Concurrently, the incidence of HPV16-positive oropharyngeal SCC increased significantly, possibly due to changes in sexual behavior [28]. Specifically, in recent decades, the number of sexual partners per individual has increased, and individuals are sexually active at a younger age [28]. From 1983 to 2002, the incidence of HPV-positive oropharyngeal SCC increased from less than 20 % to almost 70 % in economically developed countries [29]. HPV-positive oropharyngeal SCC may exceed cervical cancer, the classic HPV-induced cancer, by 2020 [29, 30]. In contrast, in developing countries, less than 10 % of oropharyngeal SCC are caused by HPV infection [31, 32].

HPV-positive and HPV-negative (tobacco- and alcohol-related) SCC are clinically distinct entities [30]. HPV-positive SCC occurs almost exclusively in the oropharynx, particularly the lingual and palatine tonsils [25, 33]. Most SCC that occur in the oral cavity (floor of mouth, anterior tongue, alveolar process, gingiva, hard palate, lip), larynx, and hypopharynx are tobacco-related and HPV negative [8]. Patients with HPV-positive oropharyngeal SCC are typically nonsmokers, nondrinkers, and younger than patients with HPV-negative SCC [25, 34]. In general, SCC occurs primarily in men. This gender predilection is amplified in HPV-positive oropharyngeal SCC [35–38]. In fact, the oropharynx is the most common site for HPV-related malignancies in men [39].

HPV-positive SCC also exhibits a racial predilection, occurring more commonly in white than black patients [25]. One-third of all SCC occurring in whites are HPV positive compared to 4 % of SCC occurring in blacks [40]. Furthermore, almost all HPV-positive tumors (97 %) and 77 % of HPV-negative tumors occur in whites [40]. The increased occurrence of oropharyngeal SCC in white compared to black patients has been attributed to the increasing incidence of HPV-positive SCC [39]. Patients with HPV-positive SCC have a higher socio-economic status and more years of education and are more likely to be married than HPV-negative patients [25]. HPV-positive HNSCC was also correlated with increasing intensity, duration, and cumulative joint years of marijuana use [23].

Biologically, HPV-positive tumors may be less aggressive lesions than stage-matched HPV-negative SCC. Patients with HPV-positive oropharyngeal SCC have a favorable prognosis compared to HPV-negative SCC [41–43], which has a 5-year survival rate of ~50 % [4]. Compared to HPV-negative SCC, patients with HPV-positive SCC have lower risk of tumor progression and better overall survival [42–47]. In fact, HPV status is the most robust independent prognostic indicator for oropharyngeal SCC [48, 49]. HPV-positive SCC often presents as a small tumor with nodal involvement [25]. Notably, nodal metastases with an unknown primary tumor are more likely to be HPV-positive than HPV-negative SCC [23, 50]. Using the AJCC staging system, the nodal involvement correlates with a later stage lesion [46, 47, 51, 52]. Even though it is detected at a late stage, HPV-positive oropharyngeal SCC has a better prognosis than similar stage HPV-negative SCC [42, 43]. Since treatment selection is guided by tumor stage, HPV-positive tumors with nodal metastases would be considered late-stage lesions and receive more aggressive treatment than early-stage lesions. HPV-positive tumors are responsive to induction chemotherapy and to chemoradiotherapy [42]. HPV16-positive oropharyngeal SCCs, even at an advanced stage, respond better to treatment than HPV-negative tumors.

Tobacco negatively affects the response of HPV-positive oropharyngeal SCC to treatment and patient survival [53, 54]. Patients with HPV-positive SCC have better survival than HPV-negative (tobacco- and alcohol-related) tumors unless they have a history of smoking [4, 43]. Survival diminishes with each additional pack-year of smoking [43].

Since patients with HPV-positive tumors are younger at diagnosis, they are less likely to have comorbidities [25]. Furthermore, patients with HPV-negative SCC are more likely to show field cancerization than HPV-positive tumors, due to the diffuse effects of carcinogens [30].

HPV positivity in oropharyngeal SCC is evaluated by in situ hybridization for genomic DNA of HPV16 and immunohistochemistry for p16 [25, 55]. Detection of E6/E7 antibodies and p16 immunostaining or HPV16 DNA are valuable biomarkers that correlate with a favorable prognosis [56]. HPV copy number in pre-treatment biopsies also appears to impact patient survival [37]. Higher copy number was correlated with better overall survival after adjustment for age, gender, past or current tobacco exposure, T-stage, N-stage, and primary site [37]. The etiologic role of HPV in oral cavity cancers has not been established [44, 57, 58]. In fact, only 5.9 % of oral cavity SCC exhibit high-risk HPV [58]. In oral cavity SCC, p16 is not recommended as a surrogate for HPV detection [58].

### Role of HPV Status in Treatment Selection

Currently, although HPV-positive SCC is associated with better prognosis, these patients are treated similarly to HPV-negative SCC [25, 59]. Unfortunately, radiation and chemotherapy, used for treatment of HPV-positive SCC, greatly impact the quality of life, including difficulties with swallowing and xerostomia after radiation [60, 61]. In a personalized medicine approach, de-escalation of therapy is being explored for patients with HPV-positive tumors with the potential to eliminate short- and long-term side effects of current therapy [30]. ECOG-E1308 is a clinical trial evaluating the efficacy of induction chemotherapy with reduced cetuximab and radiation dose (more information at clinical trials.gov; NCT01084083) [25]. Recent findings from this clinical trial are encouraging [62]. Induction chemotherapy with subsequent reduced-dose cetuximab and IMRT (intensity modulated radiation therapy) resulted in high tumor control rates and reduced toxicities [62]. Progression-free survival was 96 % for patients with HPV-positive oropharyngeal SCC with less than 10-year smoking history, T-stage one through three, and N0-2b tumors [62].

Another clinical trial, RTOG-1016 (RTOG = Radiation Therapy Oncology Group) is a clinical trial that is cetuximab or cisplatin with concurrent radiation therapy for HPV-positive SCC [63]. Cetuximab is less toxic than cisplatin [25]. However, due to the slow rate of patient accrual and the long follow-up, the results from this study may take several years [30].

While locoregional disease control is better in HPV-positive SCC, the rates of distant metastases are similar in HPV-positive and -negative SCC [64]. In fact, HPV-positive metastases may occur at multiple sites [64]. Therefore, currently, de-intensification of therapy based on tumor HPV status is not recommended outside a clinical trial [25, 65].

## Histopathology

In primary SCC, islands of malignant epithelium of surface epithelial origin invade the underlying mesenchymal tissue from where it may metastasize to distant sites. The neoplastic epithelial islands may invade adjacent structures such as blood vessels, peripheral nerves, and skeletal muscle. An inflammatory infiltrate of varying intensity is observed in proximity to the malignant epithelial islands.

Tumor histopathology may have a role in personalized medicine for oral cavity SCC by informing treatment selection. For example, in some locations, depth of invasion informs treatment selection. For floor of the mouth and tongue lesions, local control, survival rates, and nodal disease are poorer at tumor thicknesses greater than 4 mm than those that are less than 4 mm [66]. Neck dissection is advocated for tumors >2 mm depth of invasion due to association with a high rate (40 %) of occult metastatic disease [67, 68].

Currently, tumor stage dictates treatment selection. For example, surgery is the treatment of choice in early-stage oral cavity SCC [8]. In contrast, late-stage disease exhibiting metastases to lymph nodes, extracapsular spread of nodal disease, and distant metastases is treated more aggressively since these tumor characteristics are correlated with poor prognosis [69–72]. However, disease-specific mortality rates for stage I/II oral cavity SCC vary from 3 to 37 % [16–18]. These findings suggest that some patients with early-stage SCC who are at greater risk of treatment failure would benefit from aggressive initial treatment. The histologic risk model attempts to address this deficiency in selection of treatment by tumor stage. The risk assessment is based on worst pattern of invasion, perineural invasion, and lymphocytic host response at the tumor-stroma interface [19, 73–75]. Patterns of invasion are classified as broad pushing islands, fingerlike tumor islands, large islands, single-cell tumor cords, and satellite islands. Recognizing that a tumor may have multiple patterns of invasion, the worst pattern is scored. Scores for perineural invasion are based on involvement of small or large (>1 mm) nerves. The lymphocytic host response is graded as strong, intermediate, or weak. A low-risk score is correlated with a low likelihood of locoregional recurrence, whereas a high-risk score would indicate an aggressive lesion [19]. Small clusters of tumor cells or wide distances between tumor islands are predictive of regional lymph node involvement at initial presentation and locoregional recurrence [76]. Lymph node metastases at initial presentation are correlated with poor survival [77–81]. In contrast, tumors with pushing invasive fronts, solid cords, or strands of SCC cells are less likely to exhibit locoregional spread or recurrence [76].

Another risk assessment model is based on pattern of invasion at the invasive front and lymphocytic infiltration at the tumor-stroma interface, keratinization of tumor islands, nuclear pleomorphism, and mitoses per high power field [82, 83]. Essentially, the rationale for the risk assessment models that incorporate pattern of invasion is that early-stage tumors with aggressive cells at the invasive front of the tumor will behave aggressively despite the early detection [76, 82–84]. Using the risk profile, local recurrence and overall survival were correlated with pattern of invasion of SCC cells at the invasive front [76, 82, 83]. For example, the microscopic risk profile of some early-stage oral cavity SCC correlates with risk of treatment failure [19]. However, the positive predictive value for locoregional progression of low-stage oral cavity SCC with a worst pattern of invasion type 5 is 42 % [75]. Although this is not a perfect model for prediction of tumor progression in oral cavity SCC, it has been shown to have predictive value [19].

Microscopically, SCC exhibit keratinizing or nonkeratinizing histopathology, with most tumors exhibiting a keratinizing morphology [84]. The tumors may be described as well, moderately, or poorly differentiated; well-differentiated lesions exhibit prominent keratin pearl formation, intercellular bridges, and minimal nuclear pleomorphism [85]. The poorly differentiated lesions exhibit prominent nuclear pleomorphism, a high mitotic index, and atypical mitoses and may require immunohistochemical confirmation of the epithelial differentiation of tumor cells [20]. The Broder grading system, based on the extent of keratinization and cellular pleomorphism, is not strongly correlated with prognosis due to the wide variation in differentiation within the same tumor [84]. HPV-positive SCC exhibits basaloid, nonkeratinizing histopathologic features with or without central necrosis that were previously misinterpreted as poorly differentiated SCC [44, 86–88]. Recognition that the morphologic appearance of HPV-positive SCC resembles the reticulated epithelium of the tonsillar crypts, which is the epithelial origin of these tumors, led to reclassification as well-differentiated tumors [88].

The adequacy of surgical resection is evaluated by clear margins defined as tumor-free tissue ≥ 5 mm from the tumor in the fixed specimen [89]. Tumor at the surgical margins was correlated with a decrease in patient survival and an increase in locoregional recurrence [90]. However, another study reported that margin status does not independently predict local recurrence or overall survival, but in high-risk patients, clear margins in conjunction with histologic risk assessment and adjuvant radiation increased local disease-free survival [73].

Based on HPV status, pack-years of tobacco smoking, tumor stage, and nodal stage, a classification of patients as low, intermediate, or high risk of death has been proposed [43].

## Other Tumor Biomarkers

Biomarkers are likely to have an important role in selecting patients with SCC head and neck who will benefit from specific treatments while reducing morbidity in nonresponders. Chemotherapy and radiation are important treatment modalities for unresectable or locally advanced head and neck SCC, SCC in which organ preservation is important, and as adjuvant therapy in high-risk disease that has been treated with surgery [91]. Due to the critical location of these tumors, functional and cosmetic results are important issues. Unfortunately, a significant number of patients will not respond to chemotherapy and radiation but will be exposed to the toxic effects. Molecular biomarkers are studied extensively to predict response to treatment. However, given the heterogeneity of head and neck SCC, it is important to define the patient population and standardize quantification of the tissue biomarkers, to facilitate interpretation of the data. The goal of identification of a biomarker signature is to facilitate selection of patients for the most appropriate therapy, thereby enhancing survival and reducing morbidity.

### Epidermal Growth Factor Receptor (EGFR or ErbB-1 or HER1)

Epidermal growth factor receptor (*EGFR or ErbB-1 or HER1*), a transmembrane glycoprotein from the receptor tyrosine kinase family, is activated by multiple autocrine ligands, including epidermal growth factor (EGF), transforming growth factor alpha (TGFα), and amphiregulin [4, 92]. EGFRvIII is a constitutively active mutant form of EGFR with a truncated ligand-binding domain, which is the consequence of a deletion mutation in exons 2–7 [93]. EGFR, which is encoded by a gene on chromosome 7 [94], is overexpressed in SCC due to gene amplification and induction of gene transcription [4, 95]. Induction of EGFR leads to receptor dimerization, phosphorylation, and induction of downstream signaling cascades including PI3K/AKT, MAPK, and JAK/STAT (signal transducer and activator of transcription) pathways [96–98].

#### EGFR in Personalized Medicine

Head and neck cancers variably express EGFR [92]. Overexpression of EGFR, phosphorylation of EGFR, and increased gene copy number are correlated with poor prognosis [99–101]. Overexpression of EGFR or its ligand TGFα reduced disease-free survival and cause-specific survival in head and neck SCC patients [99]. In an immunohistochemical study on tissue sections, overexpression of EGFR was an independent prognostic indicator for low disease-free survival and overall survival and high locoregional recurrence [92]. SCCs with increased EGFR gene copy number (high polysomy and gene amplification) have poorer overall survival in comparison to tumors without these alterations [100]. Although overexpression of EGFR is correlated with adverse outcome, correlation between pretreatment EGFR expression and response to therapy is inconsistent [102, 103].

### p53

p53 is a tumor suppressor protein encoded by a gene on chromosome 17p13, which is frequently mutated in SCC [104, 105]. One-third to two-thirds SCC exhibit p53 mutations, usually in exons five to eight [106–108]. While the wild-type protein is rapidly degraded, the mutant protein has a prolonged half-life and can be detected in almost 70 % of SCC [85, 109, 110]. Mutations in the p53 pathway, either upstream or downstream of p53 or of p53 itself, lead to loss of p53-mediated activity and may disrupt p53-mediated cell cycle regulation and apoptosis [4]. p53 is also inactivated by E6-mediated ubiquitination; E6 is an oncoprotein encoded by the HPV16 genome [111]. Inactivation of p53 and Rb signaling pathways is common to SCC induced by HPV, tobacco, and alcohol [23]. Loss of normal function of p53, either by mutation or inactivation, disrupts the cell response to DNA damage and impairs growth control. DNA damage induces ataxia telangiectasia (ATM), which activates p53. Downstream effectors of p53 include bcl2 and bax, proteins that regulate apoptosis [112]. Thus, loss of p53 function impacts tumor growth and response to therapy.

Head and neck SCC patients with wild-type p53 have better prognosis than those with disruptive mutations that render p53 nonfunctional [113]. However, these cases were not stratified by HPV status. Therefore, the poor outcome in patients with p53 mutations may have been due to HPV-negative status. In cancers with unknown primary tumors in the head and neck region, overexpression of p53 correlated with poor disease-free survival and poor overall survival [114]. In this study, patients with HPV-positive metastases and absent or low p53 expression had better survival than patients with absent or low p53 alone.

### Bcl2 (B-Cell Lymphoma 2)

B-cell lymphoma 2 (Bcl2) is an oncogenic protein that promotes tumor growth by promoting cell survival and inhibiting apoptosis. Therefore, Bcl2 would likely impact therapies such as radiation and chemotherapy that induce cell death. In advanced oropharyngeal SCC, high expression of Bcl2 in tumor tissue of pretreatment biopsies was correlated with resistance to cisplatin and radiation treatment and tumor recurrence [115]. Moreover, in laryngeal SCC, high Bcl2 expression is correlated with resistance to radiation treatment [116] and is inversely correlated with disease-free survival and overall survival [117]. This suggests that radiation, which induces apoptosis of tumor cells, would not be an appropriate therapy for tumors overexpressing Bcl2. This is of clinical significance because in laryngeal SCC, radiation is an important treatment modality to enable voice preservation and minimize cosmetic challenges [117].

In general, HPV-positive oropharyngeal SCC respond well to treatment. However, high expression of Bcl2 was correlated with distant metastases in HPV-positive oropharyngeal SCC [118]. This suggests that high expression of Bcl2 in pretreatment biopsies is of independent prognostic significance in HPV-positive SCC

[118]. In this group of patients, more aggressive treatment may be appropriate if the findings are validated in larger studies [118].

### DNA Repair Proteins (ERCC1 and XRCC1)

ERCC1 (excision repair cross-complementing rodent repair deficiency) and XRCC1 (X-ray repair complementing defective repair in Chinese hamster cells 1) are proteins that promote DNA repair. Chemotherapy and radiation induce cell death via DNA damage; efficient DNA repair is associated with cell survival and resistance to these treatment modalities. Cisplatin, an important chemotherapeutic agent in SCC, induces DNA adduct formation with subsequent inter- and intra-strand cross-links. Radiation induces double-strand breaks in the DNA, a dangerous form of DNA damage. Significant repair pathways for these forms of DNA damage are homologous recombination, nonhomologous end joining, and the nucleotide excision pathways. Not surprisingly, proteins involved in DNA repair and survival are potential biomarkers for prediction of the response to chemotherapy and radiation. ERCC1 promotes nucleotide excision repair and removal of platinum-induced DNA adducts [119]. Low ERCC1 was correlated with responsiveness to chemotherapy and better survival [120, 121]. High ERCC1 expression in tissue specimens was inversely correlated with progression-free survival and overall survival [121]. In a more recent study on patients treated with surgery and radiation/chemoradiation, low ERCC1 was correlated with longer median survival than high ERCC1 [122].

Given its role in single-strand DNA repair and DNA base excision, XRCC1 was investigated as a predictor of resistance to chemoradiation. High XRCC1 on pretreatment biopsies was correlated with poor overall survival and progression-free survival [123]. In this study, p16 was used as a surrogate marker for HPV. Patients with HPV-positive/low XRCC1 had a better prognosis than HPV-positive SCC/high XRCC1 [123]. The significance of XRCC1 expression in patient outcome is emphasized by additional findings showing that HPV positive/high XRCC1 and HPV negative/low XRCC1 had similar survival [123].

### CCND1 and Cyclin D1

Overexpression of cyclin D1 or amplification of its gene CCND1 occurs in 17–79 % of SCC [85]. In laryngeal cancer, overexpression of cyclin D1 correlated with tumor extension, advanced stage, lymph node metastases, smoking, and alcohol consumption, all of which are negative prognostic factors [124]. Furthermore, expression of cyclin D1 correlated with reduced disease-free survival and overall survival. The cyclin-dependent kinases, cdk4 and cdk6, mediate cyclin D1-induced phosphorylation of Rb, thereby facilitating cell cycle progression to the S phase [20, 124].

### EMT (Epithelial to Mesenchymal Transition) Biomarkers

E-cadherin, a transmembrane glycoprotein, is a major component of the adherens junctions that anchor epithelial cells to each other. This calcium-dependent cell surface protein exhibits cytoplasmic and extracellular domains that mediate homophilic interactions between epithelial cells to facilitate adhesion [5]. Expression of E-cadherin is low during cancer progression [125]. E-cadherin at the cell surface is linked to the cytoskeleton via β-catenin. During malignant transformation, sequestration of E-cadherin in the nucleus or loss of expression reduces cell-cell adhesion. β-catenin is released, translocates to the nucleus, and induces transcription of EMT genes that promote invasion and metastasis of tumor cells [5]. A meta-analysis of studies investigating E-cadherin expression in SCC showed that downregulation of E-cadherin correlated with reduced disease-free survival [126]. High free β-catenin and high active rap1, a ras-like protein, were correlated with more advanced N-stage lesions [127].

SCC may occur at different sites and has multiple histopathologic presentations. Currently, the only valuable biomarker for response to treatment is HPV status. Ultimately, given the heterogeneity of SCC, it is likely that a panel of biomarkers may be the most appropriate approach to facilitate treatment selection. In fact, the favorable prognosis in HPV-positive SCC has been attributed to a molecular signature that includes low or inactive p53, low expression of cyclin D and pRb, upregulation of p16, and downregulation of EGFR [8]. Rb is a tumor suppressor protein that is inactivated by E7, the HPV16 oncoprotein.

## Targeted Therapy

Targeted therapy is treatment directed against specific molecules that promote tumor progression. Targeted therapy is different from personalized medicine since targeted therapy is not currently used in the context of selected patients. While several targeted therapies have been tested, the EGFR antagonist cetuximab is the only FDA (US Food and Drug Administration)-approved targeted therapy for SCC [4]. It is anticipated that once the appropriate subpopulations of patients are identified, targeted therapies will be clinically successful for SCC. Identification of the appropriate subpopulations may require revisiting previous studies in view of newer findings. For example, previous studies suggested that white patients have significantly better survival than black patients with SCC [128]. However, after accounting for the greater prevalence of HPV-positive SCC in white patients and HPV-negative SCC in black patients, the survival disparity is greatly reduced [40, 129]. Perhaps reevaluation of treatment response in previous clinical trials after stratification for HPV status may improve our understanding of the impact of targeted treatment in SCC.

A challenge to the development of personalized medicine for SCC is tumor heterogeneity. Multiple primary tumors may develop due to "field cancerization," which is the transformation of epithelium at multiple sites due to prolonged contact with carcinogens [130]. These multiple primary tumors may have distinct molecular lesions, such as different p53 mutations in different tumors from the same patient [131]. Therefore, the molecular lesions in each tumor would need to be characterized even if the tumors arose in the same patient.

Targeted therapy that has been tested for SCC and some promising targets will be discussed in this section. Targeted therapy evaluated for SCC includes inhibitors of EGFR and anti-angiogenic therapies [12].

### EGFR

EGFR is a receptor tyrosine kinase that is overexpressed in approximately 90 % of SCC and is correlated with poor prognosis and treatment resistance [92]. EGFR is a transmembrane receptor exhibiting three segments; the extracellular domain binds ligands, the transmembrane region is hydrophobic, and the intracellular domain has tyrosine kinase activity. Stimulation of the receptor by EGF, TGFα, or amphiregulin induces receptor dimerization and downstream signaling cascades. The signaling mechanisms induce invasion, metastasis, angiogenesis, cell survival, and proliferation, which promote tumor progression. Therefore, EGFR has been an intense focus of targeted therapy in head and neck SCC. Therapy targeting EGFR is directed against the extracellular and intracellular domains, including monoclonal antibodies and tyrosine kinase inhibitors, respectively [12].

#### Monoclonal Antibodies Targeting the Extracellular Domain of EGFR Include Cetuximab (Erbitux™) and Panitumumab (Vectibix™)

*Cetuximab* (Erbitux™) was the first (and currently only) molecular therapy to receive approval by the FDA [4, 132] for treatment of locally advanced, recurrent, and metastatic SCC. Cetuximab combined with radiation therapy is currently a standard of care [132, 133] for locally or regionally advanced SCC [132, 134–136]. It has also been approved for use in recurrent or metastatic disease as a single agent, if platinum-based therapy fails [132, 134–136]. Cetuximab can be used in combination with platinum (cisplatin or carboplatin) and 5-fluorouracil for incurable SCC [132, 134–136]. In fact, in patients with recurrent/metastatic or unresectable SCC, the combination of cetuximab, platinum, and 5-fluorouracil is a category one recommendation [59]. A category one recommendation indicates that there is NCCN (National Comprehensive Cancer Network) consensus that the treatment is appropriate due to the strong supporting evidence [59].

Cetuximab is a murine-chick chimeric monoclonal antibody that binds to EGFR with greater affinity than EGF or TGFα [137–139], thereby acting as a competitive antagonist to initiation of downstream signaling cascades and functional effects. Cetuximab also reduces EGFR expression via receptor internalization [140]. Moreover, cetuximab appears to exert its effects via immune mechanisms, including complement-mediated cytotoxicity, antibody-dependent cell-mediated cytotoxicity, and adaptive immunity [141–143].

*Panitumumab* (Vectibix™) is a fully humanized monoclonal antibody that was expected to have less hypersensitivity reactions than cetuximab [144]. Panitumumab is currently in clinical trials for use in head and neck SCC [144].

### Tyrosine Kinase Inhibitors (*Gefitinib* and *Erlotinib*)

Tyrosine kinase inhibitors including *gefitinib* (Iressa™) *and erlotinib* (Tarceva™) are small molecule antagonists that target the intracellular domain of EGFR. Tyrosine kinase inhibitors have been explored for treatment of SCC, but have not been approved for use. *Gefitinib* enhances the risk of hemorrhage, and its use in head and neck SCC is not supported [145]. In phase II studies, *erlotinib* appeared to be a promising treatment of metastatic head and neck cancer, but subsequent studies did not support its use [146].

Relative to treatments targeting EGFR, antibody-based therapy appears to be more effective than TKI-based treatment [12]. Other monoclonal antibodies (zalutumumab, Nimotuzumab) and tyrosine kinase inhibitors (afatinib, dacomitinib, and lapatinib) are in clinical trials for treatment of SCC [147].

The clinical efficacy of antibody or small molecule targeted therapy against EGFR is modest even though EGFR is highly expressed in SCC [8].

### Anti-angiogenic Therapy

Given the role of angiogenesis in SCC progression, factors that promote angiogenesis, such as vascular endothelial growth factor (VEGF), have been explored as treatment targets. High VEGF expression is correlated with poor clinical outcome [148]. Therefore, inhibitors of this cytokine and its receptor have been investigated as potential therapy for SCC. Tumor angiogenesis in recurrent or metastatic SCC has been targeted by monoclonal antibodies against VEGF (bevacizumab or Avastin™) or tyrosine kinase inhibitors (sorafenib or Nexavar™, sunitinib or Sutent™) that target VEGFR, platelet-derived growth factor receptor, and c-kit/stem cell factor [12]. The utility of anti-angiogenic therapy for treatment of SCC is unresolved; the ultimate value of these agents will depend on the severity of vascular complications [149]. Combination targeted therapy with anti-EGFR and anti-angiogenic agents appeared to have some value but require careful evaluation given the adverse effects of this combination in treatment of colon cancer [150].

### Adenovirus-p53

p53 has a critical role in cell proliferation and apoptosis. The high recurrence rate in SCC has been correlated with aberrations in p53 at histologically normal margins [151]. Intraoperative injections of adenovirus p53 were administered in a multi-institutional phase 2 trial in SCC patients [152]. Although disease control appeared to be promising, the results were inconclusive due to the small sample size. This study showed that gene therapy for p53 is technically feasible.

### Other Targeted Therapies

Several other inhibitors are at various stages of evaluation for treatment of SCC [153]. These include vorinostat (histone deacetylase inhibitor), bortezomib (proteasome inhibitor), and dasatinib (inhibitor of src kinase, c-kit and PDGFR). Due to promising results in SCC cell lines, other targets for future clinical trials are the mTOR pathway and IGF-1R (insulin-like growth factor one receptor) [149, 154], either as single or combination therapy with cetuximab.

## Personalized Medicine with Targeted Therapy

In SCC, targeted therapy inhibits tumor progression by inhibiting critical or specific molecules in signaling pathways that promote tumor growth and spread [155]. Although targeted therapy has been developed for SCC, it is not used in the context of personalized medicine. For example, cetuximab is a targeted therapy that has been approved for clinical use in head and neck cancer [4]. Biomarkers or criteria for selection of patients who will respond to this therapy have not been validated [155]. However, personalized medicine is a reasonable expectation given emerging biomarkers that will facilitate treatment selection and predict response to therapy.

Although several biomarkers have been explored in SCC, predictive biomarkers of sensitivity or resistance to cetuximab have not been validated [140, 156–158]. Overexpression of EGFR was not correlated with response to cetuximab [135]. In fact, low expression of EGFR was correlated with enhanced response to EGFR antagonists [102, 134]. Consequently, since EGFR expression is low in HPV-positive SCC [159, 160], the prediction was that these cancers would respond well to anti-EGFR treatment [6]. A clinical trial with cetuximab suggests that HPV status may have a favorable effect on response to treatment, but the HPV status was not directly investigated [6]. Patients with a profile of HPV-positive SCC (oropharyngeal SCC, male, younger age, better performance status) responded better to cetuximab than those who did not have this profile [134]. In contrast, in a phase III SPECTURM trial [161] for safety and efficacy of panitumumab in combination with cisplatin and 5-fluorouracil for treatment of recurrent or metastatic SCC, panitumumab improved overall survival in HPV-negative but not HPV-positive tumors [65]. Additional studies are required to clarify the impact of HPV status on response to anti-EGFR therapy [6].

Molecular predictive markers of response to anti-EGFR therapy include mutations and amplification of the EGFR gene [162]. Although amplification of the EGFR gene and mutant EGFR (EGFRvIII) are potential biomarkers of response to therapy, they have not been validated in the context of anti-EGFR therapy [149].

Based on gene expression patterns, head and neck SCC has been subclassified as type I or basal, type 2 or mesenchymal, type 3 or atypical, and type 4 or classical [163]. These subtypes are correlated with activation of specific genes. Currently, the individual subtypes are not correlated with prognosis. Similarly, the gene expression signatures of HPV-positive and HPV-negative SCC were elucidated [164]. Although these signatures are not correlated with prognosis, they will likely be informative in the context of targeted therapy [6].

The identification of HPV involvement in oropharyngeal SCC may lead to reevaluation of the success of targeted therapy. For example, previous studies suggested racial differences in the outcome of chemoradiotherapy treatment for SCC [40, 128, 129] However, this disparity may be linked to differences in the prevalence of the treatment-responsive HPV-positive SCC, which is more common in white patients [40, 129].

Severity of skin rash, which typically occurs on the face and upper torso, is correlated with response to anti-EGFR therapies [102, 103]. This presentation may be due to the significant role of EGFR in skin physiology [165]. A rash of grade 2 or higher severity was correlated with improved overall survival in a cetuximab plus radiation trial [134]. However, skin rash is not an independently validated marker of response to anti-EGFR therapy [149].

**Conclusions**

Personalized medicine for oral cancer, with emphasis on selection of current and future therapies, was discussed in this chapter. Specifically, treatment selection of radiation, chemotherapy, and surgery and customized strategies for selection of targeted therapy were discussed. Currently personalized medicine in oral cancer is based on tumor stage and location, but not tumor biology. Evolving approaches to customize therapy based on the biology of the individual tumor were discussed. Furthermore, targeted therapy and potential biomarkers to match therapy to patients were also discussed.

## References

1. President's Council of Advisors on Science and Technology: priorities for personalized medicine. 2008. Available at: http://www.whitehouse.gov/files/documents/ostp/PCAST/pcast_report_v2.pdf. Accessed 26 Sep 2014.
2. Leemans CR, Braakhuis BJ, Brakenhoff RH. The molecular biology of head and neck cancer. Nat Rev Cancer. 2010;11(1):9–22.
3. Singh B. Molecular pathogenesis of head and neck cancers. J Surg Oncol. 2008;97(8):634–9.
4. Klein JD, Grandis JR. The molecular pathogenesis of head and neck cancer. Cancer Biol Ther. 2010;9(1):1–7.
5. Scanlon CS, Van Tubergen EA, Inglehart RC, D'Silva NJ. Biomarkers of epithelial-mesenchymal transition in squamous cell carcinoma. J Dent Res. 2013;92(2):114–21.
6. Weiss J, Hayes DN. Classifying squamous cell carcinoma of the head and neck: prognosis, prediction and implications for therapy. Expert Rev Anticancer Ther. 2014;14(2):229–36.
7. Vaezi A, Feldman CH, Niedernhofer LJ. ERCC1 and XRCC1 as biomarkers for lung and head and neck cancer. Pharmgenomics Pers Med. 2011;4:47–63.
8. Denaro N, Russi EG, Adamo V, Merlano M. State-of-the-art and emerging treatment options in the management of head and neck cancer: News from 2013. Oncology. 2014;86(4):212–29.
9. Vokes EE, Weichselbaum RR, Lippman SM, Hong WK. Head and neck cancer. N Engl J Med. 1993;328(3):184–94.
10. Specht L. Oral complications in the head and neck radiation patient. Support Care Cancer. 2002;10(1):36–9.
11. Forastiere A, Koch W, Trotti A, Sidransky D. Head and neck cancer. N Engl J Med. 2001;345(26):1890–900.
12. Razak AR, Siu LL, Le Tourneau C. Molecular targeted therapies in all histologies of head and neck cancers: an update. Curr Opin Oncol. 2010;22(3):212–20.
13. Haddad RI, Shin DM. Recent advances in head and neck cancer. N Engl J Med. 2008;359(11):1143–54.
14. Pfister DG, Ang K-K, Brizel DM, Burtness BA, Cmelak AJ, Colevas AD, et al. Head and neck cancers. J Natl Compr Canc Netw. 2011;9(6):596–650.
15. Patel SG, Shah JP. TNM staging of cancers of the head and neck: striving for uniformity among diversity. CA Cancer J Clin. 2005;55(4):242–58.
16. Sessions DG, Spector GJ, Lenox J, Haughey B, Chao C, Marks J. Analysis of treatment results for oral tongue cancer. Laryngoscope. 2002;112(4):616–25.
17. Huang TY, Hsu LP, Wen YH, Huang TT, Chou YF, Lee CF, et al. Predictors of locoregional recurrence in early stage oral cavity cancer with free surgical margins. Oral Oncol. 2010;46(1):49–55.
18. Jerjes W, Upile T, Hamdoon Z, Mosse CA, Akram S, Hopper C. Prospective evaluation of outcome after transoral $CO_2$ laser resection of T1/T2 oral squamous cell carcinoma. Oral Surg Oral Med Oral Pathol Oral Radiol Endod. 2011;112(2):180–7.
19. Brandwein-Gensler M, Wei S. Envisioning the next WHO head and neck classification. Head Neck Pathol. 2014;8(1):1–15.
20. D'Silva NJ, Ward BB. Tissue biomarkers for diagnosis & management of oral squamous cell carcinoma. Alpha Omegan. 2007;100(4):18–9.
21. Cognetti DM, Weber RS, Lai SY. Head and neck cancer. Cancer. 2008;113(S7):1911–32.
22. Mitra RS, Goto M, Lee JS, Maldonado D, Taylor JM, Pan Q, et al. Rap1GAP promotes invasion via induction of matrix metalloproteinase 9 secretion, which is associated with poor survival in low N-stage squamous cell carcinoma. Cancer Res. 2008;68(10):3959–69.
23. Gillison ML, D'Souza G, Westra W, Sugar E, Xiao W, Begum S, et al. Distinct risk factor profiles for human papillomavirus type 16–positive and human papillomavirus type 16–negative head and neck cancers. J Natl Cancer Inst. 2008;100(6):407–20.
24. Argiris A, Karamouzis MV, Raben D, Ferris RL. Head and neck cancer. Lancet. 2008;371(9625):1695–709.
25. Benson E, Li R, Eisele D, Fakhry C. The clinical impact of HPV tumor status upon head and neck squamous cell carcinomas. Oral Oncol. 2014;50(6):565–74.
26. Carvalho AL, Nishimoto IN, Califano JA, Kowalski LP. Trends in incidence and prognosis for head and neck cancer in the United States: a site-specific analysis of the SEER database. Int J Cancer. 2005;114(5):806–16.
27. Sturgis EM, Cinciripini PM. Trends in head and neck cancer incidence in relation to smoking prevalence. Cancer. 2007;110(7):1429–35.
28. Rettig E, Kiess AP, Fakhry C. The role of sexual behavior in head and neck cancer: implications for prevention and therapy. Expert Rev Anticancer Ther. 2015;15(1):35–49.
29. Chaturvedi AK, Anderson WF, Lortet-Tieulent J, Curado MP, Ferlay J, Franceschi S, et al. Worldwide trends in incidence rates for oral cavity and oropharyngeal cancers. J Clin Oncol. 2013;31(36):4550–9.
30. Mroz EA, Forastiere AA, Rocco JW. Implications of the oropharyngeal cancer epidemic. J Clin Oncol. 2011;29(32):4222–3.
31. Herrero R, Castellsagué X, Pawlita M, Lissowska J, Kee F, Balaram P, et al. Human papillomavirus and oral cancer: the International Agency for Research on Cancer multicenter study. J Natl Cancer Inst. 2003;95(23):1772–83.
32. Ribeiro KB, Levi JE, Pawlita M, Koifman S, Matos E, Eluf-Neto J, et al. Low human papillomavirus prevalence in head and neck cancer: results from two large case–control studies in high-incidence regions. Int J Epidemiol. 2011;40(2):489–502.

33. Marur S, Burtness B. Oropharyngeal squamous cell carcinoma treatment: current standards and future directions. Curr Opin Oncol. 2014;26(3):252–8.
34. Fakhry C, Gillison ML. Clinical implications of human papillomavirus in head and neck cancers. J Clin Oncol. 2006;24(17):2606–11.
35. Ritchie JM, Smith EM, Summersgill KF, Hoffman HT, Wang D, Klussmann JP, et al. Human papillomavirus infection as a prognostic factor in carcinomas of the oral cavity and oropharynx. Int J Cancer. 2003;104(3):336–44.
36. Kumar B, Cordell KG, Lee JS, Prince ME, Tran HH, Wolf GT, et al. Response to therapy and outcomes in oropharyngeal cancer are associated with biomarkers including human papillomavirus, epidermal growth factor receptor, gender, and smoking. Int J Radiat Oncol Biol Phys. 2007;69(2):S109–11.
37. Worden FP, Kumar B, Lee JS, Wolf GT, Cordell KG, Taylor JM, et al. Chemoselection as a strategy for organ preservation in advanced oropharynx cancer: response and survival positively associated with HPV16 copy number. J Clin Oncol. 2008;26(19): 3138–46.
38. Chaturvedi AK, Engels EA, Pfeiffer RM, Hernandez BY, Xiao W, Kim E, et al. Human papillomavirus and rising oropharyngeal cancer incidence in the United States. J Clin Oncol. 2011;29(32):4294–301.
39. Jemal A, Simard EP, Dorell C, Noone AM, Markowitz LE, Kohler B, et al. Annual Report to the Nation on the Status of Cancer, 1975–2009, featuring the burden and trends in human papillomavirus (HPV)–associated cancers and HPV Vaccination coverage levels. J Natl Cancer Inst. 2013; 105(3):175–201.
40. Settle K, Posner MR, Schumaker LM, Tan M, Suntharalingam M, Goloubeva O, et al. Racial survival disparity in head and neck cancer results from low prevalence of human papillomavirus infection in black oropharyngeal cancer patients. Cancer Prev Res (Phila). 2009;2(9):776–81.
41. Licitra L, Perrone F, Bossi B, Suardi S, Mariani L, Artusi R. High-risk human papillomavirus affects prognosis in patients with surgically treated oropharyngeal squamous cell carcinoma. J Clin Oncol. 2006;24(36):5630–6.
42. Fakhry C, Westra WH, Li S, Cmelak A, Ridge JA, Pinto H, et al. Improved survival of patients with human papillomavirus–positive head and neck squamous cell carcinoma in a prospective clinical trial. J Natl Cancer Inst. 2008;100(4):261–9.
43. Ang KK, Harris J, Wheeler R, Weber R, Rosenthal DI, Nguyen-Tân PF, et al. Human papillomavirus and survival of patients with oropharyngeal cancer. N Engl J Med. 2010;363(1):24–35.
44. Gillison ML, Koch WM, Capone RB, Spafford M, Westra WH, Wu L, et al. Evidence for a causal association between human papillomavirus and a subset of head and neck cancers. J Natl Cancer Inst. 2000;92(9):709–20.
45. Mellin H, Friesland S, Lewensohn R, Dalianis T, Munck-Wikland E. Human papillomavirus (HPV) DNA in tonsillar cancer: clinical correlates, risk of relapse, and survival. Int J Cancer. 2000;89(3):300–4.
46. Weinberger PM, Yu Z, Haffty B, Kowalski D, Harigopal M, Sasaki C, et al. Prognostic significance of p16 protein levels in oropharyngeal squamous cell cancer. Clin Cancer Res. 2004;10(17):5684–91.
47. Lassen P, Eriksen JG, Hamilton-Dutoit S, Tramm T, Alsner J, Overgaard J. Effect of HPV-associated p16INK4A expression on response to radiotherapy and survival in squamous cell carcinoma of the head and neck. J Clin Oncol. 2009;27(12):1992–8.
48. Fischer C, Kampmann M, Zlobec I, Green E, Tornillo L, Lugli A, et al. p16 expression in oropharyngeal cancer: its impact on staging and prognosis compared with the conventional clinical staging parameters. Ann Oncol. 2010;21(10):1961–6.
49. O'rorke M, Ellison M, Murray L, Moran M, James J, Anderson L. Human papillomavirus related head and neck cancer survival: a systematic review and meta-analysis. Oral Oncol. 2012;48(12):1191–201.
50. Vent J, Haidle B, Wedemeyer I, Huebbers C, Siefer O, Semrau R, et al. p16 expression in carcinoma of unknown primary: diagnostic indicator and prognostic marker. Head Neck. 2013;35(11):1521–5.
51. Hong A, Dobbins T, Lee C, Jones D, Harnett G, Armstrong B, et al. Human papillomavirus predicts outcome in oropharyngeal cancer in patients treated primarily with surgery or radiation therapy. Br J Cancer. 2010;103(10):1510–7.
52. Attner P, Du J, Näsman A, Hammarstedt L, Ramqvist T, Lindholm J, et al. Human papillomavirus and survival in patients with base of tongue cancer. Int J Cancer. 2011;128(12):2892–7.
53. Fountzilas G, Kosmidis P, Avramidis V, Nikolaou A, Kalogera-Fountzila A, Makrantonakis P, et al. Long-term survival data and prognostic factors of a complete response to chemotherapy in patients with head and neck cancer treated with platinum-based induction chemotherapy: a Hellenic Co-operative Oncology Group Study. Med Pediatr Oncol. 1997; 28(6):401–10.
54. Browman GP, Mohide E, Willan A, Hodson I, Wong G, Grimard L, et al. Association between smoking during radiotherapy and prognosis in head and neck cancer: a follow-up study. Head Neck. 2002; 24(12):1031–7.
55. Jordan RC, Lingen MW, Perez-Ordonez B, He X, Pickard R, Koluder M, et al. Validation of methods for oropharyngeal cancer HPV status determination in US Cooperative Group trials. Am J Surg Pathol. 2012;36(7):945–54.
56. Liang C, Marsit CJ, McClean MD, Nelson HH, Christensen BC, Haddad RI, et al. Biomarkers of

HPV in head and neck squamous cell carcinoma. Cancer Res. 2012;72(19):5004–13.
57. De Martel C, Ferlay J, Franceschi S, Vignat J, Bray F, Forman D, et al. Global burden of cancers attributable to infections in 2008: a review and synthetic analysis. Lancet Oncol. 2012;13(6):607–15.
58. Lingen MW, Xiao W, Schmitt A, Jiang B, Pickard R, Kreinbrink P, et al. Low etiologic fraction for high-risk human papillomavirus in oral cavity squamous cell carcinomas. Oral Oncol. 2013;49(1):1–8.
59. National Comprehensive Cancer Network. NCCN clinical practice guidelines in oncology™. Head and neck cancers. 2013;V.2.2013. Available at: http://www.nccn.org/professionals/physician_gls/PDF/head-and-neck.pdf.
60. Langendijk JA, Doornaert P, Verdonck-de Leeuw IM, Leemans CR, Aaronson NK, Slotman BJ. Impact of late treatment-related toxicity on quality of life among patients with head and neck cancer treated with radiotherapy. J Clin Oncol. 2008;26(22):3770–6.
61. Francis DO, Weymuller Jr EA, Parvathaneni U, Merati AL, Yueh B. Dysphagia, stricture, and pneumonia in head and neck cancer patients: does treatment modality matter? Ann Otol Rhinol Laryngol. 2010;119(6):391.
62. Cmelak A. Abstract #LBA6006. Presented at: ASCO annual meeting; 30 May–3 Jun 2014; Chicago.
63. Radiation therapy with cisplatin or cetuximab in treating patients with oropharyngeal cancer. Available at: http://clinicaltrials.gov/ct2/show/NCT01302834.
64. Huang SH, Perez-Ordonez B, Liu FF, Waldron J, Ringash J, Irish J, et al. Atypical clinical behavior of p16-confirmed HPV-related oropharyngeal squamous cell carcinoma treated with radical radiotherapy. Int J Radiat Oncol Biol Phys. 2012;82(1):276–83.
65. Vermorken JB, Stohlmacher-Williams J, Davidenko I, Licitra L, Winquist E, Villanueva C, et al. Cisplatin and fluorouracil with or without panitumumab in patients with recurrent or metastatic squamous-cell carcinoma of the head and neck (SPECTRUM): an open-label phase 3 randomised trial. Lancet Oncol. 2013;14(8):697–710.
66. O'Brien CJ, Lauer CS, Fredricks S, Clifford AR, McNeil EB, Bagia JS, et al. Tumor thickness influences prognosis of T1 and T2 oral cavity cancer—but what thickness? Head Neck. 2003;25(11):937–45.
67. Spiro RH, Huvos AG, Wong GY, Spiro JD, Gnecco CA, Strong EW. Predictive value of tumor thickness in squamous carcinoma confined to the tongue and floor of the mouth. Am J Surg. 1986;152(4):345–50.
68. Warburton G, Nikitakis NG, Roberson P, Marinos NJ, Wu T, Sauk Jr JJ, et al. Histopathological and lymphangiogenic parameters in relation to lymph node metastasis in early stage oral squamous cell carcinoma. J Oral Maxillofac Surg. 2007;65(3):475–84.
69. Cerezo L, Millan I, Torre A, Aragon G, Otero J. Prognostic factors for survival and tumor control in cervical lymph node metastases from head and neck cancer: a multivariate study of 492 cases. Cancer. 1992;69(5):1224–34.
70. Bernier J, Domenge C, Ozsahin M, Matuszewska K, Lefèbvre JL, Greiner RH, et al. Postoperative irradiation with or without concomitant chemotherapy for locally advanced head and neck cancer. N Engl J Med. 2004;350(19):1945–52.
71. Brockstein B, Haraf D, Rademaker A, Kies M, Stenson K, Rosen F, et al. Patterns of failure, prognostic factors and survival in locoregionally advanced head and neck cancer treated with concomitant chemoradiotherapy: a 9-year, 337-patient, multi-institutional experience. Ann Oncol. 2004;15(8):1179–86.
72. Cooper JS, Pajak TF, Forastiere AA, Jacobs J, Campbell BH, Saxman SB, et al. Postoperative concurrent radiotherapy and chemotherapy for high-risk squamous-cell carcinoma of the head and neck. N Engl J Med. 2004;350(19):1937–44.
73. Brandwein-Gensler M, Teixeira MS, Lewis CM, Lee B, Rolnitzky L, Hille JJ, et al. Oral squamous cell carcinoma: histologic risk assessment, but not margin status, is strongly predictive of local disease-free and overall survival. Am J Surg Pathol. 2005;29(2):167–78.
74. Brandwein-Gensler M, Smith RV, Wang B, Penner C, Theilken A, Broughel D, et al. Validation of the histologic risk model in a new cohort of patients with head and neck squamous cell carcinoma. Am J Surg Pathol. 2010;34(5):676–88.
75. Li Y, Bai S, Carroll W, Dayan D, Dort JC, Heller K, et al. Validation of the risk model: high-risk classification and tumor pattern of invasion predict outcome for patients with low-stage oral cavity squamous cell carcinoma. Head Neck Pathol. 2013;7(3):211–23.
76. Sawair FA, Irwin CR, Gordon DJ, Leonard AG, Stephenson M, Napier SS. Invasive front grading: reliability and usefulness in the management of oral squamous cell carcinoma. J Oral Pathol Med. 2003;32(1):1–9.
77. O'Brien CJ, Smith JW, Soong S-J, Urist MM, Maddox WA. Neck dissection with and without radiotherapy: prognostic factors, patterns of recurrence, and survival. Am J Surg. 1986;152(4):456–63.
78. Tytor M, Olofsson J. Prognostic factors in oral cavity carcinomas. Acta Otolaryngol Suppl. 1992;492:75–8.
79. Jones A. Prognosis in mouth cancer: tumour factors. Eur J Cancer B Oral Oncol. 1994;30B(1):8–15.
80. Mamelle G, Pampurik J, Luboinski B, Lancar R, Lusinchi A, Bosq J. Lymph node prognostic factors in head and neck squamous cell carcinomas. Am J Surg. 1994;168(5):494–8.

81. Woolgar JA, Scott J, Vaughan E, Brown J, West C, Rogers S. Survival, metastasis and recurrence of oral cancer in relation to pathological features. Ann R Coll Surg Engl. 1995;77(5):325–31.
82. Bryne M, Koppang HS, Lilleng R, Stene T, Bang G, Dabelsteen E. New malignancy grading is a better prognostic indicator than Broders' grading in oral squamous cell carcinomas. J Oral Pathol Med. 1989;18(8):432–7.
83. Bryne M, Koppang HS, Lillen R, Kjærheim Å. Malignancy grading of the deep invasive margins of oral squamous cell carcinomas has high prognostic value. J Pathol. 1992;166(4):375–81.
84. El-Mofty SK. Histopathologic risk factors in oral and oropharyngeal squamous cell carcinoma variants: an update with special reference to HPV-related carcinomas. Med Oral Patol Oral Cir Bucal. 2014;19(4):e377–85.
85. Thomas GR, Nadiminti H, Regalado J. Molecular predictors of clinical outcome in patients with head and neck squamous cell carcinoma. Int J Exp Pathol. 2005;86(6):347–63.
86. Schwartz SR, Yueh B, McDougall JK, Daling JR, Schwartz SM. Human papillomavirus infection and survival in oral squamous cell cancer: a population-based study. Otolaryngol Head Neck Surg. 2001; 125(1):1–9.
87. Weinberger PM, Yu Z, Haffty BG, Kowalski D, Harigopal M, Brandsma J, et al. Molecular classification identifies a subset of human papillomavirus–associated oropharyngeal cancers with favorable prognosis. J Clin Oncol. 2006;24(5):736–47.
88. Westra WH. The morphologic profile of HPV-related head and neck squamous carcinoma: implications for diagnosis, prognosis, and clinical management. Head Neck Pathol. 2012;6(1):48–54.
89. Sieczka E, Datta R, Singh A, Loree T, Rigual N, Orner J, et al. Cancer of the buccal mucosa: are margins and T-stage accurate predictors of local control? Am J Otolaryngol. 2001;22(6):395–9.
90. Loree TR, Strong EW. Significance of positive margins in oral cavity squamous carcinoma. Am J Surg. 1990;160(4):410–4.
91. Burri RJ, Lee NY. Concurrent chemotherapy and radiotherapy for head and neck cancer. Expert Rev Anticancer Ther. 2009;9(3):293–302.
92. Ang KK, Berkey BA, Tu X, Zhang H-Z, Katz R, Hammond EH, et al. Impact of epidermal growth factor receptor expression on survival and pattern of relapse in patients with advanced head and neck carcinoma. Cancer Res. 2002;62(24):7350–6.
93. Sok JC, Coppelli FM, Thomas SM, Lango MN, Xi S, Hunt JL, et al. Mutant epidermal growth factor receptor (EGFRvIII) contributes to head and neck cancer growth and resistance to EGFR targeting. Clin Cancer Res. 2006;12(17):5064–73.
94. Davies RL, Grosse VA, Kucherlapati R, Bothwell M. Genetic analysis of epidermal growth factor action: assignment of human epidermal growth factor receptor gene to chromosome 7. Proc Natl Acad Sci. 1980;77(7):4188–92.
95. Kalyankrishna S, Grandis JR. Epidermal growth factor receptor biology in head and neck cancer. J Clin Oncol. 2006;24(17):2666–72.
96. Ellerbroek SM, Halbleib JM, Benavidez M, Warmka JK, Wattenberg EV, Stack MS, et al. Phosphatidylinositol 3-kinase activity in epidermal growth factor-stimulated matrix metalloproteinase-9 production and cell surface association. Cancer Res. 2001;61(5):1855–61.
97. Vivanco I, Sawyers CL. The phosphatidylinositol 3-kinase–AKT pathway in human cancer. Nat Rev Cancer. 2002;2(7):489–501.
98. Kruger JS, Reddy KB. Distinct mechanisms mediate the initial and sustained phases of cell migration in epidermal growth factor receptor-overexpressing cells11NIH grant R01 CA 83964 (to KBR). Mol Cancer Res. 2003;1(11):801–9.
99. Grandis JR, Melhem MF, Gooding WE, Day R, Holst VA, Wagener MM, et al. Levels of TGF-α and EGFR protein in head and neck squamous cell carcinoma and patient survival. J Natl Cancer Inst. 1998;90(11):824–32.
100. Temam S, Kawaguchi H, El-Naggar AK, Jelinek J, Tang H, Liu DD, et al. Epidermal growth factor receptor copy number alterations correlate with poor clinical outcome in patients with head and neck squamous cancer. J Clin Oncol. 2007;25(16): 2164–70.
101. Hama T, Yuza Y, Saito Y, Jin O, Kondo S, Okabe M, et al. Prognostic significance of epidermal growth factor receptor phosphorylation and mutation in head and neck squamous cell carcinoma. Oncologist. 2009;14(9):900–8.
102. Burtness B, Goldwasser MA, Flood W, Mattar B, Forastiere AA. Phase III randomized trial of cisplatin plus placebo compared with cisplatin plus cetuximab in metastatic/recurrent head and neck cancer: an Eastern Cooperative Oncology Group study. J Clin Oncol. 2005;23(34):8646–54.
103. Vermorken JB, Trigo J, Hitt R, Koralewski P, Diaz-Rubio E, Rolland F, et al. Open-label, uncontrolled, multicenter phase II study to evaluate the efficacy and toxicity of cetuximab as a single agent in patients with recurrent and/or metastatic squamous cell carcinoma of the head and neck who failed to respond to platinum-based therapy. J Clin Oncol. 2007; 25(16):2171–7.
104. Brachman DG, Graves D, Vokes E, Beckett M, Haraf D, Montag A, et al. Occurrence of p53 gene deletions and human papilloma virus infection in human head and neck cancer. Cancer Res. 1992;52(17):4832–6.
105. Hoffmann TK, Sonkoly E, Hauser U, van Lierop A, Whiteside TL, Klussmann JP, et al. Alterations in the p53 pathway and their association with radio-and chemosensitivity in head and neck squamous cell carcinoma. Oral Oncol. 2008;44(12):1100–9.

106. Velculescu VE, El-Deiry W. Biological and clinical importance of the p53 tumor suppressor gene. Clin Chem. 1996;42(6):858–68.
107. Olivier M, Eeles R, Hollstein M, Khan MA, Harris CC, Hainaut P. The IARC TP53 database: new online mutation analysis and recommendations to users. Hum Mutat. 2002;19(6):607–14.
108. Gasco M, Crook T. The p53 network in head and neck cancer. Oral Oncol. 2003;39(3):222–31.
109. Nogueira CP, Dolan RW, Gooey J, Byahatti S, Vaughan CW, Fuleihan NS, et al. Inactivation of p53 and amplification of cyclin D1 correlate with clinical outcome in head and neck cancer. Laryngoscope. 1998;108(3):345–50.
110. Edström S, Cvetkovska E, Westin T, Young C. Overexpression of p53-related proteins predicts rapid growth rate of head and neck cancer. Laryngoscope. 2001;111(1):124–30.
111. Chung CH, Gillison ML. Human papillomavirus in head and neck cancer: its role in pathogenesis and clinical implications. Clin Cancer Res. 2009;15(22):6758–62.
112. Chen K, Hu Z, Wang L-E, Sturgis EM, El-Naggar AK, Zhang W, et al. Single-nucleotide polymorphisms at the TP53-binding or responsive promoter regions of BAX and BCL2 genes and risk of squamous cell carcinoma of the head and neck. Carcinogenesis. 2007;28(9):2008–12.
113. Poeta ML, Manola J, Goldwasser MA, Forastiere A, Benoit N, Califano JA, et al. TP53 mutations and survival in squamous-cell carcinoma of the head and neck. N Engl J Med. 2007; 357(25):2552–61.
114. Sivars L, Näsman A, Tertipis N, Vlastos A, Ramqvist T, Dalianis T, et al. Human papillomavirus and p53 expression in cancer of unknown primary in the head and neck region in relation to clinical outcome. Cancer Med. 2014;3(2):376–84.
115. Michaud WA, Nichols AC, Mroz EA, Faquin WC, Clark JR, Begum S, et al. Bcl-2 blocks cisplatin-induced apoptosis and predicts poor outcome following chemoradiation treatment in advanced oropharyngeal squamous cell carcinoma. Clin Cancer Res. 2009;15(5):1645–54.
116. Nix P, Cawkwell L, Patmore H, Greenman J, Stafford N. Bcl-2 expression predicts radiotherapy failure in laryngeal cancer. Br J Cancer. 2005;92(12): 2185–9.
117. Gallo O, Boddi V, Calzolari A, Simonetti L, Trovati M, Bianchi S. Bcl-2 protein expression correlates with recurrence and survival in early stage head and neck cancer treated by radiotherapy. Clin Cancer Res. 1996;2(2):261–7.
118. Nichols AC, Finkelstein DM, Faquin WC, Westra WH, Mroz EA, Kneuertz P, Begum S, et al. Bcl2 and human papilloma virus 16 as predictors of outcome following concurrent chemoradiation for advanced oropharyngeal cancer. Clin Cancer Res. 2010; 16(7):2138–46.
119. Johnson SW, O'Dwyer PJ. Cisplatin and its analogues. In: DeVita VT, Rosenberg SA, editors. Principles and practice of oncology. Philadelphia: Lippincott Williams and Wilkins; 2001. p. 380–2.
120. Handra-Luca A, Hernandez J, Mountzios G, Taranchon E, Lacau-St-Guily J, Soria J-C, et al. Excision repair cross complementation group 1 immunohistochemical expression predicts objective response and cancer-specific survival in patients treated by Cisplatin-based induction chemotherapy for locally advanced head and neck squamous cell carcinoma. Clin Cancer Res. 2007;13(13):3855–9.
121. Jun H, Ahn M, Kim H, Yi S, Han J, Lee S, et al. ERCC1 expression as a predictive marker of squamous cell carcinoma of the head and neck treated with cisplatin-based concurrent chemoradiation. Br J Cancer. 2008;99(1):167–72.
122. Mehra R, Zhu F, Yang D-H, Cai KQ, Weaver J, Singh MK, et al. Quantification of excision repair cross-complementing group 1 and survival in p16-negative squamous cell head and neck cancers. Clin Cancer Res. 2013;19(23):6633–43.
123. Ang M-K, Patel MR, Yin X-Y, Sundaram S, Fritchie K, Zhao N, et al. High XRCC1 protein expression is associated with poorer survival in patients with head and neck squamous cell carcinoma. Clin Cancer Res. 2011;17(20):6542–52.
124. Pignataro L, Pruneri G, Carboni N, Capaccio P, Cesana BM, Neri A, et al. Clinical relevance of cyclin D1 protein overexpression in laryngeal squamous cell carcinoma. J Clin Oncol. 1998;16(9):3069–77.
125. Zeisberg M, Neilson EG. Biomarkers for epithelial-mesenchymal transitions. J Clin Invest. 2009;119(6): 1429–37.
126. Zhao Z, Ge J, Sun Y, Tian L, Lu J, Liu M, et al. Is E-cadherin immunoexpression a prognostic factor for head and neck squamous cell carcinoma (HNSCC)? A systematic review and meta-analysis. Oral Oncol. 2012;48(9):761–7.
127. Goto M, Mitra RS, Liu M, Lee J, Henson BS, Carey T, et al. Rap1 stabilizes β-catenin and enhances β-catenin–dependent transcription and invasion in squamous cell carcinoma of the head and neck. Clin Cancer Res. 2010;16(1):65–76.
128. Molina MA, Cheung MC, Perez EA, Byrne MM, Franceschi D, Moffat FL, et al. African American and poor patients have a dramatically worse prognosis for head and neck cancer. Cancer. 2008;113(10): 2797–806.
129. Schrank TP, Han Y, Weiss H, Resto VA. Case-matching analysis of head and neck squamous cell carcinoma in racial and ethnic minorities in the United States—possible role for human papillomavirus in survival disparities. Head Neck. 2011;33(1):45–53.
130. Slaughter DP, Southwick HW, Smejkal W. "Field cancerization" in oral stratified squamous epithelium. Clinical implications of multicentric origin. Cancer. 1953;6(5):963–8.
131. Koch WM, Boyle JO, Mao L, Hakim J, Hruban RH, Sidransky D. p53 gene mutations as markers of tumor spread in synchronous oral cancers. Arch Otolaryngol Head Neck Surg. 1994;120(9):943–7.

132. Cohen RB. Current challenges and clinical investigations of epidermal growth factor receptor (EGFR)- and ErbB family-targeted agents in the treatment of head and neck squamous cell carcinoma (HNSCC). Cancer Treat Rev. 2014;40(4):567–77.
133. Vermorken J, Specenier P. Optimal treatment for recurrent/metastatic head and neck cancer. Ann Oncol. 2010;21 Suppl 7:vii252–61.
134. Bonner JA, Harari PM, Giralt J, Azarnia N, Shin DM, Cohen RB, et al. Radiotherapy plus cetuximab for squamous-cell carcinoma of the head and neck. N Engl J Med. 2006;354(6):567–78.
135. Vermorken JB, Mesia R, Rivera F, Remenar E, Kawecki A, Rottey S, et al. Platinum-based chemotherapy plus cetuximab in head and neck cancer. N Engl J Med. 2008;359(11):1116–27.
136. Bonner JA, Harari PM, Giralt J, Cohen RB, Jones CU, Sur RK, et al. Radiotherapy plus cetuximab for locoregionally advanced head and neck cancer: 5-year survival data from a phase 3 randomised trial, and relation between cetuximab-induced rash and survival. Lancet Oncol. 2010;11(1):21–8.
137. Gill GN, Kawamoto T, Cochet C, Le A, Sato J, Masui H, et al. Monoclonal anti-epidermal growth factor receptor antibodies which are inhibitors of epidermal growth factor binding and antagonists of epidermal growth factor binding and antagonists of epidermal growth factor-stimulated tyrosine protein kinase activity. J Biol Chem. 1984;259(12):7755–60.
138. Goldstein NI, Prewett M, Zuklys K, Rockwell P, Mendelsohn J. Biological efficacy of a chimeric antibody to the epidermal growth factor receptor in a human tumor xenograft model. Clin Cancer Res. 1995;1(11):1311–8.
139. Kim ES, Khuri FR, Herbst RS. Epidermal growth factor receptor biology (IMC-C225). Curr Opin Oncol. 2001;13(6):506–13.
140. Sharafinski ME, Ferris RL, Ferrone S, Grandis JR. Epidermal growth factor receptor targeted therapy of squamous cell carcinoma of the head and neck. Head Neck. 2010;32(10):1412–21.
141. Bleeker WK, van Bueren JJL, van Ojik HH, Gerritsen AF, Pluyter M, Houtkamp M, et al. Dual mode of action of a human anti-epidermal growth factor receptor monoclonal antibody for cancer therapy. J Immunol. 2004;173(7):4699–707.
142. Dechant M, Weisner W, Berger S, Peipp M, Beyer T, Schneider-Merck T, et al. Complement-dependent tumor cell lysis triggered by combinations of epidermal growth factor receptor antibodies. Cancer Res. 2008;68(13):4998–5003.
143. Srivastava RM, Lee SC, Andrade Filho PA, Lord CA, Jie H-B, Davidson HC, et al. Cetuximab-activated natural killer and dendritic cells collaborate to trigger tumor antigen–specific t-cell immunity in head and neck cancer patients. Clin Cancer Res. 2013;19(7):1858–72.
144. Trivedi S, Concha-Benavente F, Srivastava RM, Jie HB, Gibson SP, Schmitt NC, et al. Immune biomarkers of anti-EGFR monoclonal antibody therapy. Ann Oncol. 2015;26(1):40–7.
145. Mahipal A, Kothari N, Gupta S. Epidermal growth factor receptor inhibitors: coming of age. Cancer Control. 2014;21(1):74–9.
146. Soulieres D, Senzer NN, Vokes EE, Hidalgo M, Agarwala SS, Siu LL. Multicenter phase II study of erlotinib, an oral epidermal growth factor receptor tyrosine kinase inhibitor, in patients with recurrent or metastatic squamous cell cancer of the head and neck. J Clin Oncol. 2004;22(1):77–85.
147. Roskoski Jr R. The ErbB/HER family of protein-tyrosine kinases and cancer. Pharmaco Res. 2014;79:34–74.
148. Lothaire P, de Azambuja E, Dequanter D, Lalami Y, Sotiriou C, Andry G, et al. Molecular markers of head and neck squamous cell carcinoma promising signs in need of prospective evaluation. Head Neck. 2006;28(3):256–69.
149. Le Tourneau C, Siu LL. Molecular-targeted therapies in the treatment of squamous cell carcinomas of the head and neck. Curr Opin Oncol. 2008;20(3):256–63.
150. Tol J, Koopman M, Cats A, Rodenburg CJ, Creemers GJ, Schrama JG, et al. Chemotherapy, bevacizumab, and cetuximab in metastatic colorectal cancer. N Engl J Med. 2009;360(6):563–72.
151. Brennan JA, Boyle JO, Koch WM, Goodman SN, Hruban RH, Eby YJ, et al. Association between cigarette smoking and mutation of the p53 gene in squamous-cell carcinoma of the head and neck. N Engl J Med. 1995;332(11):712–7.
152. Yoo GH, Moon J, LeBlanc M, Lonardo F, Urba S, Kim H, et al. A phase 2 trial of surgery with perioperative INGN 201 (Ad5CMV-p53) gene therapy followed by chemoradiotherapy for advanced, resectable squamous cell carcinoma of the oral cavity, oropharynx, hypopharynx, and larynx: report of the Southwest Oncology Group. Arch Otolaryngol Head Neck Surg. 2009;135(9):869–74.
153. Selzer E, Kornek G. Targeted drugs in combination with radiotherapy for the treatment of solid tumors: current state and future developments. Expert Rev Clin Pharmacol. 2013;6(6):663–76.
154. Dorsey K, Agulnik M. Promising new molecular targeted therapies in head and neck cancer. Drugs. 2013;73(4):315–25.
155. Worsham MJ, Ali H, Dragovic J, Schweitzer VP. Molecular characterization of head and neck cancer. Mol Diagn Ther. 2012;16(4):209–22.
156. Egloff AM, Grandis JR. Improving response rates to EGFR-targeted therapies for head and neck squamous cell carcinoma: candidate predictive biomarkers and combination treatment with src inhibitors. J Oncol. 2009;2009:896407.
157. Argiris A, Lee SC, Feinstein T, Thomas S, Branstetter IV BF, Seethala R, et al. Serum biomarkers as potential predictors of antitumor activity of cetuximab-containing therapy for locally advanced head and neck cancer. Oral Oncol. 2011;47(10):961–6.
158. Licitra L, Mesia R, Rivera F, Remenar E, Hitt R, Erfan J, Rottey S, Kawecki A, Zabolotnyy D, Benasso M. Evaluation of EGFR gene copy number as a predictive biomarker for the efficacy of

cetuximab in combination with chemotherapy in the first-line treatment of recurrent and/or metastatic squamous cell carcinoma of the head and neck: EXTREME study. Ann Oncol. 2011;22(5):1078–87.
159. Reimers N, Kasper HU, Weissenborn SJ, Stützer H, Preuss SF, Hoffmann TK, Speel EJM, Dienes HP, Pfister HJ, Guntinas-Lichius O. Combined analysis of HPV-DNA, p16 and EGFR expression to predict prognosis in oropharyngeal cancer. Int J Cancer. 2007;120(8):1731–8.
160. Kumar B, Cordell KG, Lee JS, Worden FP, Prince ME, Tran HH, Wolf GT, Urba SG, Chepeha DB, Teknos TN. EGFR, p16, HPV Titer, Bcl-xL and p53, sex, and smoking as indicators of response to therapy and survival in oropharyngeal cancer. J Clin Oncol. 2008;26(19):3128–37.
161. Study of Panitumumab Efficacy in Patients with Recurrent and/or Metastatic Head and Neck Cancer (SPECTRUM). Available at: http://clinicaltrials.gov/show/NCT00460265.
162. Forastiere AA, Burtness BA. Epidermal growth factor receptor inhibition in head and neck cancer—more insights, but more questions. J Clin Oncol. 2007;25(16):2152–5.
163. Walter V, Yin X, Wilkerson MD, Cabanski CR, Zhao N, Du Y, et al. Molecular subtypes in head and neck cancer exhibit distinct patterns of chromosomal gain and loss of canonical cancer genes. PLoS One. 2013;8(2):e56823.
164. Martinez I, Wang J, Hobson KF, Ferris RL, Khan SA. Identification of differentially expressed genes in HPV-positive and HPV-negative oropharyngeal squamous cell carcinomas. Eur J Cancer. 2007;43(2):415–32.
165. Lacouture ME. Mechanisms of cutaneous toxicities to EGFR inhibitors. Nat Rev Cancer. 2006;6(10):803–12.

# Clinical Diagnostics and Patient Stratification for Use in the Dental Office

5

Alexandra B. Plonka and William V. Giannobile

**Abstract**

Diagnostics and prognostics in dentistry can be applied to stratify patients according to risk for individualized disease forecasting and, ultimately, targeting resources to maximize health outcomes. Traditional clinical measures of periodontal disease show a history of tissue destruction but are unable to determine biologic onset or initiation of inflammation and fail to predict susceptibility to or progression of disease. The state of the art in periodontal diagnostics is point-of-care (POC) periodontal methods (use of microbial, protein biomarker, and genetic measures). POC methods may use lab-on-a-chip (LOC) devices to analyze oral fluids such as saliva. This technology can be applied for patient risk stratification and predictive modeling to optimize personalized care in the dental office to target healthcare resources to those at highest risk.

## Introduction

Developing a personalized dental treatment plan begins with a diagnosis, which is the identification of all conditions or diseases. Diagnoses are driven from medical and dental histories, patient-reported symptoms, and clinical and radiographic exam findings [1, 2]. A step further is prognosis—predicting the progress, course, and outcome of a disease [3]. Diagnostics and prognostics in dentistry can be applied to stratify patients according to risk for individualized disease, forecasting, and ultimately targeting resources to maximize health outcomes. This chapter will highlight state-of-the-art point-of-care (POC) periodontal diagnostics (use of microbial, protein biomarker,

A.B. Plonka, DDS
Department of Periodontics and Oral Medicine, University of Michigan School of Dentistry, Ann Arbor, MI, USA
e-mail: aplonka@umich.edu

W.V. Giannobile, DDS, DMedSc (✉)
Department of Periodontics and Oral Medicine, University of Michigan School of Dentistry, Ann Arbor, MI, USA

Department of Biomedical Engineering, College of Engineering, Ann Arbor, MI, USA
e-mail: wgiannob@umich.edu



P.J. Polverini (ed.), *Personalized Oral Health Care: From Concept Design to Clinical Practice*,
DOI 10.1007/978-3-319-23297-3_5

and genetic measures) and their application for patient risk stratification to optimize personalized care in the dental office.

## Diagnostics in Periodontics: Limitations of Traditional Diagnostics

Periodontal disease is a chronic host-inflammatory response to polymicrobial infection (Fig. 5.1). In addition to its breadth of contributing factors, variety of diagnostic signs, and systemic health associations, it is a leading cause of tooth loss and affects almost 50 % of the US population [5]. These characteristics and resulting multidisciplinary treatment ramifications allow the use of periodontics as a key prototype for dental diagnostics. Periodontal diagnosis and prognosis are primarily based upon clinical information such as periodontal probing, clinical attachment levels, bleeding or suppuration upon probing, radiographic bone loss, furcation involvement, and tooth mobility.

The common limitation of physical and radiographic measures is their primarily historic illustration of tissue destruction rather than current display of active inflammation or prediction of

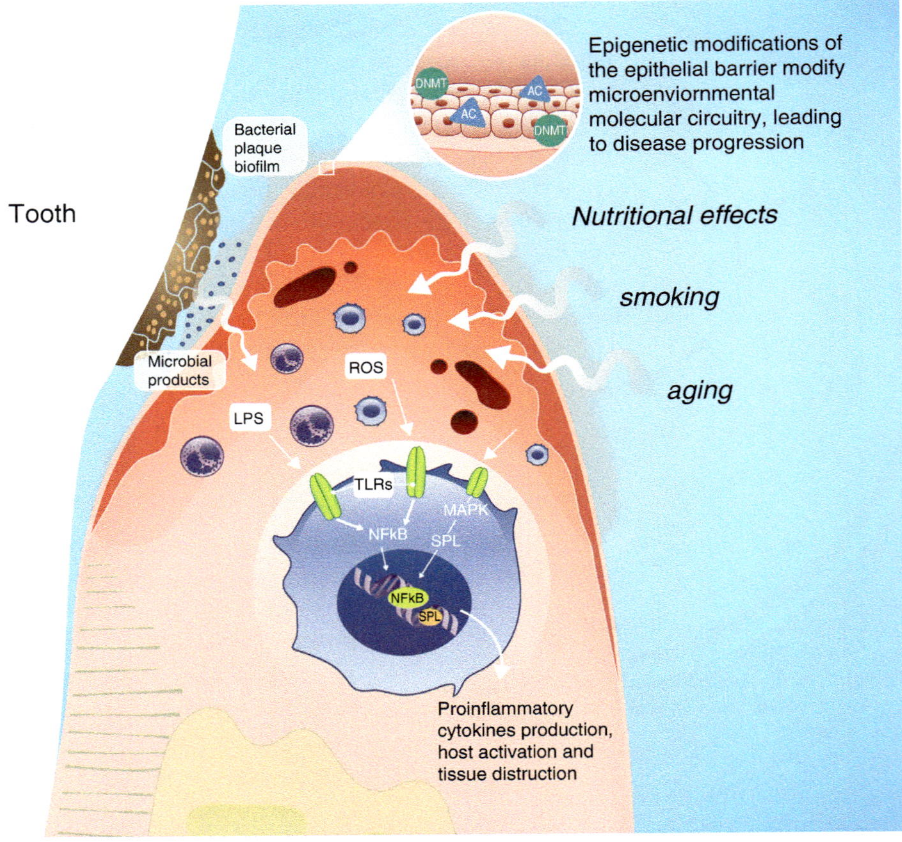


**Fig. 5.1** Periodontal disease is initiated by bacterial plaque biofilm and its components such as lipopolysaccharide (*LPS*), to which the host responds with a proinflammatory cascade, involving immune cell reactive oxygen species (*ROS*). The host interacts with these components via toll-like-receptors (*TLRs*), effecting downstream mediators nuclear-factor kappa beta (*NFkb*), mitogen-activated protein kinase (*MAPK*), and sphingosine-1-phosphate lyase (*SPL*). Susceptibility and tissue destruction are modified by environmental, genetic, and epigenetic factors, such as alterations to epithelial cell adenylate cyclase (*AC*) and DNA methyltransferase (*DNMT*) (From Larsson et al. [4]. Reproduced with permission from the American Academy of Periodontology)

future disease [6]. Periimplantitis is further hampered by a lack of consensus on disease identification and classification [7, 8]. A personalized approach to patient management would allow for subclinical disease detection, prior to the onset of potentially irreversible clinical signs of tissue loss. Subclinical disease may be identified by one or a combination of genetic changes or predispositions, microbial tests, and host markers, as shown in Fig. 5.2 [9]. Genetic (single-gene), genomic (gene-gene-interaction), or epigenetic (altered gene expression) tests can identify inherited or acquired risk factors to predict susceptibility to periodontal disease, as well as allow more accurate diagnosis, prognosis, and treatment planning [4, 10, 11]. The onset of periodontal infection can be determined by testing for pathogens and their genes [9]. Biomarkers are proteins that indicate host-response to disease or tissue breakdown. Saliva is an easily accessible medium to identify genetic and microbial biomarkers to allow for the use of rapid point-of-care (POC) diagnostics. Traditional laboratory-based tests such as enzyme-linked immunosorbent assays (ELISA) to detect proteins and polymerase chain reaction (PCR) to identify RNA and DNA are now being adapted in miniaturized systems as handheld or chairside devices [12].

The goal of implementing POC salivary diagnostics to the clinic is to identify, at the chairside, the onset of inflammation and determine which patients are at highest risk for disease progression in order to develop personalized treatment plans tailored to the needs of each individual patient. In addition to identifying disease or risk at earlier stages of the disease timeline, these methods may be faster, easier to obtain, and require less training and personnel than conventional clinical parameters using "signatures of periodontal disease" [12–14].

## Risk Stratification: What Is It?

In addition to identification of disease, treatment planning, and monitoring, biologic information may be used as risk factors to determine the likelihood of disease occurrence or progression. Risk stratification involves assessing a patient's susceptibility to disease and targeting resources toward groups at highest risk and limiting unnecessary treatment recommendations for patients at minimal or zero risk. The goals of risk stratification, listed in Table 5.1, include using diagnostic information to forecast health risks, prioritize and target treatment interventions, and mitigate adverse outcomes.

Ultimately, risk stratification aims to correctly identify and appropriately funnel healthcare efforts toward the classic "Pareto's principle," in which 20 % of the population require 80 % of the resources [15].

The highest-level information for risk stratification is the implementation of clinical, biologic, or genetic risk factors. Risk factors have been verified in longitudinal studies to be associated

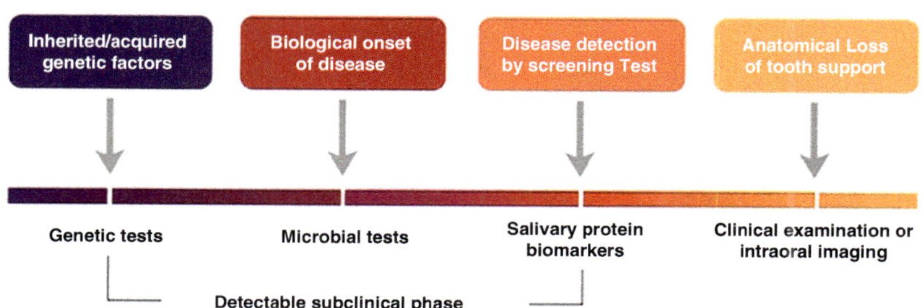


**Fig. 5.2** Timeline of periodontal disease progression. Genetic tests can elucidate inherited periodontal disease risk factors. Periodontal disease is initiated by pathogen infection, which can be detected at onset by microbial tests. Protein biomarkers found in saliva can allow for screening of disease activity and progression. Clinical diagnostic methods show destruction to the periodontal attachment apparatus (Reprinted from Giannobile [9]. Copyright © 2012, with permission from Elsevier)

**Table 5.1** Risk stratification applied to periodontal disease management

| Goal | Application |
|---|---|
| Forecast patient health risks | Periodontal diseases |
| | Tooth loss |
| Prioritize treatment interventions | Initial and advanced periodontal therapy |
| | Periodontal maintenance |
| | Nonsurgical debridement |
| | Periodontal surgery |
| Mitigate adverse outcomes | Oral infection |
| | Gingival inflammation |
| | Periodontal bone loss |
| | Tooth loss |

with a patient's increased predilection for disease and can be environmental, biologic, or behavioral in nature [16, 17]. Proven risk factors for periodontal disease include tobacco smoking, diabetes mellitus, and specific pathogens [18–20].

*Risk determinants*, or background characteristics, are risk factors that are not modifiable, such as age, genetics, or gender [21–24]. Risk indicators are possible risk factors that have been identified in cross-sectional but not longitudinal studies. Examples of *risk indicators* for periodontal disease are the systemic conditions osteoporosis, rheumatoid arthritis, and obesity [25, 26]. *Risk predictors* are associated with, but do not cause, disease. Finally, *risk markers* include a previous history of periodontal disease and bleeding on probing [27–29].

Patients may be stratified according to biologic or metabolic phenotypes ("metabotypes"), or disease presentations [30]. Such phenotypes may be determined by a combination of oral-fluid biomarkers, microbiologic profiles, and clinical features of disease [9, 31, 32]. Metabotypes are caused by the same epigenetic processes that are responsible for susceptibility to disease occurrence, progression, and therapeutic outcomes and are directly related to disease risk factors [33]. They provide a compilation of the effects of an individual's environmental exposure, biochemical and physiologic processes, and microbiome [30]. Increased understanding of phenotypes may improve disease classification, diagnosis, and treatment effectiveness. Phenotypes may be based on a variety of information modalities; other examples include transcriptomes, or gene expression signatures [34].

Predictive modeling may be used to optimize risk stratification and clinical decision making and allow cost-benefit analysis of treatment recommendations for a given patient group [30]. Predictive modeling involves applying historical associations between risk factors and target disease events to predict future outcomes based on mathematical formulae. These formulae can be applied to populations to rank (or stratify) persons according to risk and prioritize target interventions, resulting in increased efficiency, cost savings, and improved overall health [35]. Building a predictive model requires identifying a target outcome, such as healthcare costs or disease status, followed by the time interval until which the prediction is desired. Thirdly, health data is used as predictive information. Finally, data is tested and weighted according to its influence on the target outcome, until the most effective combination of risk factors is reached. Models are assessed based on their performance at maximizing true positives and true negatives, indicating identification of those at highest risk. Similarly, the model's false positive/negative rates should approach 0 % [15].

## Application of Saliva Diagnostics to Periodontology

Historically, treatment recommendations have derived from mean data from large epidemiologic studies [15]. Key to personalized medicine is assessing all available and specific risk factors on an individual level, to maximize the quality and quantity of information to be used for risk stratification [15]. A potentially simple and rapid way in which potential risk factors may be identified chairside in the dental office setting is through the application of salivary diagnostics. Information gleaned from such tests (most currently in various stages of development) may preempt traditional clinical signs and provide information on patient risk at the biochemical, molecular, and/or genetic levels [36, 37]. Salivary and gingival crevicular fluid (GCF) are rich sources of biomarkers in the oral cavity, which are quantifiable biologic parameters that have been validated to be signs of disease processes, provide information regarding pharmacologic interventions, and verify health status [14, 38]. Ideally, biomarkers provide information prior to the onset of potentially irreversible clinical sequelae and allow for prevention or early intervention with personalized treatment recommendations.

Salivary and GCF biomarkers can be used to address elements along the spectrum of periodontal disease development. Biomarkers may provide information on oral microbes, host immune response factors, and tissue breakdown products [39]. Analyzing "clusters" of biomarkers can provide enhanced information regarding disease status and effects of treatment [14, 40]. Biomarkers must be validated as accurate for disease detection and proven to have utility beyond traditional microscopic analytic methods (Fig 5.3) [10]. For a given sample media, such as saliva, an appropriate laboratory method is selected based on the biochemical mechanism to be evaluated. After the biomarker identification and quantification test has been validated, the role of the biomarker within the biologic or pathologic process is analyzed and compared with current accepted diagnostic practices. When treatment algorithms are developed for the clinician, biomarkers could be easily applied to personalized medicine or a variety of other healthcare applications [9].

Key biomarkers for risk assessment of periodontal and peri-implant disease progression are the use of periodontal pathogens (such as red complex bacteria of *Porphyromonas gingivalis*, *Treponema denticola*, and *Tanerella forsythia*) [42–44], matrix metalloproteinase-8 (MMP-8) [45], and interleukin-1 beta (IL-1) [46], for example.

## Microbial Assessment and Periodontal Diagnostics

Generally, an empirical approach to periodontal therapy involves initial mechanical scaling and root planing followed by reevaluation and potential surgical intervention. For special patient populations, microbial analysis such as DNA probes, PCR-based testing, and culture and sensitivity analysis can provide an added benefit to select and determine effectiveness of adjunctive antibiotics; for example, in patients refractory to treatment, medically compromised, or with aggressive disease or acute infections. Microbial testing methods are limited in their ability to culture or otherwise detect bacterial species. Microbial testing may also be performed to assess response to therapy [47–50] or potential antibiotic resistance [51]. When associated with improvements in clinical parameters, microbial testing may be used in clinical trials to assess effectiveness of treatment modalities, such as combination antibi-

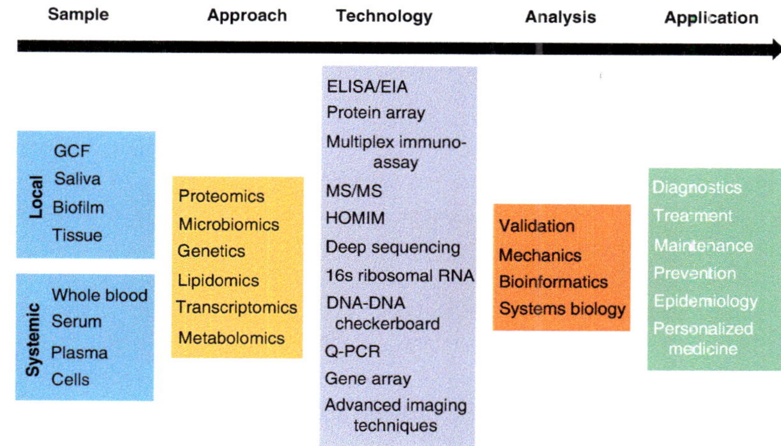


**Fig. 5.3** Process of biomarker identification and validation. Biomarkers may be obtained from biologic fluids. Selection of assay technology is guided by the scientific approach. Analysis determines the accuracy of the biomarker in predicting disease and clinical value compared with traditional methods. Personal and global healthcare applications are possible (From Kantarci [41]. Printed with the permission of Quintessence)

otic therapy, laser or photodynamic therapy, or implant technology [52–56]. The importance of microbial profiling alone or in combination with other biomarkers in diagnostics is to intercept patients susceptible to disease [37, 57–59] or at risk of progression or recurrence of chronic or aggressive periodontal disease [14, 60–62] or periimplantitis [51, 63–65] In addition to localized periodontal disease applications, salivary tests can also identify systemic infections such as H1N1 virus or HIV [66, 67].

The most important pathogens contributing to the development and progression of periodontal disease were initially identified by DNA probes and DNA-DNA checkerboard hybridization and grouped into complexes by Socransky and colleagues [20]. The "red complex" bacteria, Gram-negative obligate anaerobes *P. gingivalis, T. denticola, and T. forsythia*, are significantly associated with increased probing depth and BOP. Another common feature of these bacteria is their ability to hydrolyze the substrate N-benzoyl-DL-arginine-2-naphthylamide (BANA) using a trypsin-like enzyme, which can be detected by a chairside test for periodontal disease [68]. Currently, the field of microbial biomarker analysis is evolving with the development of detection methods, as many species have yet to be identified. In the intersection of microbiology and genetics, the human microbiome consists of all microorganisms inhabiting the oral cavity and their corresponding genome. Identification of the human oral microbiome, made possible by "high-throughput" methods, such as 16S rRNA or 454 pyrosequencing, allows for comparison between states of health and disease [69, 70].

## Host-Response Factors

The inflammatory component of periodontal disease can be captured by host-response biomarkers, which consist of immune system cell products and inflammatory mediators. These products tend to increase as the body responds to active infection and in instances of chronic inflammation and with treatment ideally resolve towards baseline levels. Examples include cytokines, such as interleukin-1 beta (IL-1β), and host-cell enzymes, such as polymorphonuclear lymphocyte (PMN) cell collagenase MMP-8. Periodontal pathogens initially elicit a non-specific inflammatory response. Subsequently, T- and B-lymphocytes produce cell signaling cytokines. Interleukins are cytokines that facilitate interactions between leukocytes and host epithelial cells, endothelial cells, and fibroblasts. Some cytokines, such as interleukin-1β (IL-1β), interleukin-6 (IL-6), and tumor necrosis factor (TNF)-α, may induce bone resorption. Specific interleukin-1 gene variants *IL1A* and *IL1B* are significantly associated with chronic periodontitis in Caucasian individuals [71]. Salivary IL-1β has been implicated in peri-implant inflammation [72]. Other host cells act as chemokines to recruit additional proinflammatory cells such as PMNs and macrophages. Continuing the inflammatory cascade, PMNs and macrophages secrete proinflammatory and tissue-destructive mediators that can be monitored in saliva and GCF. Such host-derived enzymes, like matrix-metalloproteinases (MMPs), degrade the periodontal attachment apparatus.

These host-response components can be monitored in saliva and GCF. PMN-derived MMP-8 (gelatinase) significantly decreases after periodontal therapy and maintenance, but persistently elevated MMP-8 may indicate a refractory site at risk of further breakdown, both applicable to monitoring, one goal of risk stratification [73–75]. Salivary MMP-8 may also be applied to risk stratification by discriminating between periodontitis patients with severe versus slight alveolar bone loss [76]. Peri-implant disease may have biomarker expression profiles similar to or unique from periimplantitis [77, 78].

## Tissue Breakdown Products

Osteocalcin (OCN), the main non-collagenous protein in bone matrix, may promote osteoclast differentiation and bone resorption and is a marker for bone turnover and when increased in oral fluids may predict periodontal bone loss [79]. A collagen degradation product, pyridinoline cross-linked carboxyterminal telopeptide of type I collagen (ICTP), is specific to bone, and its serum levels are elevated in bone resorptive diseases [39]. More so than OCN, GCF ICTP may have potential in predicting periodontal breakdown and response to treatment; however, reports vary [76, 80]. Salivary OCN and ICTP may be decreased, while can be MMP-8 increased in smokers [81–83].

Independently, biomarkers may be limited with respect to their ability to predict disease progression. Combining host-response and microbial oral-fluid biomarkers with clinical measures may allow for determination of characteristic profiles with higher sensitivity and specificity for periodontal disease progression [13, 37, 71]. This information can also be used to explore peri-implant health and disease [42].

## Application of Personalized Medicine and Risk Stratification in Clinical Practice

Personalized medicine has been an area of intense research focus over the past years and a strategic initiative of the National Institute of Dental and Craniofacial Research. Biomarkers may be detected chairside through POC saliva or GCF collection and analyzed using microfluidic lab-on-a-chip (LOC) technology [12, 84–86]. Microfluidic technology involves the processing of small fluid samples within precisely controlled "microscale" channels. Microfluidic platforms can improve test sensitivity, collection, and analysis speed and efficiency, and device portability, while minimizing sample size, material quantity, and cost [87]. Biomarkers like salivary MMP-8 are prototypes in the development of microfluidic assays for POC technology [88]. Other chairside technology includes "test sticks" which have been developed for detection of MMP-8 in periodontitis diagnosis [89].

Saliva has the advantage of ease and speed of collection over GCF sampling and, in addition to periodontal disease, has been applied for detection of systemic diseases such as oral cancer, breast cancer, and Sjogren's syndrome [90, 91]. Although simpler to collect than GCF, challenges facing the use of saliva as a diagnostic media include its variations in flow rate and overall quantity, which can be affected by medications, time of day, and other patient-related factors [9].

Microfluidic devices have also been developed to detect salivary bacteria [37]. Combining host-response biomarkers with microbial analysis addresses multiple components of the periodontal disease process and may optimize diagnosis of disease progression or stability [14, 37, 92, 93]. Application of biomarker technology within clinical research is guided by the desired study outcome and could improve the quality of study findings and translation to personalized medicine approaches (Fig. 5.4) [41].

Risk stratification has been applied in dentistry as recently illustrated in the *Michigan Periodontal Prevention Study*. The goal of this investigation was to determine the benefit of the biannual preventive care model in preventing tooth loss over the long term. In this retrospective cohort study of 5117 patients, individuals were divided into high or low risk based on presence or absence of at least one of the following risk factors: history of periodontal disease, current or recent cigarette smoking, and/or presence of interleukin-1 genotype polymorphisms. Assessing insurance claims information, the results of the study found no difference in tooth loss outcomes based on recall interval for low-risk patients (possessing no risk factors); however, high-risk patients demonstrated significantly less tooth loss over the 16-year observation period when the preventive recall was more frequent (twice yearly versus once yearly). Further, the study applied predictive modeling to show a healthcare-cost savings of over $2.2 million when risk stratification was applied to the study population. Application of this strategy to the US insured adult population could lead to significant healthcare savings [85, 94, 95].

Risk for periodontal disease can be combined with that for caries and oral cancer to tailor recall intervals during treatment and maintenance [96]. Risk stratification could be applied to many oral and systemic diseases with the increased breadth of information that genome-wide sequencing provides, strengthening dentistry's integration into primary care for large healthcare impact [95, 97].

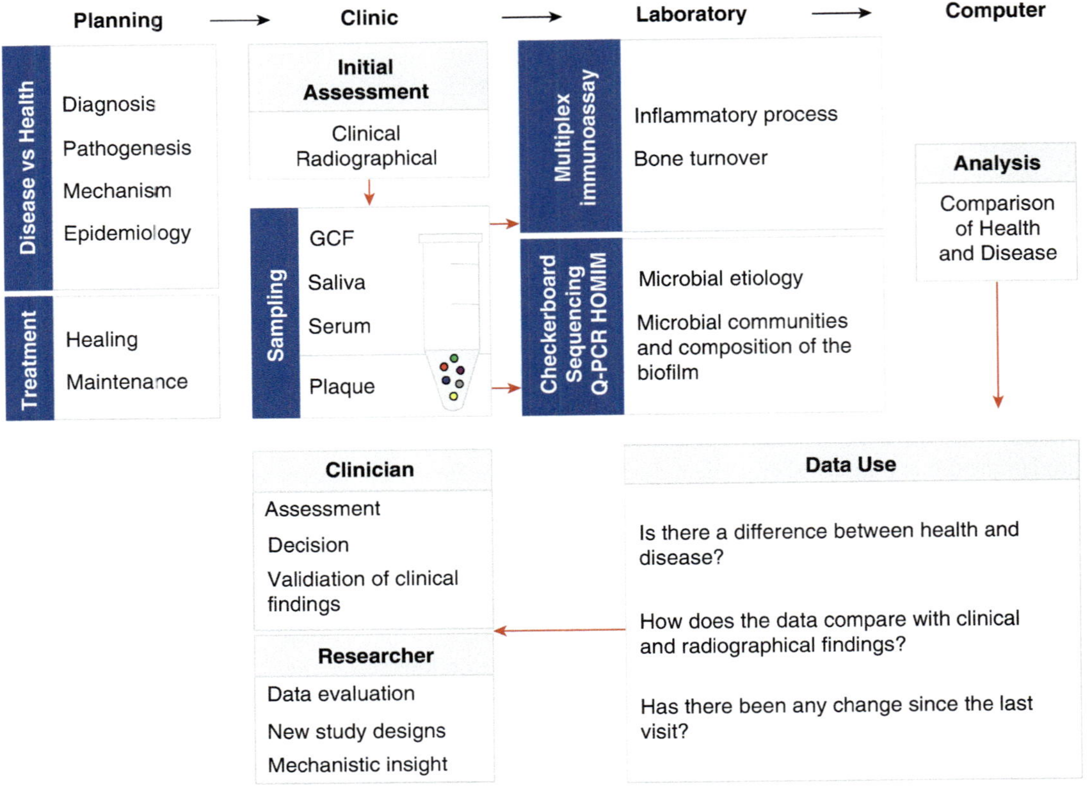


**Fig. 5.4** Biomarker technology improves translational clinical research. Study designs are selected by desired outcome comparisons, such as disease and health (cross-sectional) or wound healing (longitudinal). Optimization of biomarker selection facilitates translation to clinical applications (From Kantarci [41]. Printed with the permission of Quintessence)

## Conclusions

The field of clinical diagnostics and prognostics for the customization of patient care has advanced considerably over the past two decades (Fig. 5.5) [98]. The emerging utility of specific biomarkers of periodontal diseases has shown value in identifying early pathologic progression phases of the disease. However, the clinical regulatory path of biomarker selection to measure bone destruction or loss of clinical attachment is plagued on endpoints fraught with low sensitivity. The use of "signatures" of multiple biomarkers to predict disease progression offers stronger promise, given the pleotropic nature of periodontitis. The use of LOC diagnostics allows for real-time assessment of disease status with potential POC chairside application. Lastly, the use of prognostic measures for predicting or forecasting of disease activation offers strong potential. The implementation of patient stratification in dentistry allows for the better identification of low-risk and high-risk patients in an era of limited resources to use "one-size-fits-all" protocols that waste precious resources available to our patients.

**Acknowledgments** This work has been supported by NIH UL1RR024986, Colgate-Palmolive, and Renaissance Healthcare Corporation to WVG. WVG has licensed technology to Microsystemic Health, LLC on the use of saliva diagnostics.

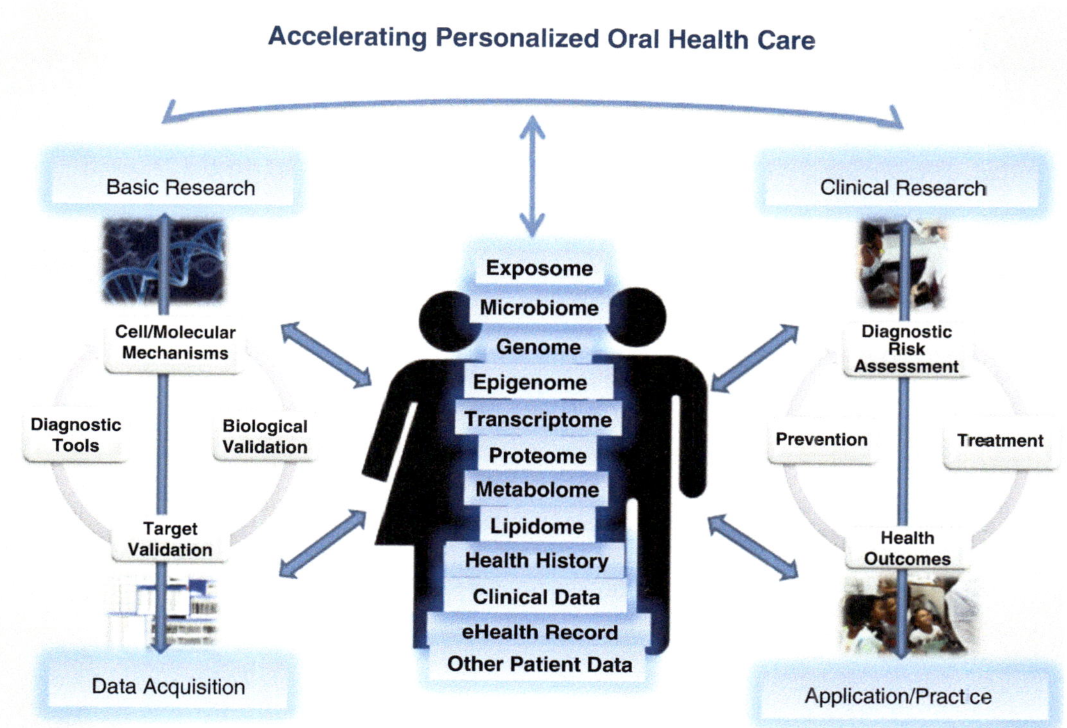


**Fig. 5.5** Integration of biologic information allows translation of personalized oral healthcare from basic science to clinical practice (From: Garcia et al. [98]; copyright © 2013 by SAGE Publications. Reprinted by permission of SAGE Publications)

## References


1. Armitage GC. Periodontal diagnoses and classification of periodontal diseases. Periodontol 2000. 2004;34:9–21.
2. American Academy of Periodontology. Parameter on comprehensive periodontal examination. J Periodontol. 2000;71(5 Suppl):847–8.
3. American Academy of Periodontology. Glossary of periodontal terms. 4th ed. Chicago: American Academy of Periodontology; 2001. p. 53–6.
4. Larsson L, Castilho RM, Giannobile WV. Epigenetics and its role in periodontal diseases – a state-of-the-art review. J Periodontol. 2015;86:556–68.
5. Eke PI, Thornton-Evans G, Dye B, Genco R. Advances in surveillance of periodontitis: the Centers for Disease Control and Prevention periodontal disease surveillance project. J Periodontol. 2012;83(11):1337–42.
6. Mdala I, Olsen I, Haffajee AD, Socransky SS, Thoresen M, de Blasio BF. Comparing clinical attachment level and pocket depth for predicting periodontal disease progression in healthy sites of patients with chronic periodontitis using multi-state Markov models. J Clin Periodontol. 2014;41(9):837–45.
7. Tomasi C, Derks J. Clinical research of peri-implant diseases – quality of reporting, case definitions and methods to study incidence, prevalence and risk factors of peri-implant diseases. J Clin Periodontol. 2012;39 Suppl 12:207–23.
8. Koldsland OC, Scheie AA, Aass AM. Prevalence of peri-implantitis related to severity of the disease with different degrees of bone loss. J Periodontol. 2010;81(2):231–8.
9. Giannobile WV. Salivary diagnostics for periodontal diseases. J Am Dent Assoc. 2012;143(10 Suppl):6S–11.
10. Eng G, Chen A, Vess T, Ginsburg GS. Genome technologies and personalized dental medicine. Oral Dis. 2012;18(3):223–35.
11. Razzouk S, Termechi O. Host genome, epigenome, and oral microbiome interactions: toward personalized periodontal therapy. J Periodontol. 2013;84(9):1266–71.
12. Giannobile WV, McDevitt JT, Niedbala RS, Malamud D. Translational and clinical applications of salivary diagnostics. Adv Dent Res. 2011;23(4):375–80.

13. Kinney JS, Morelli T, Oh M, Braun TM, Ramseier CA, Sugai JV, et al. Crevicular fluid biomarkers and periodontal disease progression. J Clin Periodontol. 2014;41(2):113–20.
14. Kinney JS, Morelli T, Ramseier CA, Herr A, Shelburne C, Rayburn LA, et al. Saliva/pathogen biomarker signatures and periodontal disease progression. J Dent Res. 2011;90(6):752–8.
15. Kornman KS, Duff GW. Personalized medicine: will dentistry ride the wave or watch from the beach? J Dent Res. 2012;91(7 Suppl):8S–11.
16. Genco RJ. Current view of risk factors for periodontal diseases. J Periodontol. 1996;67(10 Suppl):1041–9.
17. Genco RJ, Borgnakke WS. Risk factors for periodontal disease. Periodontol 2000. 2013;62(1):59–94.
18. Tomar SL, Asma S. Smoking-attributable periodontitis in the United States: findings from NHANES III. National Health and Nutrition Examination Survey. J Periodontol. 2000;71(5):743–51.
19. Grossi SG, Zambon JJ, Ho AW, Koch G, Dunford RG, Machtei EE, et al. Assessment of risk for periodontal disease. I. Risk indicators for attachment loss. J Periodontol. 1994;65(3):260–7.
20. Socransky SS, Haffajee AD, Cugini MA, Smith C, Kent Jr RL. Microbial complexes in subgingival plaque. J Clin Periodontol. 1998;25(2):134–44.
21. Kornman KS, Crane A, Wang HY, di Giovine FS, Newman MG, Pirk FW, et al. The interleukin-1 genotype as a severity factor in adult periodontal disease. J Clin Periodontol. 1997;24(1):72–7.
22. Michalowicz BS, Aeppli D, Virag JG, Klump DG, Hinrichs JE, Segal NL, et al. Periodontal findings in adult twins. J Periodontol. 1991;62(5):293–9.
23. Burt BA. Periodontitis and aging: reviewing recent evidence. J Am Dent Assoc. 1994;125(3):273–9.
24. Albandar JM, Brunelle JA, Kingman A. Destructive periodontal disease in adults 30 years of age and older in the United States, 1988–1994. J Periodontol. 1999;70(1):13–29.
25. Bartold PM, Marshall RI, Haynes DR. Periodontitis and rheumatoid arthritis: a review. J Periodontol. 2005;76(11 Suppl):2066–74.
26. von Wowern N, Klausen B, Kollerup G. Osteoporosis: a risk factor in periodontal disease. J Periodontol. 1994;65(12):1134–8.
27. Page RC, Beck JD. Risk assessment for periodontal diseases. Int Dent J. 1997;47(2):61–87.
28. Lang NP, Adler R, Joss A, Nyman S. Absence of bleeding on probing. An indicator of periodontal stability. J Clin Periodontol. 1990;17(10):714–21.
29. Lang NP, Joss A, Orsanic T, Gusberti FA, Siegrist BE. Bleeding on probing. A predictor for the progression of periodontal disease? J Clin Periodontol. 1986;13(6):590–6.
30. Nicholson JK, Holmes E, Kinross JM, Darzi AW, Takats Z, Lindon JC. Metabolic phenotyping in clinical and surgical environments. Nature. 2012;491(7424):384–92.
31. Offenbacher S, Barros SP, Singer RE, Moss K, Williams RC, Beck JD. Periodontal disease at the biofilm-gingival interface. J Periodontol. 2007;78(10):1911–25.
32. Morelli T, Stella M, Barros SP, Marchesan JT, Moss KL, Kim SJ, et al. Salivary biomarkers in a biofilm overgrowth model. J Periodontol. 2014;85(12):1770–8.
33. Holmes E, Wilson ID, Nicholson JK. Metabolic phenotyping in health and disease. Cell. 2008;134(5):714–7.
34. Kebschull M, Demmer RT, Grun B, Guarnieri P, Pavlidis P, Papapanou PN. Gingival tissue transcriptomes identify distinct periodontitis phenotypes. J Dent Res. 2014;93(5):459–68.
35. Cousins LM, Bander JA. An introduction to predictive modeling for disease management risk stratification. Dis Manag. 2002;5(3):157–67.
36. Nie S, Henley WH, Miller SE, Zhang H, Mayer KM, Dennis PJ, et al. An automated integrated platform for rapid and sensitive multiplexed protein profiling using human saliva samples. Lab Chip. 2014;14(6):1087–98.
37. Salminen A, Gursoy UK, Paju S, Hyvarinen K, Mantyla P, Buhlin K, et al. Salivary biomarkers of bacterial burden, inflammatory response, and tissue destruction in periodontitis. J Clin Periodontol. 2014;41(5):442–50.
38. Biomarkers Definitions Working Gruop. Biomarkers and surrogate endpoints: preferred definitions and conceptual framework. Clin Pharmacol Ther. 2001;69(3):89–95.
39. Taba Jr M, Kinney J, Kim AS, Giannobile WV. Diagnostic biomarkers for oral and periodontal diseases. Dent Clin North Am. 2005;49(3):551–71, vi.
40. Miller CS, King Jr CP, Langub MC, Kryscio RJ, Thomas MV. Salivary biomarkers of existing periodontal disease: a cross-sectional study. J Am Dent Assoc. 2006;137(3):322–9.
41. Kantarci A. Biomarkers and molecular biological methods in diagnostic, preventive and regenerative dental research. In: Giannobile WV, Lang NP, Tonetti MS, editors. Osteology guidelines for oral and maxillofacial regeneration: clinical research. London/Chicago: Quintessence; 2014. p. 318.
42. Tatarakis N, Kinney JS, Inglehart M, Braun TM, Shelburne C, Lang NP, et al. Clinical, microbiological, and salivary biomarker profiles of dental implant patients with type 2 diabetes. Clin Oral Implants Res. 2014;25(7):803–12.
43. Ito T, Yasuda M, Kaneko H, Sasaki H, Kato T, Yajima Y. Clinical evaluation of salivary periodontal pathogen levels by real-time polymerase chain reaction in patients before dental implant treatment. Clin Oral Implants Res. 2014;25(8):977–82.
44. Liljestrand JM, Gursoy UK, Hyvarinen K, Sorsa T, Suominen AL, Kononen E, et al. Combining salivary pathogen and serum antibody levels improves their diagnostic ability in detection of periodontitis. J Periodontol. 2014;85(1):123–31.
45. Rathnayake N, Akerman S, Klinge B, Lundegren N, Jansson H, Tryselius Y, et al. Salivary biomarkers of

oral health: a cross-sectional study. J Clin Periodontol. 2013;40(2):140–7.
46. Ebersole JL, Schuster JL, Stevens J, Dawson 3rd D, Kryscio RJ, Lin Y, et al. Patterns of salivary analytes provide diagnostic capacity for distinguishing chronic adult periodontitis from health. J Clin Immunol. 2013;33(1):271–9.
47. Parameter on "refractory" periodontitis. American Academy of Periodontology. J Periodontol. 2000; 71(5 Suppl):859–60.
48. Slots J, Research S, Therapy C. Systemic antibiotics in periodontics. J Periodontol. 2004;75(11): 1553–65.
49. Socransky SS, Haffajee AD, Teles R, Wennstrom JL, Lindhe J, Bogren A, et al. Effect of periodontal therapy on the subgingival microbiota over a 2-year monitoring period. I. Overall effect and kinetics of change. J Clin Periodontol. 2013;40(8):771–80.
50. Listgarten MA, Loomer PM. Microbial identification in the management of periodontal diseases. A systematic review. Ann Periodontol. 2003;8(1):182–92.
51. Charalampakis G, Leonhardt A, Rabe P, Dahlen G. Clinical and microbiological characteristics of peri-implantitis cases: a retrospective multicentre study. Clin Oral Implants Res. 2012;23(9):1045–54.
52. Chui C, Aoki A, Takeuchi Y, Sasaki Y, Hiratsuka K, Abiko Y, et al. Antimicrobial effect of photodynamic therapy using high-power blue light-emitting diode and red-dye agent on Porphyromonas gingivalis. J Periodontal Res. 2013;48(6):696–705.
53. Nagahara A, Mitani A, Fukuda M, Yamamoto H, Tahara K, Morita I, et al. Antimicrobial photodynamic therapy using a diode laser with a potential new photosensitizer, indocyanine green-loaded nanospheres, may be effective for the clearance of Porphyromonas gingivalis. J Periodontal Res. 2013;48(5):591–9.
54. Benavides E, Rios HF, Ganz SD, An CH, Resnik R, Reardon GT, et al. Use of cone beam computed tomography in implant dentistry: the International Congress of Oral Implantologists consensus report. Implant Dent. 2012;21(2):78–86.
55. Soares GM, Mendes JA, Silva MP, Faveri M, Teles R, Socransky SS, et al. Metronidazole alone or with amoxicillin as adjuncts to non-surgical treatment of chronic periodontitis: a secondary analysis of microbiological results from a randomized clinical trial. J Clin Periodontol. 2014;41(4):366–76.
56. Mdala I, Olsen I, Haffajee AD, Socransky SS, de Blasio BF, Thoresen M. Multilevel analysis of bacterial counts from chronic periodontitis after root planing/scaling, surgery, and systemic and local antibiotics: 2-year results. J Oral Microbiol. 2013;5, doi: 10.3402/jom.v5i0.20939.
57. Lee A, Ghaname CB, Braun TM, Sugai JV, Teles RP, Loesche WJ, et al. Bacterial and salivary biomarkers predict the gingival inflammatory profile. J Periodontol. 2012;83(1):79–89.
58. Saygun I, Nizam N, Keskiner I, Bal V, Kubar A, Acikel C, et al. Salivary infectious agents and periodontal disease status. J Periodontal Res. 2011;46(2):235–9.
59. Haubek D, Johansson A. Pathogenicity of the highly leukotoxic JP2 clone of Aggregatibacter actinomycetemcomitans and its geographic dissemination and role in aggressive periodontitis. J Oral Microbiol. 2014;6, doi: 10.3402/jom.v6.23980. eCollection 2014. Review. PMID: 25206940.
60. Divaris K, Monda KL, North KE, Olshan AF, Lange EM, Moss K, et al. Genome-wide association study of periodontal pathogen colonization. J Dent Res. 2012;91(7 Suppl):21S–8.
61. Hoglund Aberg C, Kwamin F, Claesson R, Dahlen G, Johansson A, Haubek D. Progression of attachment loss is strongly associated with presence of the JP2 genotype of Aggregatibacter actinomycetemcomitans: a prospective cohort study of a young adolescent population. J Clin Periodontol. 2014;41(3):232–41.
62. Meyer-Baumer A, Eick S, Mertens C, Uhlmann L, Hagenfeld D, Eickholz P, et al. Periodontal pathogens and associated factors in aggressive periodontitis: results 5–17 years after active periodontal therapy. J Clin Periodontol. 2014;41(7):662–72.
63. Kumar PS, Mason MR, Brooker MR, O'Brien K. Pyrosequencing reveals unique microbial signatures associated with healthy and failing dental implants. J Clin Periodontol. 2012;39(5):425–33.
64. Botero JE, Gonzalez AM, Mercado RA, Olave G, Contreras A. Subgingival microbiota in peri-implant mucosa lesions and adjacent teeth in partially edentulous patients. J Periodontol. 2005;76(9):1490–5.
65. Hultin M, Gustafsson A, Hallstrom H, Johansson LA, Ekfeldt A, Klinge B. Microbiological findings and host response in patients with peri-implantitis. Clin Oral Implants Res. 2002;13(4):349–58.
66. Bilder L, Machtei EE, Shenhar Y, Kra-Oz Z, Basis F. Salivary detection of H1N1 virus: a clinical feasibility investigation. J Dent Res. 2011;90(9):1136–9.
67. Reynolds SJ, Muwonga J. OraQuick ADVANCE Rapid HIV-1/2 antibody test. Expert Rev Mol Diagn. 2004;4(5):587–91.
68. Schmidt EF, Bretz WA, Hutchinson RA, Loesche WJ. Correlation of the hydrolysis of benzoyl-arginine naphthylamide (BANA) by plaque with clinical parameters and subgingival levels of spirochetes in periodontal patients. J Dent Res. 1988;67(12): 1505–9.
69. Chen H, Jiang W. Application of high-throughput sequencing in understanding human oral microbiome related with health and disease. Front Microbiol. 2014;5:508.
70. Zarco MF, Vess TJ, Ginsburg GS. The oral microbiome in health and disease and the potential impact on personalized dental medicine. Oral Dis. 2012;18(2): 109–20.
71. Karimbux NY, Saraiya VM, Elangovan S, Allareddy V, Kinnunen T, Kornman KS, et al. Interleukin-1 gene polymorphisms and chronic periodontitis in adult whites: a systematic review and meta-analysis. J Periodontol. 2012;83(11):1407–19.
72. Rocha FS, Jesus RN, Rocha FM, Moura CC, Zanetta-Barbosa D. Saliva versus peri-implant inflammation:

quantification of IL-1 beta in partially and totally edentulous patients. J Oral Implantol. 2014;40(2):169–73.

73. Mantyla P, Stenman M, Kinane D, Salo T, Suomalainen K, Tikanoja S, et al. Monitoring periodontal disease status in smokers and nonsmokers using a gingival crevicular fluid matrix metalloproteinase-8-specific chair-side test. J Periodontal Res. 2006;41(6):503–12.
74. Kinane DF, Darby IB, Said S, Luoto H, Sorsa T, Tikanoja S, et al. Changes in gingival crevicular fluid matrix metalloproteinase-8 levels during periodontal treatment and maintenance. J Periodontal Res. 2003;38(4):400–4.
75. Sexton WM, Lin Y, Kryscio RJ, Dawson 3rd DR, Ebersole JL, Miller CS. Salivary biomarkers of periodontal disease in response to treatment. J Clin Periodontol. 2011;38(5):434–41.
76. Gursoy UK, Kononen E, Huumonen S, Tervahartiala T, Pussinen PJ, Suominen AL, et al. Salivary type I collagen degradation end-products and related matrix metalloproteinases in periodontitis. J Clin Periodontol. 2013;40(1):18–25.
77. Casado PL, Canullo L, de Almeida Filardy A, Granjeiro JM, Barboza EP, Leite Duarte ME. Interleukins 1 beta and 10 expressions in the periimplant crevicular fluid from patients with untreated periimplant disease. Implant Dent. 2013;22(2):143–50.
78. Guncu GN, Akman AC, Gunday S, Yamalik N, Berker E. Effect of inflammation on cytokine levels and bone remodelling markers in peri-implant sulcus fluid: a preliminary report. Cytokine. 2012;59(2):313–6.
79. Giannobile WV, Lynch SE, Denmark RG, Paquette DW, Fiorellini JP, Williams RC. Crevicular fluid osteocalcin and pyridinoline cross-linked carboxyterminal telopeptide of type I collagen (ICTP) as markers of rapid bone turnover in periodontitis. A pilot study in beagle dogs. J Clin Periodontol. 1995;22(12):903–10.
80. Kinney JS, Ramseier CA, Giannobile WV. Oral fluid-based biomarkers of alveolar bone loss in periodontitis. Ann N Y Acad Sci. 2007;1098:230–51.
81. Ozcaka O, Nalbantsoy A, Buduneli N. Salivary osteocalcin levels are decreased in smoker chronic periodontitis patients. Oral Dis. 2011;17(2):200–5.
82. Gurlek O, Lappin DF, Buduneli N. Effects of smoking on salivary C-telopeptide pyridinoline cross-links of type I collagen and osteocalcin levels. Arch Oral Biol. 2009;54(12):1099–104.
83. Heikkinen AM, Sorsa T, Pitkaniemi J, Tervahartiala T, Kari K, Broms U, et al. Smoking affects diagnostic salivary periodontal disease biomarker levels in adolescents. J Periodontol. 2010;81(9):1299–307.
84. Christodoulides N, Floriano PN, Miller CS, Ebersole JL, Mohanty S, Dharshan P, et al. Lab-on-a-chip methods for point-of-care measurements of salivary biomarkers of periodontitis. Ann N Y Acad Sci. 2007;1098:411–28.
85. Giannobile WV, Kornman KS, Williams RC. Personalized medicine in dentistry. What will this mean for clinical practice? J Am Dent Assoc. 2013;144:874–6.
86. Yager P, Edwards T, Fu E, Helton K, Nelson K, Tam MR, et al. Microfluidic diagnostic technologies for global public health. Nature. 2006;442(7101):412–8.
87. Nahavandi S, Baratchi S, Soffe R, Tang SY, Nahavandi S, Mitchell A, et al. Microfluidic platforms for biomarker analysis. Lab Chip. 2014;14(9):1496–514.
88. Herr AE, Hatch AV, Throckmorton DJ, Tran HM, Brennan JS, Giannobile WV, et al. Microfluidic immunoassays as rapid saliva-based clinical diagnostics. Proc Natl Acad Sci U S A. 2007;104(13):5268–73.
89. Mantyla P, Stenman M, Kinane DF, Tikanoja S, Luoto H, Salo T, et al. Gingival crevicular fluid collagenase-2 (MMP-8) test stick for chair-side monitoring of periodontitis. J Periodontal Res. 2003;38(4):436–9.
90. Liu J, Duan Y. Saliva: a potential media for disease diagnostics and monitoring. Oral Oncol. 2012;48(7):569–77.
91. Wang Q, Gao P, Wang X, Duan Y. The early diagnosis and monitoring of squamous cell carcinoma via saliva metabolomics. Sci Rep. 2014;4:6802.
92. Teles R, Sakellari D, Teles F, Konstantinidis A, Kent R, Socransky S, et al. Relationships among gingival crevicular fluid biomarkers, clinical parameters of periodontal disease, and the subgingival microbiota. J Periodontol. 2010;81(1):89–98.
93. Ramseier CA, Kinney JS, Herr AE, Braun T, Sugai JV, Shelburne CA, et al. Identification of pathogen and host-response markers correlated with periodontal disease. J Periodontol. 2009;80(3):436–46.
94. Giannobile WV, Braun TM, Caplis AK, Doucette-Stamm L, Duff GW, Kornman KS. Patient stratification for preventive care in dentistry. J Dent Res. 2013;92(8):694–701.
95. Slavkin HC. From phenotype to genotype: enter genomics and transformation of primary health care around the world. J Dent Res. 2014;93(7 suppl):3S–6.
96. Teich ST. Risk Assessment-Based Individualized Treatment (RABIT): a comprehensive approach to dental patient recall. J Dent Educ. 2013;77(4):448–57.
97. Wong DT. Salivaomics. J Am Dent Assoc. 2012;143(10 Suppl):19S–24.
98. Garcia I, Kuska R, Somerman MJ. Expanding the foundation for personalized medicine: implications and challenges for dentistry. J Dent Res. 2013;92(7 Suppl):3S–10.

# Metabolomics and Oral Disease Diagnosis

6

Yvonne L. Kapila

**Abstract**

The view of personalized care has evolved with the advent of modern molecular and genomic science, the completion of the Human Genome Project, the launching of the Human Microbiome Project, the focus on the individual in western societies, the explosion of Big Data, and business models and political systems becoming interwoven with health care. Dentistry is embracing this new paradigm that focuses on health care that is personalized, predictive, preventive, and participatory. Whether using "omic" technology, handheld devices, or sampling of various body substances, health and dental care are poised to write the next chapter in our historical text of personalization of oral health care. Notable advances in personalization of oral care include knowledge gained in oral cancer, periodontal disease, and caries. These advances, with an emphasis on metabolomics, will be discussed within the framework of the current status of these diseases, their limitations, and the emerging opportunities in these fields in terms of disease diagnosis.

## Introduction

The personalization of oral and general health care has reached a new zenith. For some, personalized care may summon visions of a dentist or doctor paying a house call. In historical and religious texts, we learn that essential oils and botanicals were at the heart of personalized healing practices used by ancient healers including the Egyptians, Chinese, and Greeks. In present times, the view of personalized care has evolved with the advent of modern molecular and genomic science, the completion of the Human Genome Project, the launching of the Human Microbiome Project, the focus on the individual in western societies, the explosion of Big Data, and business models and political systems becoming interwoven with health care. Dentistry is embracing this new paradigm that focuses on

Y.L. Kapila, DDS, PhD
Department of Periodontics and Oral Medicine, University of Michigan, School of Dentistry, Ann Arbor, MI, USA
e-mail: ykapila@umich.edu





P.J. Polverini (ed.), *Personalized Oral Health Care: From Concept Design to Clinical Practice*,
DOI 10.1007/978-3-319-23297-3_6

health care that is personalized, predictive, preventive, and participatory. Whether using "omic" technology, handheld devices, or sampling of various body substances, health and dental care are poised to write the next chapter in our historical text of personalization of oral health care. Notable advances in personalization of oral care include knowledge gained in oral cancer, periodontal disease, and caries. These advances will be discussed within the framework of the current status of these diseases, the limitations, and the emerging opportunities in these fields in terms of disease diagnosis.

## Current Status of Personalized Approaches to the Diagnosis of Oral Diseases and Their Limitations

Current diagnostic strategies for oral diseases are based on knowledge gained from somewhat subjective interpretation of clinical observations, clinical examination, radiographic examination, and, in some cases, histological examination. Borrowing from historical knowledge, much of what we espouse in oral and physical diagnosis has not changed much from our early origins and dates back to Grecian medicine, Hippocrates, Egypt, Crete, and Babylonia. In the *Iliad* (ca 1200 B.C.), Homer had 150 anatomic terms to describe 141 wounds. Hippocrates and his contemporaries were masters of observation, and this ability of observation is still our most powerful tool. However, this approach is changing with the advent of personalized health.

In the field of periodontology, diagnosis of periodontal disease is based on a radiographic examination and clinical examination that requires the use of a periodontal probe to measure and diagnose historical or past disease. These diagnostic aids are simple and easy to use. They are cost-effective and relatively noninvasive. Therefore, clinicians frequently employ them to make diagnoses and predict the destructive activity of periodontal disease. Markers that have been used to evaluate periodontal status, both to determine diagnosis or prognosis, include probing depth, clinical attachment level, bleeding on probing, suppuration, gingival redness, and plaque accumulation. These vary in terms of their sensitivity and specificity, yet changes in probing depth; clinical attachment levels; bleeding on probing and its absence, especially when recorded continuously over time; and plaque represent the best available markers of disease with good specificity and good positive and negative predictive values [1,2].

The value of a diagnostic test or biomarker is determined based on its sensitivity, specificity, positive predictive value, and negative predictive value. Sensitivity is the probability of the test being positive when the disease is truly present. A test with a sensitivity of 1.0 would detect the disease in all cases with no false negatives. Specificity is the probability of the test being negative when the disease is not present. A test with a specificity of 1.0 would detect disease in all cases with no false positives. Positive predictive value is the probability that the disease is present when the test is positive. Negative predictive value is the probability that the disease is absent when the test is negative. Predictive values are influenced by the prevalence of disease in a population. A higher prevalence of a disease within a particular population will lead to a higher predictive value compared to a population with a lower prevalence of the disease. Given the high prevalence of periodontal disease in the US population and around the world [3,4], biomarkers with good predictive values can potentially be developed for this disease.

However, the current diagnostic markers for periodontal disease are inherently limited. For example, clinical attachment loss readings obtained with a periodontal probe and radiographic evaluations of alveolar bone loss only measure damage from past episodes of disease and not current or active disease. In addition, a minimum threshold of 2- to 3-mm change is required before a site can be identified as having experienced a breakdown (i.e., low sensitivity) and longer monitoring periods (2–5 years) may be needed before markers of disease reach a higher level of sensitivity and meaningful diagnostic value [1,5,6]. Furthermore, probing pressure and inflammation can influence the measurements obtained [7–13].

Significant efforts have been made to identify risk indicators or biomarkers of subclinical periodontal disease or biomarkers that can predict disease progression and that have a higher sensitivity. A biomarker is a substance that is measured objectively and evaluated as an indicator of normal biologic processes, pathogenic processes, or pharmacologic responses to a therapeutic intervention [14]. These biomarkers are generally derived from site-specific dental plaque or gingival crevicular fluid (GCF) or from saliva or serum for whole-mouth/body analyses. Periodontal disease biomarkers attempt to capture subclinical aspects of the disease or the initiation of the periodontal lesion and thus have focused on examining the initiating microbiological flora, the inflammatory reaction to these pathogens, the extracellular matrix breakdown components that ensue, or the cellular damages that result from these insults. In-depth reviews of biomarkers obtained from GCF and saliva have been described for periodontal disease diagnosis, disease progression, and disease susceptibility [15–17]. Over 65 GCF components have been reported as potential markers for diagnosis and progression of periodontal disease. A problem with these biomarkers includes the inability to distinguish gingivitis from periodontitis, since most of these are based on general inflammatory proteins or enzymes or nonspecific tissue breakdown products. Those markers that focus on bone breakdown may hold greater promise in distinguishing between gingivitis and periodontitis, and thus the need for longitudinal studies to evaluate their diagnostic potential is warranted.

Periodontal diseases are initiated by bacterial species living in polymicrobial biofilms at or below the gingival margin, and disease progression ensues largely as a result of the inflammation initiated by specific subgingival species in a susceptible host. Thus, microbiological sampling using traditional culture methods and various identification approaches have been used to identify a series of bacteria that are associated with periodontal diseases. Classic studies that focused on analyses of subgingival plaque samples have identified bacterial complexes that are associated with severe forms of periodontal disease and increased pocket depths and bleeding on probing [18]. One such complex, the red or first complex of bacteria, is comprised of *Porphyromonas gingivalis, Treponema denticola, and Tannerella forsythia*. Longitudinal monitoring of these complex biofilms reveals the effects of treatment on the dynamic composition of these biofilm communities [19]. Oral biofilms are one of the best-studied biofilms of the human body, and thus many lessons have been learned in periodontal microbiology from their years of study [20].

Currently, academic-based commercial laboratories offer microbial analyses of patient samples to assist with disease diagnosis. These analytical platforms use conventional culturing methods for limited sets of periodontal/oral pathogens from plaque samples [21,22]. Thus, one of the limitations of these culturing and identification approaches is the limited numbers of species that can be identified using these methods. Furthermore, it is becoming apparent that oral biofilms and companion salivary constituents are exquisitely complex, containing members of methanogenic Archaea and bacteriophages that have been previously missed due to the limited methods used for their identification [23–25]. Given this emerging knowledge about the complexity of the oral biome, caution is being advised about disturbing the long-term community residents of these ecological niches with the use of antibiotics and probiotics [26].

## Emerging Opportunities for the Application of a Personalized Approach to Dental or Craniofacial Disease Diagnostics

Emerging opportunities for the application of a personalized approach to dental and craniofacial diseases are largely reliant on the development of "omics" technology. Integrating omics technology, including genomics, proteomics, transcriptomics, and metabolomics, provides a more complete picture of a functional signature of a cell or organism. With the completion of the human genome and microbiome projects, advancements in the identification of disease signatures and biomarkers have been made [27]. An integrative personal omics profile that is based on genomic, transcriptomic, proteomic, metabolomic, and autoantibody data, such as a circos plot, may someday be used as a "RiskOGram," for early diagnosis of subclinical disease, for disease monitoring, or for treatment follow-up [28].

Novel systems biology approaches hold promise for unraveling new details about the pathogenesis of periodontal disease. For example, with emerging data on the human microbiome, great advances can be made in understanding the synergistic interactions between humans and the normal flora of the human body and the oral cavity. This is a vast area that remains largely unexplored yet holds great promise, given that there are ten times more bacteria than the number of human cells in our body. We need to understand the delicate ecology that exists between the symbiotic, commensal, and pathologic microbes that share our body space.

With the advent of the human microbiome project, detailed profiles of the uncultivable and hard-to-detect microbes that comprise the polymicrobial biofilms of the oral cavity and that may be associated with periodontal disease or caries are now becoming possible. Commercial laboratories and research-focused laboratories have taken a lead role in this area. One such laboratory provides personalized human oral microbe identification using next generation sequencing [29]. The human oral microbe identification microarray, known as HOMIN can detect about 270 of the most prevalent cultivated and not-yet-cultivated oral bacterial species from plaque samples. HOMIN technology has been used by investigators and teams from academic and private institutions, government, and industry and presented in numerous publications. Another commercial lab provides testing of saliva using PCR-based approaches for detection of a set of four periodontal pathogens [30].

However, microbial examination requires sampling and submission of a sample to a distant site that requires time for analyses. This is not optimum in a clinical setting, especially when clinical probing and bleeding on probing provide information about the quality of the disease. Thus, novel point-of-care diagnostics are still needed to address this shortcoming.

In addition to the microbiome, expressed genome, and proteome, scientists can now study a substantial component of the expressed metabolome. Such an analysis demands an in-depth understanding of how metabolic pathways may be involved in the pathogenesis of different diseases. Mass spectrometry- and NMR-based metabolomics offer innovative, noninvasive platforms for the development of marker panels that are characteristic of disease phenotypes or cellular processes that are readily measured in biofluids/biospecimens/tissues (tissue biopsy, plasma/serum, urine, saliva, breath). Metabolomic profiling yields a signature set of functional metabolites of disease phenotypes.

Analyses of the various "omes" (metabolome, proteome, genome) are complementary, but identifying a panel of key metabolites that defines a given condition or disease provides an accurate readout of the cellular physiology of this process. Individual metabolites play an important role in representing endpoints of molecular pathways perturbed by events in the other "omes." Importantly, the metabolome is relatively small (~3200 compounds), highly conserved, and highly defined. Thus, metabolomic data sets are more computationally approachable, more amenable to interpretation, and more precise in characterization. The metabolome can be integrated into systems biology or with other omics datasets.

Metabolomics, which is based on mass spectroscopy and nuclear magnetic resonance spectroscopy, measures changes in small molecules or metabolites. The human metabolome contains approximately 5000 discrete metabolites. Metabolomic analyses have been applied to chronic disease including diabetes, obesity, cardiovascular disease, cancer, mental disorders, and drug toxicity.

Within dentistry, metabolomic approaches have been applied to a few disease conditions including head and neck cancer diagnosis, periodontal disease diagnosis, and caries. Although diagnosis of head and neck cancer has been traditionally based on histological examination of a tissue biopsy specimen, metabolomic approaches offer new possibilities. Within dentistry, head and neck cancer diagnosis has been the most extensively studied in terms of metabolomic approaches (Table 6.1). A 2002 study explored the diagnostic potential of $^{1}$H magnetic resonance spectroscopy in head and neck squamous cell carcinoma (HNSCC) tissues from 40 subjects (135 specimens) and found that the resonance from taurine, choline, glutamic acid, lactic acid, and lipid had diagnostic potential [31].

A 2008 study proposed a metabolomic-based diagnostic approach for oral squamous cell carcinoma (OSCC) ($n=20$) and its precancerous lesions, including oral lichen planus ($n=20$) and oral leukoplakia ($n=7$), using saliva samples and HPLC/MS analysis. Statistical analysis of the metabolomic data distinguished these different pathologic conditions [32].

Using NMR-based approaches, two studies in 2009 examined the metabolomic profiles of HNSCC and OSCC. One group, which examined serum from 15 OSCC patients and 10 healthy controls, was able to discriminate between the two groups and between different stages of disease. Metabolites that were differentially altered in the OSCC group compared to the healthy controls, included metabolites in choline pathways, glucose/Krebs cycle, the urea cycle, and acetoacetate pathways [33]. The other NMR-based study examined plasma from patients who had OSCC ($n=33$), oral leukoplakia ($n=5$), and healthy controls ($n=28$) and found that they could differentiate the OSCC patients from those with oral leukoplakia and controls based on differential metabolites, including tyrosine, aspartic acid, glucose, myoinositol, taurine, arginine, choline, creatinine, lipids, glutamic acid, proline, arginine, 3-hydroxybutyrate, valine, and isoleucine [34].

A study that analyzed a variety of conditions, including, oral cancer ($n=69$), breast cancer ($n=30$), pancreatic cancer ($n=18$), periodontal disease ($n=11$), and healthy controls ($n=87$), performed metabolomic analysis using capillary electrophoresis time-of-flight mass spectroscopy and found that 57 principal metabolites could predict the probability of being affected by each disease [35].

A 2010 study used ultraperformance liquid chromatography coupled with quadrupole/time-of-flight mass spectrometry (LC/Q-TOF MS) to explore its diagnostic potential in distinguishing between OSCC ($n=37$), oral leukoplakia ($n=32$), and healthy controls ($n=34$) using saliva samples [37]. This study found that these groups have characteristic salivary metabolic signatures and that a panel of three metabolites (valine, lactic acid, and phenylalanine) in combination yielded satisfactory accuracy (0.89, 0.97), sensitivity (86.5 and 94.6 %), specificity (82.4 and 84.4 %), and positive predictive value (81.6 and 87.5 %) in distinguishing OSCC from the controls or oral leukoplakia, respectively.

A 2011 study used LC/MS to examine the metabolomic energy profile of 15 HNSCC cell lines and found that glucose is required for survival and glutamine is needed for maximal proliferation for these cells [38]. They found that glucose deprivation triggers increased glutamate, glutathione, and 5-oxoproline, whereas normal DMEM/media leads to increased glucose, 6-phosphogluconate, mannose-6-phosphate, inosine, and adenine. They also reported that inhibition of glucose catabolism inhibited cell proliferation and anchorage-independent growth across a range of HNSCC cell lines. They suggested that the presence of wild-type p53 was a potential mechanism conferring relative resistance to antiglycolytic strategies in HNSCC.

Another study used high-resolution magic angle spinning (HR-MAS) to explore the metabolic signatures of HNSCC, which included matched normal adjacent tissue (NAT) and primary tumor originating from the tongue, lip, larynx, and the oral cavity and associated lymph node metastatic tissues (LN-Met) [36]. A total of 43 tissues (18 NAT, 18 tumor, and 7 LN-Met) from 22 HNSCC patients were analyzed. This study found NMR metabolic profiles that could differentiate normal from tumor tissues. Furthermore, primary and metastatic tumor tissues showed elevated levels of lactate, amino acids (including leucine, isoleucine, valine, alanine, glutamine, glutamate, aspartate, glycine, phenylalanine, and tyrosine), choline-containing compounds, creatine, taurine, glutathione, and decreased

**Table 6.1** Metabolomic analyses of head and neck and oral cancer specimens

| Study | Subjects | Cancer types | Tissue/fluid sampled | Methods used | Metabolites/pathways altered |
|---|---|---|---|---|---|
| El-Sayed et al. [31] | 40 HNSCC subjects (135 specimens) | HNSCC | Tissues | $^{1}$H MRS | 5 differential metabolites:<br>↑taurine<br>↑choline<br>↑glutamic Acid<br>↑lactic Acid<br>↑lipid |
| Yan et al. [32] | 20 0SCC<br>20 Lichen planus<br>7 Leukoplakia | OSCC<br>Oral<br>Leukoplakia<br>Oral lichen planus | Saliva | HPLC/MS | Metabolomic data distinguished different pathologic conditions |
| Tziani et al. [33] | 15 OSCC<br>10 Healthy controls | OSCC | Serum | ID $^{1}$H and 2D $^{1}$H J-resolved NMR | 19 differential metabolites:<br>↑2-hydroxybutyrate, 3-hydroxybutyrate, acetone, acetate, acetoacetate, creatinine, asparagine, glucose, dimethylglycine, betaine, choline in late vs. early stage<br>↓Valine, lactate, alanine, pyruvate, lysine, creatine, acetyl-L-carnitine, carnitine in late vs. early stage<br>Altered pathways: coline pathways, Krebs cycle, glucose pathways, urea cycle, acetoacetate pathways |
| Zhou et al. [34] | 33 OSCC<br>5 Oral leukoplakia<br>28 Healthy Controls | OSCC<br>Oral<br>Leukoplakia<br>Healthy | Plasma | $^{1}$H NMR | 17 differential metabolites:<br>Separate the 3 subject groups; tyrosine, aspartic acid, glucose, myo-inositol, taurine, arginine, choline, creatinine, lipids, glutamic acid, proline, arginine, 3-hydroxybutyrate, valine, isoleucine |
| Sugimoto et al. [35] | 69 Oral cancer subjects<br>87 Healthy controls (oral, breast, and pancreatic cancer, perio disease) | Oral cancer | Saliva | CE-TOF-MS | 2 differential metabolites:<br>Taurine and piperidine specific for oral cancer<br>57 principal metabolites predict probability of each disease |

| | | | | | |
|---|---|---|---|---|---|
| Somashekar et al. [36] | 22 HNSCC subjects<br>43 Tissues (matched tissue sets)<br>18 Normal adjacent tumor<br>18 Primary tumor<br>7 Lymph node metastases | HNSCC | Tissues | HR-MAS $^{1}$H NMR | 16 differential metabolites: lactate, amino acids (leucine, isoleucine, valine, alanine, glutamine, glutamate, aspartate, glycine, phenylalanine, and tyrosine), choline containing compounds, creatine, taurine, glutathione, and decreased levels of triglycerides<br>Altered pathways: glycolysis, increased amino acid influx (anaplerosis) into TCA cycle, altered energy metabolism, membrane choline phospholipid metabolism, oxidative/osmotic defense mechanisms |
| Wei et al. [37] | 37 OSCC<br>32 Oral leukoplakia<br>34 Healthy subjects | OSCC<br>Oral leukoplakia | Saliva | LC/Q-TOF MS | 3 differential metabolites: valine, lactic acid, phenylalanine; combined metabolites distinguish OSCC from OL and healthy controls |
| Sandaluche et al. [38]) | 15 HNSCC cell lines | HNSCC | Cells | LC/MS | Glucose deprivation triggers increased glutamate, glutathione, 5-oxoproline<br>Normal media increases glucose, 6-phosphogluconate, mannose-6-phosphate, inosine, adenine |
| Tripathi et al. [39] | 5 HNSCC cell lines<br>3 Primary normal human oral keratinocytes from different patients | HNSCC | Cells | $^{1}$H NMR | 21 differential metabolites:<br>Isoleucine, valine, lactate, alanine, acetate, glutamine, aspartate, creatine, choline, phosphocholine, glycerophosphocholine, taurine, myo-inositol, glutathione, tyrosine, phenylalanine, glycine, fumarate, udp-sugars, nad, axp<br>Altered pathways: Warburg effect, oxidative phosphorylation, energy metabolism, TCA cycle anaplerotic flux, glutaminolysis, hexosamine pathway, osmoregulatory, anti-oxidant mechanism, membrane choline phospholipid metabolism, PLA2 activity |
| Yonezawa et al. [40] | 25 HNSCC subjects (17 serum) (19 tissues) | HNSCC | Serum tissues | GC/MS | 4 differential metabolites:<br>↑glycolysis (serum)<br>↓amino acids(serum)<br>↓glycolysis (tissues)<br>↑amino acids (serum) |
| Wang et al. [41] | 2 Cell lines (altered culture transfection conditions) | HNSCC | Cells | Cap IC and Orbitrap MS | Differential metabolites in energy metabolism pathways, including glycolysis and TCA cycle |

**Table 6.2** Metabolomic analyses of cariogenic-associated specimens

| Study | Subjects | Samples | Method | Metabolites |
|---|---|---|---|---|
| Takahashi et al. [42] | 5 Healthy subjects | Oral plaque and oral cariogenic bacteria (*Streptococcus*, *Actinomyces*) | Capillary Electrophoresis MS | Similar profiles for plaque and oral bacteria; EMP, pentose phosphate pathway, TCA cycle |
| Foxman et al. (2013) | 25 Sibling pairs | Saliva | LC/MS GC/MS | Profile of metabolites in children with decayed teeth more similar than those with healthy teeth |

levels of triglycerides. These elevated metabolites were associated with highly active glycolysis, increased amino acid influx (anaplerosis) into the TCA cycle, altered energy metabolism, membrane choline phospholipid metabolism, and oxidative and osmotic defense mechanisms. Also, decreased levels of triglycerides suggested active lipolysis followed by β-oxidation of fatty acids that may exist to deliver bioenergy for rapid tumor cell proliferation and growth.

Another study by the same group used 1H NMR-based metabolic profiling of HNSCC cells from five different patients that were derived from various sites of the upper aerodigestive tract, including the floor of mouth, tongue, and larynx [39]. Primary cultures of normal human oral keratinocytes (NHOK) from three different donors were used for comparison. HNSCC cells exhibited significantly altered levels of various metabolites that clearly revealed dysregulation in multiple metabolic processes, including the Warburg effect, oxidative phosphorylation, energy metabolism, TCA cycle anaplerotic flux, glutaminolysis, hexosamine pathway, osmoregulatory, and antioxidant mechanisms. In addition, significant alterations in the ratios of phosphatidylcholine/lysophosphatidylcholine and phosphocholine/glycerophosphocholine and elevated arachidonic acid observed in HNSCC cells reveal an altered membrane choline phospholipid metabolism (MCPM). Furthermore, significantly increased activity of phospholipase A2 (PLA2) especially cytosolic PLA2 (cPLA2) observed in all the HNSCC cells confirmed an altered MCPM. Thus, cPLA2 may serve as a potential therapeutic target for anticancer therapy of HNSCC.

Recently, a 2013 study used GC/MS to perform metabolomic analyses of serum and tissue samples from 25 HNSCC subjects (17 serum, 19 tissues) and found opposing results between tissues and serum samples with respect to certain metabolites [40]. In serum, several metabolites related to the glycolytic pathway, like glucose, were elevated, whereas the levels of several amino acids were lower in HNSSC patients. In contrast to serum, the levels of many metabolites related to the glycolytic pathway were lower in tumor tissues compared to control tissues, and the levels of several amino acids, such as valine, tyrosine, serine, and methionine, were higher. The metabolites with the greatest fold change between oral cancer/HNSCC and normal tissues included uracil (6.28/6.2), glutamic acid (5.9/4.2), aspartic acid (5.5/3.9), and asparagine (5.5/4.7).

Another recent study explored the metabolomic profile of anionic metabolites in head and neck cancer cells by capillary ion chromatography with orbitrap mass spectrometry and found that these methods were highly sensitive allowing for excellent separation of polar metabolites [41].

Thus, metabolomic studies of HNSCC indicate that while examination of tissues and cells can distinguish between disease states, salivary diagnostics offer a new noninvasive platform to aid in the diagnosis of this disease and its different states and therefore warrant further study.

Limited studies on metabolomic analyses of plaque and saliva related to caries have also been conducted (Table 6.2). A study of five healthy subjects used capillary electrophoresis-mass spectrometry (Human Metabolome Technologies) to examine the metabolome present in oral plaque and oral cariogenic bacteria, including *Streptococcus mutans*, *Streptococcus sanguinis*, *Actinomyces oris*, and *Actinomyces naeslundii* [42]. Similar profiles were identified for the oral plaque and oral bacteria, which

**Table 6.3** Metabolomic analyses of periodontitis-associated specimens

| Study | Subjects | Disease | Tissue/fluid | Method | Metabolites |
|---|---|---|---|---|---|
| Barnes et al. [44] | 22 subjects with chronic perio (330 sites) | Healthy, gingivitis, periodontitis sites | GCF | GC/MS<br>LC/MS | ↑inosine, hypoxanthine, xanthine, guanosine, guanine at diseased sites=↑purine degradation pathway (ROS)<br>↑amino acids= degradation host components<br>↑bacterial products (cadaverine)<br>↓anti-oxidants (glutathione, ascorbic acid, uric acid) |
| Barnes et al. [45] | 39 subjects with chronic perio | Healthy, gingivitis, periodontitis sites | GCF | GC/MS; UHLC/MS/MS; basic and acidic species | Tricolsan-containing dentifrice reduces inosine, lysine, putrescine, and xanthine at gingivitis sites |
| Sugimoto et al. [35] | 11 subjects (oral, breast, and pancreatic cancer, and periodontal disease) | 11 Disease<br>87 Healthy | Saliva | CE-TOF-MS | 57 metabolites can predict each disease |
| Barnes et al. [46] | 68 subjects | 34 Disease<br>34 Healthy | Saliva | UHPLC/MS/tandem MS | ↑lipids, peptides, amino acids, carbohydrates (glucose), nucleotides (macromolecular degradation) in disease |

consisted of increased metabolites in the Embden-Meyerhof-Parnas (EMP) pathway and pentose phosphate pathway, but decreased metabolites in the tricarboxylate acid (TCA) cycle. Another study of 25 sibling pairs used LC/MS and GC/MS (Metabolon, Inc.) to examine the metabolome present in saliva of these children [43]. The profiles of metabolites in children with decayed teeth were more similar than those with healthy teeth; however, there was also a strong effect of sibship on the metabolite profiles.

Metabolomic approaches have also been applied to periodontal disease diagnosis (Table 6.3). A metabolomic study of gingival crevicular fluid (GCF) from periodontitis, gingivitis, and healthy sites from 22 individuals with chronic periodontitis was performed using GC/MS and LC/MS (Metabolon, Inc.) [44]. This study found elevated levels of inosine, hypoxanthine, xanthine, guanosine, and guanine at diseased sites, indicating an increased purine degradation pathway, which yields reactive oxygen species (ROS). This suggests that diseased sites exhibit oxidative stress. In diseased sites, they also found increased levels of amino acids, indicative of degradation of host cellular components, plus increased levels of bacterial products, including cadaverine, and a decrease in antioxidants, including glutathione, ascorbic acid, and uric acid. Thus, metabolomic analyses of periodontally diseased sites reflect the host-bacterial interactions within and highlight a depletion of antioxidants, degradation of host cellular components, and a buildup of bacterial products in GCF. These metabolites may serve as biomarkers of periodontal diseases.

A related study by the same group selected a panel of ten markers from their previous metabolomic study for further exploration [45]. These ten markers were examined in GCF from healthy, gingivitis, and periodontitis sites from 39 chronic periodontitis subjects who were assigned to a triclosan-containing dentifrice group or a control dentifrice group. The GCF samples were analyzed using three approaches: gas chromatrography/mass spectrometry (GC/MS), ultrahigh performance liquid chromatography/tandem mass spectrometry (UHPLD/MS/MS) optimized for basic species, and UHPLD/MS/MS optimized for acidic species (Metabolon, Inc.). The study found that ten markers (cadaverine, lysine, putrescine, isoleucine, leucine, phenylalanine, choline, hypoxanthine, xanthine, inosine) were elevated in the diseased sites, and the triclosan-containing dentrifice reduced the level of inosine, lysine, putrescine, and xanthine at gingivitis sites by 1 week.

Another study by the same group evaluated 34 periodontally diseased and 34 healthy subjects using untargeted metabolomic analysis of saliva employing ultrahigh performance liquid chromatography/tandem mass spectrometry (UHPLD/MS/MS) optimized for basic species, UHPLD/MS/MS optimized for acidic species, and gas chromatrography/mass spectrometry (GC/MS) (Metabolon, Inc.) [46]. With this approach, a total of 390 metabolites were detected in these samples. High levels of lipids plus altered peptides, amino acids, carbohydrates, and nucleotides were detected in samples from periodontitis patients, indicating macromolecular degradation. In addition, this study found altered levels of triacylglycerol, glycerolphospholipids, polysaccharides, and polynucleotides in individuals with periodontal disease, partially reflecting the enhanced host-bacterial interactions in the diseased state as further evidenced by increased levels of bacterially modified amino acids and carnitine metabolites.

A final study of 87 healthy and 11 diseased subjects that analyzed a variety of conditions, including periodontal disease, oral cancer, breast cancer, and pancreatic cancer, performed metabolomic analysis using capillary electrophoresis time-of-flight mass spectroscopy and found that 57 metabolites could predict each disease [35].

Thus, metabolomic approaches hold promise for advancing periodontal disease diagnosis. Combining these methods with other current diagnostic methods may enhance clinicians' ability to diagnose and predict periodontal disease progression.

## Conclusions

Predicting periodontal disease progression relies on clinical and radiographic examinations and a thorough medical history, since conditions, such as uncontrolled diabetes, immune and vascular deficiencies, and smoking, can contribute to disease pathogenesis and increase the risk for progression. Several studies evaluating the relationship between smoking and periodontal disease indicate increased risk for tooth loss, reduction in clinical outcomes, and dose effects from smoking [47–49]. Meta-analyses and literature reviews similarly show that diabetes increases the risk for periodontal disease, and the two have a bidirectional relationship, such that periodontal treatment may improve glycemic control [50–52]. In addition, genetic information could help determine risk or susceptibility for periodontal disease, since studies conducted on twins revealed that 50 % of the clinical severity of periodontal disease can be explained by genetics [53,54]. Specific genetic information, such as the presence of genetic polymorphisms in the inflammatory cytokine, IL-1, can also provide predictive information about the risk of periodontal disease [47,55]. A patient's DNA can be captured with a saliva-saline matrix oral rinse sample (MyPerioID) [30], which is sent to a laboratory for rapid analysis of genotypic status for IL-1. This test is based on the premise that a single nucleotide polymorphism of the IL-1 gene is a susceptibility factor for periodontal disease [56]. IL-1 polymorphisms indicate risk of tooth loss [47] and advancing periodontal diseases [57]. Genome-wide association studies of periodontal disease have also identified potential genetic polymorphisms associated with chronic periodontitis-related phenotypes and warrant additional study [58]. In the future, these approaches can be complemented by laboratory tests for microbial plaque biofilm (MyPerioPath; http://www.oraldna.com/periodontal-testing.html) [59]. Coupled with these tests, the use of salivary- or GCF-based OMIC technologies to identify disease-specific biomarker profiles can help rank or stratify a patient's risk for disease progression based on a combination of risk factors.

Thus, OMIC-based biomarkers, including those obtained from metabolomics, can aid or be used to identify baseline risk, preclinical progression, and disease initiation and progression along the continuum of a disease. These can also assist in monitoring treatment and for treatment follow-up. Coupling the OMICs with big data and data management systems are other emerging areas that afford new opportunities for personalized general and oral health care. The use of handheld devices and point-of-care diagnostics are other future areas that hold great promise for personalized care. Handheld devices can be used to monitor health status [60–62]. These devices, like a glucometer for monitoring blood glucose levels in diabetics, may use a finger-prick, or saliva, or a breath sample to analyze DNA mutations, proteins, metabolites, or other body components to monitor health or disease control. Thus, these might serve as a personalized or remote monitoring device. These individual DNA sequences, proteins, or metabolites would be part of a patient's medical and dental record and would be used to track health history, optimize wellness, or track potential disease. Coupling of these OMIC approaches with smartphone devices could personalize health care even further and could reach global or underserved communities that do not have access to care. One could envision receiving individualized health-related text messages based on readouts from breath, saliva, or finger-prick sampling to help in health management. With a wellness focus in mind, these approaches could also be used to tailor and optimize nutrition and preventive approaches for the individual patient. Furthermore, big data and systems approaches could be used to design drugs to target individual disease networks. The future looks bright for improving oral disease diagnosis and prognosis with the application of metabolomics and other OMIC technologies to saliva, serum, or breath analyses for the individual patient.

## References


1. Haffajee AD, Socransky SS, Goodson JM. Clinical parameters as predictors of destructive periodontal disease activity. J Clin Periodontol. 1983;10:257–65.
2. Lang NP, Joss A, Orsanic T, Gusberti FA, Siegrist BE. Bleeding on probing. A predictor for the progression of periodontal disease? J Clin Periodontol. 1986;13:590–6.
3. Eke PI, Dye BA, Wei L, Thornton-Evans GO, Genco RJ, Beck J, et al. Prevalence of periodontitis in adults in the United States: 2009 and 2010. J Dent Res. 2012;91:914–20.
4. Petersen PE, Ogawa H. The global burden of periodontal disease: towards integration with chronic disease prevention and control. Periodontol 2000. 2012; 60:15–39.
5. Greenstein G, Caton J. Periodontal disease activity: a critical assessment. J Periodontol. 1990;61:543–52.
6. Goodson JM. Conduct of multicenter trials to test agents for treatment of periodontitis. J Periodontol. 1992;63:1058–63.
7. Armitage GC, Svanberg GK, Loe H. Microscopic evaluation of clinical measurements of connective tissue attachment levels. J Clin Periodontol. 1977;4: 173–90.
8. Hancock EB, Wirthlin MR. The location of the periodontal probe tip in health and disease. J Periodontol. 1981;52:124–9.
9. van der Velden U. Influence of probing force on the reproducibility of bleeding tendency measurements. J Clin Periodontol. 1980;7:421–7.
10. van der Velden U, de Vries JH. The influence of probing force on the reproducibility of pocket depth measurements. J Clin Periodontol. 1980;7:414–20.
11. van der Velden U, Jansen J. Probing force in relation to probe penetration into the periodontal tissues in dogs. A microscopic evaluation. J Clin Periodontol. 1980;7:325–7.
12. Fowler C, Garrett S, Crigger M, Egelberg J. Histologic probe position in treated and untreated human periodontal tissues. J Clin Periodontol. 1982;9 373–85.
13. Jeffcoat MK, Reddy MS. A comparison of probing and radiographic methods for detection of periodontal disease progression. Curr Opin Dent. 1991;1:45–51.
14. Biomarkers Definitions Working Group. Biomarkers and surrogate endpoints: preferred definitions and conceptual framework. Clin Pharmacol Ther. 2001; 69:89–95.
15. Armitage GC. Analysis of gingival crevice fluid and risk of progression of periodontitis. Periodontol 2000. 2004;34:109–19.
16. Lamster IB, Ahlo JK. Analysis of gingival crevicular fluid as applied to the diagnosis of oral and systemic diseases. Ann N Y Acad Sci. 2007;1098:216–29.
17. Giannobile WV. Salivary diagnostics for periodontal diseases. J Am Dent Assoc. 2012;143:6S–11.
18. Socransky SS, Haffajee AD, Cugini MA, Smith C, Kent Jr RL. Microbial complexes in subgingival plaque. J Clin Periodontol. 1998;25:134–44.
19. Socransky SS, Haffajee AD, Teles R, Wennstrom JL, Lindhe J, Bogren A, et al. Effect of periodontal therapy on the subgingival microbiota over a 2-year monitoring period. I. Overall effect and kinetics of change. J Clin Periodontol. 2013;40:771–80.

20. Teles R, Teles F, Frias-Lopez J, Paster B, Haffajee A. Lessons learned and unlearned in periodontal microbiology. Periodontol 2000. 2013;62:95–162.
21. Herman Ostrow School of Dentistry of USC. Oral microbiology testing. Available at: https://dentists.usc.edu/dental-practitioners/oral-microbiology.
22. Kornberg School of Dentistry, Temple University. Oral Microbiology Testing Service (OMTS) Laboratory. Available at: http://dentistry.temple.edu/departments/periodontology-and-oral-implantology/omts-laboratory.
23. Lepp PW, Brinig MM, Ouverney CC, Palm K, Armitage GC, Relman DA. Methanogenic Archaea and human periodontal disease. Proc Natl Acad Sci U S A. 2004;101:6176–81.
24. Bik EM, Long CD, Armitage GC, Loomer P, Emerson J, Mongodin EF, et al. Bacterial diversity in the oral cavity of 10 healthy individuals. ISME J. 2010;4:962–74.
25. Pride DT, Salzman J, Haynes M, Rohwer F, Davis-Long C, White 3rd RA, et al. Evidence of a robust resident bacteriophage population revealed through analysis of the human salivary virome. ISME J. 2012;6:915–26.
26. Lemon KP, Armitage GC, Relman DA, Fischbach MA. Microbiota-targeted therapies: an ecological perspective. Sci Transl Med. 2012;4:137rv5.
27. Chan IS, Ginsburg GS. Personalized medicine: progress and promise. Annu Rev Genomics Hum Genet. 2011;12:217–44.
28. Chen R, Mias GI, Li-Pook-Than J, Jiang L, Lam HY, Chen R, et al. Personal omics profiling reveals dynamic molecular and medical phenotypes. Cell. 2012;148:1293–307.
29. Homings Forsyth. Human oral microbe identification using next generation sequencing. Available at: http://homings.forsyth.org/index2.html.
30. Oral DNA Labs. Periodontal testing. Available at: http://www.oraldna.com/periodontal-testing.html.
31. El-Sayed S, Bezabeh T, Odlum O, Patel R, Ahing S, MacDonald K, et al. An ex vivo study exploring the diagnostic potential of 1H Magnetic resonance spectroscopy in squamous cell carcinoma of the head and neck region. Head Neck. 2002;24:766–72.
32. Yan S-K, Wei B-J, Lin Z-Y, Yang Y, Zhou Z-T, Zhang W-D. A metabonomic approach to the diagnosis of oral squamous cell carcinoma, oral lichen planus, and oral leukoplakia. Oral Oncol. 2008;44:477–83.
33. Tziani S, Lopex V, Günther UL. Early stage diagnosis or oral cáncer using $^{1}$H NMR-based metabolomics. Neoplasia. 2009;11:269–76.
34. Zhou J, Xu B, Huang J, Jia X, Xue J, Shi X, et al. $^{1}$H NMR-based metabonomic and pattern recognition analysis for detection of oral squamous cell carcinoma. Clin Chim Acta. 2009;401:8–13.
35. Sugimoto M, Wong DT, Hirayama A, Soga T, Tomita M. Capillary electrophoresis mass spectrometry-based saliva metabolomics identified oral, breast and pancreatic cancer-specific profiles. Metabolom. 2010;6:78–95.
36. Somashekar BS, Kamarajan P, Danciu T, Kapila YL, Chinnaiyan AM, Rajendiran TM, et al. Magic angle spinning NMR-based metabolic profiling of head and neck squamous cell carcinoma tissues. J Proteome Res. 2011;10:5232–41.
37. Wei J, Xie G, Zhou Z, Shi P, Qui Y, Zheng X, et al. Salivary metabolite signatures of oral cancer and leukoplakia. Int J Cancer. 2011;129:2207–17.
38. Sandaluche VC, Ow TJ, Pickering CR, Frederick MJ, Zhou G, Fokt I, et al. Glucose, not glutamine, is the dominant energy source required for proliferation and survival of head and neck squamous carcinoma cells. Cancer. 2011;117:2926–38.
39. Tripathi P, Kamarajan P, Somashekar BS, MacKinnon N, Chinnaiyan AM, Kapila YL, et al. Delineating metabolic signatures of head and neck squamous cell carcinoma: phospholipase A2, a potential therapeutic target. Int J Biochem Cell Biol. 2012;44:1852–61.
40. Yonezawa K, Nishiumii S, Kitamoto-Matsuda J, Fujita T, Morimoto K, Yamashita D, et al. Serum and tissue metabolomics of head and neck cancer. Cancer Genom Proteom. 2013;10:233–8.
41. Wang J, Christison TT, Misuno K, Lopez L, Huhmer AF, Huang Y, et al. Metabolomic profiling of anionic metabolites in head and neck cancer cells by capillary ion chromatography with Orbitrap mass spectrometry. Anal Chem. 2014;86:5116–24.
42. Takahashi N, Washio J, Mayanagi G. Metabolomics of supragingival plaque and oral bacteria. J Dent Res. 2010;89:1383–8.
43. Foxman B, Srinivasan U, Wen A, Zhang L, Marrs CF, Goldberg D, et al. Exploring the effect of dentition, dental decay and familiality on oral health using metabolomics. Infect Genet Evol. 2014;22:201–7.
44. Barnes VM, Teles R, Trivedi HM, Devizio W, Xu T, Mitchell MW, et al. Acceleration of purine degradation by periodontal diseases. J Dent Res. 2009;88:851–5.
45. Barnes VM, Teles R, Trivedi HM, Devizio W, Xu T, Lee DP, et al. Assessment of the effects of dentifrice on periodontal disease biomarkers in gingival crevicular fluid. J Periodontol. 2010;81:1273–9.
46. Barnes VM, Ciancio SG, Shibly O, Xu T, Devizio W, Trivedi HM, et al. Metabolomics reveals elevated macromolecular degradation in periodontal disease. J Dent Res. 2011;90:1293–7.
47. McGuire MK, Nunn ME. Prognosis versus actual outcome. IV. The effectiveness of clinical parameters and IL-1 genotype in accurately predicting prognoses and tooth survival. J Periodontol. 1999;70:49–56.
48. Krall EA, Dietrich T, Nunn ME, Garcia RI. Risk of tooth loss after cigarette smoking cessation. Prev Chronic Dis. 2006;3:A115.
49. Kotsakis GA, Javed F, Hinrichs JE, Karoussis IK, Romanos GE. Impact of cigarette smoking on clinical outcomes of periodontal flap surgical procedures: a systematic review and meta-analysis. J Periodontol. 2014;9:1–17.
50. Taylor GW. Bidirectional interrelationships between diabetes and periodontal diseases: an epidemiologic perspective. Ann Periodontol. 1991;6:99–112.

51. Salvi GE, Carollo-Bittel B, Lang NP. Effects of diabetes mellitus on periodontal and peri-implant conditions: update on associations and risks. J Clin Periodontol. 2008;35:398–409.
52. Darré L, Vergnes JN, Gourdy P, Sixou M. Efficacy of periodontal treatment on glycaemic control in diabetic patients: a meta-analysis of interventional studies. Diabetes Metab. 2008;34:497–506.
53. Michalowicz BS, Aeppli D, Virag JG, Klump DG, Hinrichs JE, Segal NL, et al. Periodontal findings in adult twins. J Periodontol. 1991;62:293–9.
54. Michalowicz BS, Diehl SR, Gunsolley JC, Sparks BS, Brooks CN, Koertge TE, et al. Evidence of a substantial genetic basis for risk of adult periodontitis. J Periodontol. 2000;71:1699–707.
55. Karimbux NY, Saraiya VM, Elangovan S, Allareddy V, Kinnunen T, Kornman KS, et al. Interleukin-1 gene polymorphisms and chronic periodontitis in adult whites: a systematic review and meta-analysis. J Periodontol. 2012;83:1407–19. Erratum in: J Periodontol 2013 84:273.
56. Kornman KS, Crane A, Wang HY, di Giovine FS, Newman MG, Pirk FW, et al. The interleukin-1 genotype as a severity factor in adult periodontal disease. J Clin Periodontol. 1997;24:72–7.
57. Eickholz P, Kaltschmitt J, Berbig J, Reitmeir P, Pretzl B. Tooth loss after active periodontal therapy. 1: patient-related factors for risk, prognosis, and quality of outcome. J Clin Periodontol. 2008;35:165–74.
58. Shaffer JR, Polk DE, Wang X, Feingold E, Weeks DE, Lee MK, et al. Genome-wide association study of periodontal health measured by probing depth in adults ages 18–49 years. G3 (Bethesda). 2014;4(2):307–14.
59. Nabors TW, McGlennen RC, Thompson D. Salivary testing for periodontal disease diagnosis and treatment. Dent Today. 2010;29:53–4, 56, 58–60.
60. Wang J. Electrochemical biosensors: towards point-of-care cancer diagnostics. Biosens Bioelectron. 2006;21:1887–92.
61. Khalili B, Boggs PB, Bahna SL. Reliability of a new hand-held device for the measurement of exhaled nitric oxide. Allergy. 2007;62:1171–4.
62. Metters JP, Kampouris DK, Banks CE. Electrochemistry provides a point-of-care approach for the marker indicative of Pseudomonas aeruginosa infection of cystic fibrosis patients. Analyst. 2014;139:3999–4004.

# Genomics of Dental Caries and Caries Risk Assessment

7

J. Tim Wright

**Abstract**

Our understanding of dental caries was transformed over the past century to recognize that this chronic disease is an infectious and complex condition involving host, biofilm, and environmental factors. The severity and distribution of dental caries, or its clinical phenotype, is highly variable in the population. During the past 20 years, the genomic era has provided new insights into the interactions of host, oral flora, and environmental factors that make dental caries similar to many other complex hereditary conditions. Our knowledge of the contributions of an individual's genome to their risk and resistance to dental caries has grown tremendously over the past decade. New insights continue to be gained as our understanding of the interactions between our genome, oral microbiome, microbial metabolomics, and environmental influences advances. Knowledge of, and the ability to predict, these underlying determinants of disease and health will ultimately provide approaches to accurately predict risk and activity of dental caries in an individual, allowing personalized approaches to preventing and managing this common disease of humans.

## Introduction

The transformation in medicine over the past 120 years has been remarkable, with medical education and patient care becoming based on a foundation of science. The scientific foundation that unpins our understanding of dental caries also changed during this period. In 1891 W.D. Miller published his observations that tooth decay or dental caries was caused by infection of the oral cavity with bacteria that produced acid, thereby leading to destruction of the mineralized dental tissues [1]. Much of the research since these early observations has focused on understanding and treating dental caries. There has been tremendous effort to understand the microbiological contributions of dental caries since Keyes classic experiments in the 1960s showed that specific organisms

J.T. Wright, DDS, MS
Department of Pediatric Dentistry, University of North Carolina School of Dentistry, Chapel Hill, NC, USA
e-mail: Tim_wright@unc.edu





P.J. Polverini (ed.), *Personalized Oral Health Care: From Concept Design to Clinical Practice*,
DOI 10.1007/978-3-319-23297-3_7

were associated with dental caries [2]. With advances in technologies to interrogate the oral microbiome, we are now coming to realize that the complexity and diversity of the oral flora appears to be critical in imparting resistance and risk for having dental caries. It is well known that dental caries is a complex disease involving factors related to the host, the oral biofilm, the environment, and the interactions of these three key elements over time. Since sequencing of the human genome, elucidation of the human microbiome, the human and microbial metabolomes, and the explosion in biotechnology and bioinformatics, the complexity of these key elements and intricacies of their interactions are changing the way we think about dental caries as a disease. Our ability to examine the human genome, microbiome, and interactions between these genomic, microbiomic, and environmental factors is providing new knowledge of the pathogenesis of dental caries and novel approaches to advance health care. Consequently, our approaches to assessing an individual's risk/resistance to develop dental caries and how focused and individualized interventions might be applied also are changing.

Dental caries is the most common chronic disease afflicting humans. Industrialized countries are spending 5–10 % of their public health expenditures on oral health [3]. Despite extensive research, our ability to accurately predict those likely to develop disease before they have clinical symptoms remains suboptimal. This chapter reviews our current understanding of genetically determined risk and resistance for dental caries in humans and how this knowledge is currently used and could potentially be used in the management of dental caries.

## Dental Caries Phenotypes

Dental caries is the clinical presentation that results from the imbalance of tooth mineral content and oral biofilm acid production. The recurring cyclical demineralization of the mineralized dental tissues by bacterially produced acids is the disease mechanism that can result in the destruction of the dentition. Clinically, dental caries is typically measured using the decayed, missing, and filled teeth or surfaces (DMFT and DMFS for permanent dentition and dmft and dmfs for the primary dentition) caries index tool. More refined measurements of dental caries also exist, such as the International Caries Detection and Assessment System (ICDAS) [4]. Studies to identify the genetic contributions to a disease process are hampered by having clinical phenotype measures that are difficult for even experienced clinicians to consistently arrive at similar diagnoses [5, 6]. Caries diagnostics remain problematic for ideally characterizing genetic contributions to this complex disease. Pit and fissure caries is still best diagnosed by visual appearance, and there are not systems with good sensitivity and specificity to evaluate differences between developmentally hypomineralized enamel and early stages of dental caries [7, 8]. Improved caries detection systems and diagnostics remain an important area for future research. Having objective and accurate diagnostic tools for dental caries will help advance our understanding of heredity and its role in this complex disease and its pathogenesis.

Clinicians are well aware that there are differences in the way dental caries manifests in patients. Pit and fissure caries can have a different significance than smooth-surface caries when considering caries risk. Risk factors for dental caries are not uniformly distributed across all teeth and tooth surfaces (Fig. 7.1a, b). The presence of enamel defects is known to be strongly associated with the presence and progression of dental caries [9, 10].

Enamel defects promote colonization by oral bacteria associated with dental caries [11] and compromise the tooth's surface resistance to caries. The etiology of enamel defects is known to be extremely diverse, with nearly 100 genetic [12] and over 100 environmental causes of enamel defects having been documented [13, 14].

It is not surprising that protective and risk factors differ from site to site given differences in tooth morphology, location of salivary gland ducts, clearance of food, exposure differences for different tooth surfaces, and many other factors

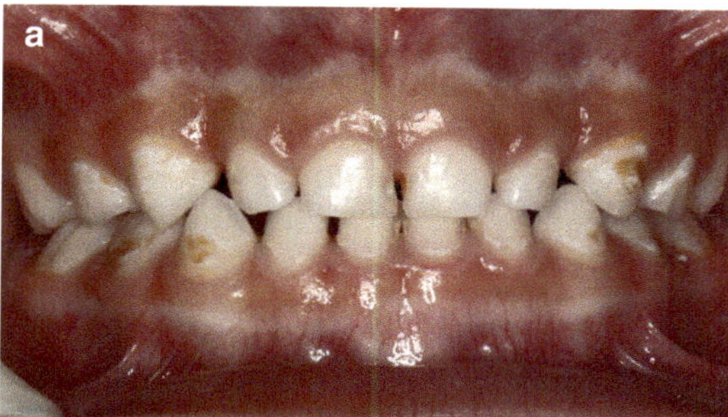


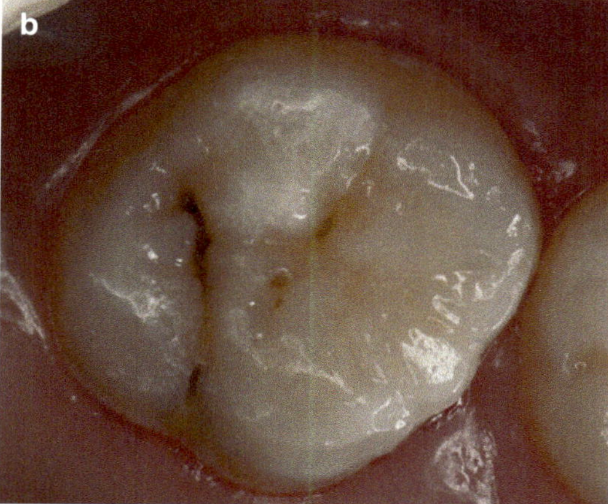


**Fig. 7.1** (**a**, **b**) Caries patterns or phenotypes vary tremendously, as illustrated in these contrasting clinical disease levels. The child (**a**) has enamel defects and caries in the facial surfaces of the primary canines and molars as well as the proximal surfaces of the maxillary anterior teeth and cervical areas. In contrast, (**b**) limited pit and fissure caries of the 6-year molars was the only disease seen in this individual (image **b** courtesy Andrea Zandona). The genetic contributions to the risk of dental caries is likely quite different in these two individuals, as are the management approaches

that are not uniform throughout the mouth. The distribution of caries on different teeth also is known to be associated with differing levels of future risk for disease, although current caries risk assessment tools typically do not take these factors into account. For example, an individual with carious lesions on the mandibular incisor teeth is usually thought to be affected by a high caries attack rate and level of disease because these teeth tend to be protected from caries due to their physical location anterior to the mandibular salivary ducts.

While differences in pit and fissure and smooth-surface caries have long been considered as different types of disease patterns, it is only relatively recently that distinct patterns of dental caries in the primary and permanent dentitions and at the tooth and surface level have been associated with heritability [15]. These studies indicate that some caries patterns have a greater heritable contribution compared with others. Recent studies by Schaffer et al. using hierarchical analyses indicate there are multiple distinct clusters of teeth that differ in their caries experience. They found that these groups could be classified as (C1) pit and fissure molar surfaces, (C2) mandibular anterior surfaces, (C3) posterior non-pit and fissures surfaces, (D4) maxillary anterior surfaces, and (C5) mid-dentition surfaces [16]. Furthermore, they found that the heritability and environmental factors contributing to caries in these various clusters differed. So while caries in the mandibular anterior teeth appear to have a considerable heritability factor, caries in the maxillary anterior teeth appear to have a much stronger environmental determinant. A genome-wide association study (GWAS) examining possible loci in the genome associated with dental caries in the permanent dentition showed different loci for pit and fissure caries and smooth-surface caries [17, 18]. Collectively, these studies show that the observed patterns of dental caries, or dental caries phenotypes, are associated with different protective and risk factors. There also is evidence suggesting that different suites of genes, having varying levels of effect, likely explain a portion of the variation seen between heritability in the primary and permanent dentitions [19]. Understanding the differing contributions of these factors could allow better disease risk assessment and individualized interventions that can address the genetic and environmental factors associated with the specific disease phenotype or clinical presentation.

## Heritability of Dental Caries

Dental caries is typically referred to as an infectious and transmissible disease and not as a hereditary disease [20, 21]. Frequently, when dental practitioners think about the heritability of dental caries and the potential magnitude of that genetics contributes to this disease, it is commonly believed that genetics plays a role, but that it is not as great a determinant as environmental interactions. Dental school curricula traditionally focus on environmental factors such as the oral biofilm and specific bacterial species (e.g., *Streptococcus mutans* and *lactobacillus*), fluoride exposure, and diet when reviewing the etiology of dental caries [22, 23]. While current caries risk assessments do evaluate an individual's caries experience, they tend not to evaluate an individual's family history of this disease to determine if heritability might be playing a contributing role to the disease [23, 24]. Caries risk assessments of pediatric patients do address if the caregiver has active caries or has had caries in the past 12 months [25]. The rationale for assessing caregiver caries is because there is an association between caregiver and infant caries, and this is especially strong when the mothers have untreated dental caries [26]. The assessment of caregiver caries is primarily directed at assessing the potential risk of transmissibility of the microbes associated with caries, and not heritability of the disease [25]. Interestingly, a study assessing caries status in 32-year-olds showed that self-reported poor maternal health when the children were young continued to be associated with higher caries levels in offspring as they became adults [27]. This suggests that assessing the family history for dental caries could be of benefit for determining risk of developing dental caries even in adults.

The concept that genetics plays a role in dental caries is certainly not a new one. Many animal and human studies have shown the importance genetics as a determinant of dental caries [28, 29]. Twin studies have been used for over 50 years to evaluate the potential role of heredity in dental caries [30, 31]. Adequately powered studies show a higher concordance of caries in monozygotic twins compared with dizygotic twins or siblings, supporting the role of genetics as a dental caries determinant [32–34]. The specific factors proposed as being influenced by genetics are varied and include such factors as taste preference, salivary factors, immune response, tooth morphology, enamel composition and structure, and behavior. Other hereditary factors that can affect oral function and food clearance also can be associated with increased dental caries risk. For example, individuals who have generalized recessive dystrophic epidermolysis bullosa (OMIM # 226600) tend to consume a soft diet and typically eat very slowly due to the oral ulcerations and oral scarring caused by fragile skin and mucosal surfaces due to mutations in their type VII collagen genes (*COL7A1*). They also suffer from oral mucosal scarring due to recurrent ulceration that results in binding and immobility of the tongue and oral vestibules, further hampering oral clearance. Consequently, many individuals with this condition suffer from rampant tooth decay (Fig. 7.2) that has an unusual clinical pattern, with caries often starting around the cervical area of the teeth adjacent to the scared and abnormal soft tissue [35]. The following sections will evaluate each of these risk factors and what is known related to their genetic determinants.

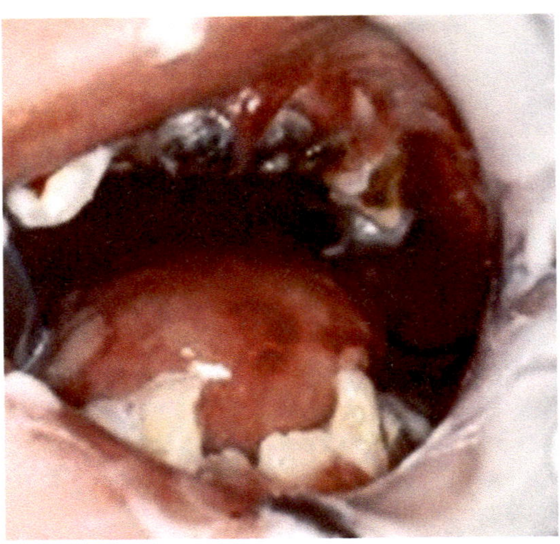

**Fig. 7.2** This child with generalized recessive dystrophic epidermolysis bullosa suffers from severe mucosal fragility and intraoral soft tissue scarring that contribute greatly to her caries risk due to consumption of a high-carbohydrate and soft diet that is difficult to clear from the oral cavity

## Diet and Taste Related To Caries

The relationship of diet and genetics related to dental caries has been assessed by a number of approaches. Several different hereditary conditions that cause dietary modifications have been associated with decreased and increased caries risk. Human studies have investigated caries levels in people with hereditary fructose intolerance (HIF) (OMIM #22960), a rare autosomal recessive hereditary condition caused by mutations in the gene coding for aldose B. Individuals with HIF greatly restrict their intake of fructose and sucrose, resulting in a marked reduction in dental caries experience [36]. As mentioned earlier, individuals affected with generalized recessive dystrophic epidermolysis bullosa (OMIM# 22660) have marked fragility of the skin and mucosa and have a need for high caloric intake due to problems with eating and uptake of nutrients, as well as high energy expenditures directed at tissue repair [37]. Consequently, affected individuals tend to eat slowly, have a delayed oral clearance of food, consume carbohydrate-rich diets with high calorie foods to achieve adequate intake, and suffer from a high caries attack rate [37].

Taste preference for an individual is determined by genetics and environmental exposures, and the possible association of taste preference differences to caries is not a new concept [38]. The sense of taste evolved to assist humans in detecting important sources of nutrients (e.g., sugars, salts, amino acids) and to protect them from possible poisonous substances like acids and alkyloids [39]. Environmental exposures that influence taste preference begin in utero as the developing fetus is subjected to different nutrient components derived from the mother through the amniotic fluid [40]. These exposures continue through contact with components from foods the mother eats being passed to the infant while nursing on the mother's breast milk [41]. As the infant diet changes and there are new exposures to different flavors and textures, food preferences continue to develop. Interestingly, a number of taste genes have been associated with differing levels of dental caries.

Many taste buds reside in the oral cavity and largely on the tongue in the fungiform, foliate, and circumvallate papillae. While these oral taste buds are critical in taste sensation, there is now great interest in the role of taste receptors in other tissues such as the airway and GI tract [39]. There are many known taste receptors that exist on taste bud cells. These receptors are coded for by families of genes that reside in clusters in the human genome [39]. The receptors are G-coupled protein receptors that are characterized by their 7-alpha helical transmembrane domains [39]. Searching Online Mendelian Inheritance in Man® (OMIM) [42] using the term "taste" results in 95 separate entries, with most of these being descriptions of the genes coding for the different known taste receptors such taste receptor type 1 member 1 (gene: *TAS1R1*; OMIM #606225). Recent studies indicate there are associations of differing caries levels in people with genetic variations in their taste genes [43, 44]. The *TAS1R1* gene codes for a receptor whose protein product forms a heterotrimer with the protein TAS1R3 that then mediates umami (distinct form of saltiness) perception. The *TAS1R1*gene is located on chromosome 1p36 and is associated with a cluster of other taste receptor genes such as *TAS1R2* that codes for a receptor involved in sweet perception. The *TASR38* taste receptor gene that is involved in perception of glucosinolates has been associated with lower caries rates [43]. Other genes that may be involved in dietary preference that are associated with caries include the guanine nucleotide-binding protein, alpha transducing 3 *(GNAT3)* gene [43]. Gustaducin is the protein product of the *GNAT3* gene and is present in all forms of taste buds. Gustaducin is thought to play a role in transduction of taste perception. Evaluation of caries and sucrose taste preference in twins reveals that both are associated with genetic determinants and understanding the heritability of these traits may add to our ability to assess an individual's caries risk [45].

## Saliva and Caries

Saliva has long been known to be a key host defense mechanism to dental caries development, providing a vehicle for fluoride, calcium, and phosphate ions; an aqueous medium to allow diffusion of these ions to the dental tissues; buffering; lubrication; digestive capacity of food substrates; and immunological factors, to name just a few critical salivary functions. Individuals with xerostomia, due to a lack of saliva formation, are at increased risk for developing dental caries. There are several hereditary conditions associated with abnormal saliva, such as aplasia of the lacrimal and salivary gland (OMIM # 180920). This autosomal dominant condition, caused by mutations in the *FGF10* gene that is a growth factor critical for development of these exocrine glands, causes marked aplasia in the lacrimal and salivary gland development and, consequently, a drastic reduction in salivary formation and flow. Individuals with this condition typically suffer from markedly increase levels of dental caries. Not surprisingly, multiple genes coding for saliva have been associated with dental caries [46].

The proline-rich salivary proteins have long been considered as protective against the formation of dental caries [47]. Genetic variations in alleles coding for the protein-rich protein, HaeIII subfamily 1 *(PRH1)* gene are associated with both *Streptococcus mutans* colonization and dental caries risk [48]. In addition to genes that are critical to salivary gland development, such as *FGF10*, there are many genes important in normal salivary formation and rate of flow. Variation in one such gene, Aquaporin 5 (*AQP5*), has been shown to be protective against caries [49]. Saliva has a complex buffering system that is considered critical in helping regulate the oral environment to a healthy pH level. There are a number of salivary carbonic anhydrase genes that play a role in buffering capacity, and studies suggest that polymorphisms in some these genes, suca as *CA6*, are associated with differing levels of this enzyme in saliva [50]. While these polymorphisms do appear associated with differences in buffering capacity in saliva, they have not been associated with differing risk or protection levels to dental caries [51]. It seems likely, given the many different functions of saliva, that suites genes and genetic variations in saliva formation, flow, and function will be associated with differing levels of risk and protection for caries. Salivary proteomics offers another potentially valuable tool for caries risk assessment in addition to the more traditional salivary flow rate and buffering capacity. Proteomics could assess the presence and differing levels of function in salivary protein variants that could influence caries risk and resistance.

## Immune System and Caries

A certain segment of the population is considered to be immune from dental caries, and part of this resistance to disease is thought to emanate from the immune system. Saliva provides a rich medium to support the oral cavities' immune response and does so with many different genes that have antimicrobial properties such as the salivary peroxidase system. Several genes coding for salivary proteins with antimicrobial properties have been associated with caries susceptibility such as Lactotransferrin *(LTF)* [52]. Others have failed to confirm this association in different populations [53]. Variations in the salivary protein T-cell receptor alpha chain variable 4 and the gene that codes for this protein *(TRAV4)* are associated with low caries experience [54]. Individuals having a missense mutation in *TRAV4* had higher caries levels, and it was predicted that this mutation caused a diminution in the possible protective role of this protein in caries resistance [54]. The protein beta defensin 1 (DEFB1) is an antimicrobial peptide secreted in saliva that is implicated in antimicrobial defense of epithelia surfaces and has been both dental caries and periodontal disease. Haplotype studies of *DEFB1* indicate that different allelic variants are associated with increased DMFT scores, while other allelic variants are associated with a low DMFT score suggesting these functional polymorphisms are possible markers for caries risk [55]. Other salivary proteins that appear to play a role in oral immunity, such as the mucins, have been implicated in dental caries, but the role of genetics and genetic variability contributing to caries risk and the immune system remains to be defined [56, 57].

## Tooth-Associated Factors and Caries

The mineralized tissues of the tooth are the primary defense against the development of dental caries. Tooth development is the culmination of exquisitely orchestrated processes that are under strict molecular control. These developmental processes are affected by a variety of environmental influences such as diet, infection, trauma, and other factors. There also is evidence that an individual's response to different environmental exposures, such as fluoride that can result in enamel fluorosis, can vary depending on genetic constitution [58]. There are thousands of genes expressed by the cells that form the human enamel, the ameloblasts, so it is not surprising that there are over 90 conditions with enamel defects that are known to be hereditary [12]. The ameloblasts must differentiate into highly specialized cells that secrete a unique extracellular matrix, process this matrix in a highly controlled fashion, regulate the microenvironment with regard to pH and ion content, and are motile moving away from the dentin enamel junction. The genes participating in these many different enamel-forming processes have been identified through a variety of approaches. Numerous genes participating in enamel development are now known to be associated with hereditary defects of enamel such as the various forms of amelogenesis imperfecta. Clinical studies indicate that enamel defects are strongly associated with early and greater colonization with streptococcus mutations and with the formation of dental caries [9, 11]. It has been proposed that certain cases of early childhood caries are the direct result of enamel hypoplasia that causes early development and progression of a severe disease phenotype [10]. So while there are many environmental exposures that can affect the quantity and quality of enamel, there are many enamel defects directly caused by genetic mutations, and there are likely to be many gene-environment interactions involved in abnormal enamel formation. For example, individuals with X-linked nephrogenic diabetes insipidus (OMIM # 304800) suffer from dental fluorosis due to their polydipsia and renal dysfunction [59]. First permanent molars frequently have enamel hypomineralization (about 5–30 % of populations around the world are affected) [60] and also are frequently affected with dental caries. The condition known as molar incisor hypomineralization has traditionally been thought to be environmental in etiology, while more recent studies indicate there are possibly gene variants that contribute to the condition [14, 61, 62].

Genes involved in producing and processing the enamel extracelluar matrix proteins amelogenin *(AMELX)*, enamelin *(ENAM)*, matrix metalloproteinase 20 *(MMP20)*, and kallikrein 4 *(KLK4)* have all been shown to cause different forms of amelogenesis imperfecta [63]. Variations in the genetic code of these genes – which are not causative of amelogenesis imperfecta – have been associated with either increased or decreased levels of dental caries in different populations in a number of studies [49, 64, 65]. Not surprisingly, the influence these genes have on dental caries in a population can be modified by environmental factors such as fluoride exposure [66].

Humans with mutations in genes coding for laminin type V (i.e., *LAMA3*) can have junctional epidermolysis bullosa that is associated with fragility of the skin and blistering, as well as enamel hypoplasia due to abnormal cell-cell attachment of the ameloblasts [67]. Individuals with this autosomal recessive trait are at markedly increased risk for developing dental caries, primarily due to their defective enamel [35]. Although not well understood, the genetic determinants of the pits and fissures of teeth also are likely involved in contributing to the heritability of dental caries. Studies have mapped pit and fissure caries in families, showing there can be strong similarities in the caries patterns over multiple generations in certain families. Other enamel-associated genes including ameloblastin *(AMBN)*, tuftelin *(TUFT1)*, and tuftelin-interacting protein 11 *(TFIP11)* also have been associated with variation in caries rates.

Given that dental development is so controlled at the molecular level, there will likely be many additional genes involved in tooth formation that are discovered to be associated with caries risk and resistance. The shape and size of teeth, cuspal pattern, pit and fissure morphology, and enamel composition and structure are all genetically determined traits that likely play a role in the risk and resistance to dental caries. Future studies, in large populations, are needed to decipher the diversity and magnitude of contributions that these different genes and genetic variants involved in determining tooth level traits have toward the formation of dental caries.

## Oral Microbiome

The Human Microbiome Project has been gathering information for over a decade to study the role of microbes in human health and disease and has characterized the microbial communities inhabiting different body surfaces including the oral cavity. Over the past two decades, new technologies, such as 16S rRNA gene sequencing, have allowed a more comprehensive understanding of the oral microbiome and its relationship to caries and health. The human oral microbiome is extremely diverse, with over 600 taxa and likely twice that many microbial species [68, 69]. Maintaining a stable and healthy oral microbiota that is associated with oral health, in contrast to dysbiosis or a microbial shift toward disease and how this shift occurs, is a concept that is not fully understood [70]. Metagenomics, or the genomic study of uncultured microorganisms, allows the investigation of the diverse microbiota in the oral cavity and how it changes in conditions of health and disease and is likely to contribute to developing personalized dental medicine for the management of dental caries [70]. Knowledge gained using these approaches indicates that the caries-associated microorganisms are more diverse than previously believed and that greater microbial diversity is seen in children without dental caries and better oral health compared with children who have dental caries [71].

Another approach to understanding the possible pathological mechanisms involved in dental caries involves evaluation of the metabolomics profile of the biofilm, taken from either plaque or saliva samples or microbial cultures [72]. Initial studies suggest that the oral microbial metabolites associated with acid production, such as pyruvate, and the pentose-phosphate pathway can be measured and that these pathways show increased activity (more metabolites produced) when bacteria such as *Streptococcus* are challenged with glucose [73]. Combining information about the diversity and types of microbes in the biofilm and its metabolic activity provides a new approach and potentially powerful tool for evaluating an individual's caries risk. While some early prototype devices have been developed to measure the oral biofilms' metabolic activity, there are no commercially available systems to evaluate the microbiome and/or its metabolomics as part of a validated caries risk assessment. One commercially available system measures plaque ATP levels that is indicative of microbial metabolic activity, but has not been shown to be predictive of caries activity risk.

### Conclusions

At this time, the most informative factor in caries risk assessment is the presence of caries activity. Those with dental caries or a history of disease are more likely to develop disease in the future. Other factors, such as environmental exposures to fluoride and carbohydrates, have value in predicting caries risk. In the United States, dental caries is disproportionately represented in populations of lower socioeconomic status. Lower socioeconomic status is associated with many different potential risk factors for dental caries including access to care, dental literacy, ability to purchase oral health-care products, and diet, to name a few. It also is possible that differences in genetics and the oral microbiome exist in lower socioeconomic populations and that these differences contribute to their risk of developing dental caries. We know that there are differences in the dental anatomy and tooth size in different populations and differences in the prevalence of missing teeth and malocclusions, so it would not seem unreasonable that there are genetic differences that could contribute to dental caries risk or resistance.

As our knowledge of the human genome and epigenetics continues to evolve and is integrated with our understanding of the microbiome and its metabolome, there is tremendous opportunity for advancing risk assessment and management of dental caries (Fig. 7.3). It seems likely that there will be many different genes and many different genetic variants that will contribute to an individual's risk and resistance for developing dental caries. Some of these genetic variants are already known and recommendations have been developed. For example, individuals with conditions such as generalized recessive dystrophic epidermolysis bullosa or salivary flow insufficiency should receive early and aggressive oral health-care and dietary counseling. Understanding the genomic and microbiomic contributions to an individual's caries risk would increase our ability to develop more targeted or personalized treatment approaches. If there is a family history of pit and fissure caries and genetic risk factors were identified to support this, then specific preventive approaches such as pit and fissure sealants could be applied. The familial and genetic information could even help determine which teeth would benefit most from sealants. Alternatively, if an individual's genomic and microbiomic assessments indicated a risk for smooth-surface and proximal caries, then other preventive measures could be taken, such as fluorides and dietary measures. It may be possible in the future to evaluate patient compliance with dietary measures by evaluating the microbiome and the level of dysbiosis that is contributing to the development of dental caries.

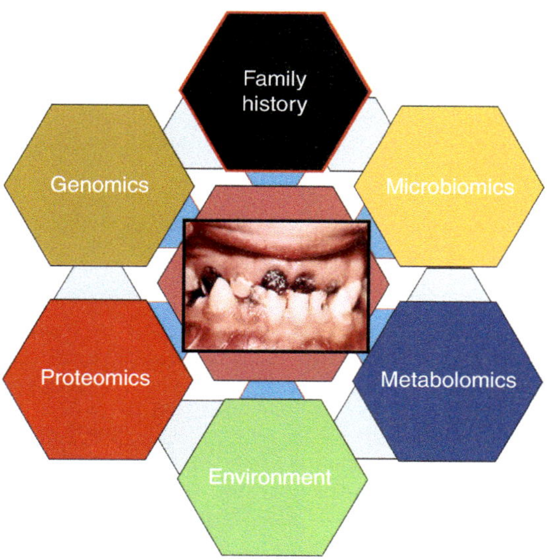


**Fig. 7.3** Personalized oral health care can become increasingly targeted as we add information from the different and interacting domains that help determine dental caries risk and activity for an individual. Anchoring this caries risk assessment paradigm are family history and environmental factors, with genomics, microbiomics, metabolomics, and salivary proteomics adding new knowledge that could improve the sensitivity and specificity of our caries risk assessment tools

Population-based caries management approaches such as water fluoridation are very successful, but they do not require any assessment of the disease risk in the population. The challenge is to identify the individuals in the population who have disproportionately high dental caries attack rates and apply targeted interventions. In the near future, it will be possible to evaluate an individual's genome and to study specific gene sets that contribute to their risk or resistance to dental caries. It may also be possible to have relatively inexpensive approaches to evaluate the microbiome and or its metabolome to add further information to their caries risk assessment. These new technological approaches will allow earlier and more accurate risk assessments and the ability to individualize the management of dental caries. Future studies on the cost and necessary resources to implement these types of assessments at the population level are needed as we move forward into these new areas of diagnostics, disease prediction, and personalized intervention.

## References

1. Miller W. The human mouth as a focus of infection. Dent Cosmos. 1891;33:689–789.
2. Keyes PH. The infectious and transmissible nature of experimental dental caries. Findings and implications. Arch Oral Biol. 1960;1:304–20. PubMed.
3. Petersen PE, Bourgeois D, Ogawa H, Estupinan-Day S, Ndiaye C. The global burden of oral disease and

risks to oral health. Bull World Health Organ. 2005;83:661–9.
4. Pitts NB, Ekstrand KR, Foundation I. International Caries Detection and Assessment System (ICDAS) and its International Caries Classification and Management System (ICCMS) – methods for staging of the caries process and enabling dentists to manage caries. Community Dent Oral Epidemiol. 2013;41(1):e41–52. PubMed.
5. Jablonski-Momeni A, Stachniss V, Ricketts DN, Heinzel-Gutenbrunner M, Pieper K. Reproducibility and accuracy of the ICDAS-II for detection of occlusal caries in vitro. Caries Res. 2008;42(2):79–87. PubMed.
6. Oliveira MD, Tedesco TK, Lenzi TL, Guedes Pinto AC, Rocha RO. Comparison of validation methods for the diagnosis of occlusal caries in primary molars. Eur Arch Paediatr Dent. 2012;13(2):91–3. PubMed.
7. Kuhnisch J, Berger S, Goddon I, Senkel H, Pitts N, Heinrich-Weltzien R. Occlusal caries detection in permanent molars according to WHO basic methods, ICDAS II and laser fluorescence measurements. Community Dent Oral Epidemiol. 2008;36(6):475–84. PubMed.
8. Sinanoglu A, Ozturk E, Ozel E. Diagnosis of occlusal caries using laser fluorescence versus conventional methods in permanent posterior teeth: a clinical study. Photomed Laser Surg. 2014;32(3):130–7. PubMed.
9. Seow WK, Clifford H, Battistutta D, Morawska A, Holcombe T. Case-control study of early childhood caries in Australia. Caries Res. 2009;43(1):25–35. PubMed.
10. Caufield PW, Li Y, Bromage TG. Hypoplasia-associated severe early childhood caries – a proposed definition. J Dent Res. 2012;91(6):544–50. PubMed Pubmed Central PMCID: 3348067.
11. Li Y, Navia JM, Caufield PW. Colonization by mutans streptococci in the mouths of 3- and 4-year-old Chinese children with or without enamel hypoplasia. Arch Oral Biol. 1994;39(12):1057–62. PubMed.
12. Wright JT, Carrion IA, Morris C. The molecular basis of hereditary enamel defects in humans. J Dent Res. 2014 Nov 11. PubMed
13. Murray JJ, Shaw L. Classification and prevalence of enamel opacities in the human deciduous and permanent dentitions. Arch Oral Biol. 1979;24(1):7–13. PubMed.
14. Jalevik B, Noren JG. Enamel hypomineralization of permanent first molars: a morphological study and survey of possible aetiological factors. Int J Paediatr Dent. 2000;10(4):278–89. PubMed.
15. Shaffer JR, Wang X, Desensi RS, Wendell S, Weyant RJ, Cuenco KT, et al. Genetic susceptibility to dental caries on pit and fissure and smooth surfaces. Caries Res. 2012;46(1):38–46. PubMed Pubmed Central PMCID: 3304515.
16. Shaffer JR, Feingold E, Wang X, Weeks DE, Weyant RJ, Crout R, et al. Clustering tooth surfaces into biologically informative caries outcomes. J Dent Res. 2013;92(1):32–7. PubMed Pubmed Central PMCID: 3521447.
17. Zeng Z, Shaffer JR, Wang X, Feingold E, Weeks DE, Lee M, et al. Genome-wide association studies of pit-and-fissure- and smooth-surface caries in permanent dentition. J Dent Res. 2013;92(5):432–7. PubMed Pubmed Central PMCID: 3627505.
18. Zeng Z, Feingold E, Wang X, Weeks DE, Lee M, Cuenco DT, et al. Genome-wide association study of primary dentition pit-and-fissure and smooth surface caries. Caries Res. 2014;48(4):330–8. PubMed Pubmed Central PMCID: 4043868.
19. Wang X, Shaffer JR, Weyant RJ, Cuenco KT, DeSensi RS, Crout R, et al. Genes and their effects on dental caries may differ between primary and permanent dentitions. Caries Res. 2010;44(3):277–84. PubMed Pubmed Central PMCID: 2919434.
20. Tanzer JM. Dental caries is a transmissible infectious disease: the Keyes and Fitzgerald revolution. J Dent Res. 1995;74(9):1536–42. PubMed.
21. Caufield PW. Dental caries: an infectious and transmissible disease where have we been and where are we going? N Y State Dent J. 2005;71(2):23–7. PubMed.
22. Brown JP. A new curriculum framework for clinical prevention and population health, with a review of clinical caries prevention teaching in U.S. and Canadian dental schools. J Dent Educ. 2007;71(5):572–8. PubMed.
23. Pitts N, Melo P, Martignon S, Ekstrand K, Ismail A. Caries risk assessment, diagnosis and synthesis in the context of a European Core Curriculum in Cariology. Eur J Dent Educ. 2011;15 Suppl 1:23–31. PubMed.
24. Domejean S, White JM, Featherstone JD. Validation of the CDA CAMBRA caries risk assessment – a six-year retrospective study. J Calif Dent Assoc. 2011;39(10):709–15. PubMed.
25. Ramos-Gomez FJ, Crystal YO, Ng MW, Crall JJ, Featherstone JD. Pediatric dental care: prevention and management protocols based on caries risk assessment. J Calif Dent Assoc. 2010;38(10):746–61. PubMed Pubmed Central PMCID: 3470809.
26. Dye BA, Vargas CM, Lee JJ, Magder L, Tinanoff N. Assessing the relationship between children's oral health status and that of their mothers. J Am Dent Assoc. 2011;142(2):173–83. PubMed.
27. Shearer DM, Thomson WM, Broadbent JM, Poulton R. Maternal oral health predicts their children's caries experience in adulthood. J Dent Res. 2011;90(5):672–7. PubMed Pubmed Central PMCID: 3144114.
28. Kurihara Y, Naito T, Obayashi K, Hirasawa M, Kurihara Y, Moriwaki K. Caries susceptibility in inbred mouse strains and inheritance patterns in F1 and backcross (N2) progeny from strains with high and low caries susceptibility. Caries Res. 1991;25(5):341–6. PubMed.
29. Vieira AR, Modesto A, Marazita ML. Caries: review of human genetics research. Caries Res. 2014;48(5):491–506. PubMed Pubmed Central PMCID: 4167926.
30. Horowitz SL, Osborne RH, Degeorge FV. Caries experience in twins. Science. 1958;128(3319):300–1. PubMed.

31. Finn SB, Caldwell RC. Dental caries in twins – I. a comparison of the caries experience of monozygotic twins, dizygotic twins and unrelated children. Arch Oral Biol. 1963;8:571–85. PubMed.
32. Boraas JC, Messer LB, Till MJ. A genetic contribution to dental caries, occlusion, and morphology as demonstrated by twins reared apart. J Dent Res. 1988;67(9):1150–5. PubMed.
33. Conry JP, Messer LB, Boraas JC, Aeppli DP, Bouchard Jr TJ. Dental caries and treatment characteristics in human twins reared apart. Arch Oral Biol. 1993;38(11):937–43. PubMed.
34. Bretz WA, Corby PM, Hart TC, Costa S, Coelho MQ, Weyant RJ, et al. Dental caries and microbial acid production in twins. Caries Res. 2005;39(3):168–72. PubMed.
35. Wright JT, Fine JD, Johnson L. Dental caries risk in hereditary epidermolysis bullosa. Pediatr Dent. 1994;16(6):427–32. PubMed.
36. Newbrun E, Hoover C, Mettraux G, Graf H. Comparison of dietary habits and dental health of subjects with hereditary fructose intolerance and control subjects. J Am Dent Assoc. 1980;101(4):619–26. PubMed.
37. Haynes L. Nutrition for children with epidermolysis bullosa. Dermatol Clin. 2010;28(2):289–301. x. PubMed.
38. Chung CS, Witkop CJ, Henry JL. A genetic study of dental caries with special reference to Ptc taste sensitivity. Am J Hum Genet. 1964;16:231–45. PubMed Pubmed Central PMCID: 1932310.
39. Kinnamon SC. A plethora of taste receptors. Neuron. 2000;25(3):507–10. PubMed.
40. Ventura AK, Worobey J. Early influences on the development of food preferences. Curr Biol. 2013;23(9):R401–8. PubMed.
41. Mennella JA. Ontogeny of taste preferences: basic biology and implications for health. Am J Clin Nutr. 2014;99(3):704S–11. PubMed Pubmed Central PMCID: 3927698.
42. OMIM—Online Mendelian Inheritance in Man®. An Online Catalog of Human Genes and Genetic Disorders. Updated 28 November 2014.http://omim.org/.
43. Wendell S, Wang X, Brown M, Cooper ME, DeSensi RS, Weyant RJ, et al. Taste genes associated with dental caries. J Dent Res. 2010;89(11):1198–202. PubMed Pubmed Central PMCID: 2954250.
44. Kulkarni GV, Chng T, Eny KM, Nielsen D, Wessman C, El-Sohemy A. Association of GLUT2 and TAS1R2 genotypes with risk for dental caries. Caries Res. 2013;47(3):219–25. PubMed.
45. Bretz WA, Corby PM, Melo MR, Coelho MQ, Costa SM, Robinson M, et al. Heritability estimates for dental caries and sucrose sweetness preference. Arch Oral Biol. 2006;51(12):1156–60. PubMed.
46. Wang X, Shaffer JR, Zeng Z, Begum F, Vieira AR, Noel J, et al. Genome-wide association scan of dental caries in the permanent dentition. BMC Oral Health. 2012;12:57. PubMed Pubmed Central PMCID: 3574042.
47. Yu PL, Bixler D, Goodman PA, Azen EA, Karn RC. Human parotid proline-rich proteins: correlation of genetic polymorphisms to dental caries. Genet Epidemiol. 1986;3(3):147–52. PubMed.
48. Zakhary GM, Clark RM, Bidichandani SI, Owen WL, Slayton RL, Levine M. Acidic proline-rich protein Db and caries in young children. J Dent Res. 2007;86(12):1176–80. PubMed.
49. Wang X, Willing MC, Marazita ML, Wendell S, Warren JJ, Broffitt B, et al. Genetic and environmental factors associated with dental caries in children: the Iowa Fluoride Study. Caries Res. 2012;46(3):177–84. PubMed Pubmed Central PMCID: 3580152.
50. Aidar M, Marques R, Valjakka J, Mononen N, Lehtimaki T, Parkkila S, et al. Effect of genetic polymorphisms in CA6 gene on the expression and catalytic activity of human salivary carbonic anhydrase VI. Caries Res. 2013;47(5):414–20. PubMed.
51. Peres RC, Camargo G, Mofatto LS, Cortellazzi KL, Santos MC, Nobre-dos-Santos M, et al. Association of polymorphisms in the carbonic anhydrase 6 gene with salivary buffer capacity, dental plaque pH, and caries index in children aged 7–9 years. Pharmacogenom J. 2010;10(2):114–9. PubMed.
52. Azevedo LF, Pecharki GD, Brancher JA, Cordeiro Jr CA, Medeiros KG, Antunes AA, et al. Analysis of the association between lactotransferrin (LTF) gene polymorphism and dental caries. J Appl Oral Sci. 2010;18(2):166–70. PubMed.
53. Volckova M, Linhartova PB, Trefna T, Vlazny J, Musilova K, Kukletova M, et al. Lack of association between lactotransferrin polymorphism and dental caries. Caries Res. 2014;48(1):39–44. PubMed.
54. Briseno-Ruiz J, Shimizu T, Deeley K, Dizak PM, Ruff TD, Faraco Jr IM, et al. Role of TRAV locus in low caries experience. Hum Genet. 2013;132(9):1015–25. PubMed Pubmed Central PMCID: 3744616.
55. Ozturk A, Famili P, Vieira AR. The antimicrobial peptide DEFB1 is associated with caries. J Dent Res. 2010;89(6):631–6. PubMed.
56. Pol J. [Association of the polymorphism of MUC7 gene encoding the low-molecular-weight mucin MG2 with susceptibility to caries]. Article in Polish. Ann Acad Med Stetin. 2011;57(2):85–91. PubMed.
57. Gabryel-Porowska H, Gornowicz A, Bielawska A, Wojcicka A, Maciorkowska E, Grabowska SZ, et al. Mucin levels in saliva of adolescents with dental caries. Med Sci Monit. 2014;20:72–7. PubMed Pubmed Central PMCID: 3907531.
58. Everett ET, Yin Z, Yan D, Zou F. Fine mapping of dental fluorosis quantitative trait loci in mice. Eur J Oral Sci. 2011;119 Suppl 1:8–12. PubMed Pubmed Central PMCID: 3402502.
59. Seow WK, Thomsett MJ. Dental fluorosis as a complication of hereditary diabetes insipidus: studies of six affected patients. Pediatr Dent. 1994;16(2):128–32. PubMed.
60. Allazzam SM, Alaki SM, El Meligy OA. Molar incisor hypomineralization, prevalence, and etiology. Int

J Dent. 2014;2014:234508. PubMed Pubmed Central PMCID: 4034724.

61. Kuhnisch J, Thiering E, Heitmuller D, Tiesler CM, Grallert H, Heinrich-Weltzien R, et al. Genome-wide association study (GWAS) for molar-incisor hypomineralization (MIH). Clin Oral Investig. 2014;18(2):677–82. PubMed.

62. Jeremias F, Koruyucu M, Kuchler EC, Bayram M, Tuna EB, Deeley K, et al. Genes expressed in dental enamel development are associated with molar-incisor hypomineralization. Arch Oral Biol. 2013;58(10):1434–42. PubMed Pubmed Central PMCID: 3769477.

63. Wright JT, Torain M, Long K, Seow K, Crawford P, Aldred MJ, et al. Amelogenesis imperfecta: genotype-phenotype studies in 71 families. Cells Tissues Organs. 2011;194(2–4):279–83. PubMed Pubmed Central PMCID: 3178091.

64. Deeley K, Letra A, Rose EK, Brandon CA, Resick JM, Marazita ML, et al. Possible association of amelogenin to high caries experience in a Guatemalan-Mayan population. Caries Res. 2008;42(1):8–13. PubMed Pubmed Central PMCID: 2814012.

65. Chaussain C, Bouazza N, Gasse B, Laffont AG, Opsahl Vital S, Davit-Beal T, et al. Dental caries and enamelin haplotype. J Dent Res. 2014;93(4):360–5. PubMed.

66. Shaffer JR, Carlson JC, Stanley BO, Feingold E, Cooper M, Vanyukov MM, et al. Effects of enamel matrix genes on dental caries are moderated by fluoride exposures. Hum Genet. 2015;134:159–67. PubMed.

67. Wright JT. Oral manifestations in the epidermolysis bullosa spectrum. Dermatol Clin. 2010;28(1):159–64. PubMed Pubmed Central PMCID: 2787479.

68. Jenkinson HF. Beyond the oral microbiome. Environ Microbiol. 2011;13(12):3077–87. PubMed.

69. Chen T, Yu WH, Izard J, Baranova OV, Lakshmanan A, Dewhirst FE. The Human Oral Microbiome Database: a web accessible resource for investigating oral microbe taxonomic and genomic information. Database. 2010;2010:baq013. PubMed Pubmed Central PMCID: 2911848.

70. Zarco MF, Vess TJ, Ginsburg GS. The oral microbiome in health and disease and the potential impact on personalized dental medicine. Oral Dis. 2012;18(2):109–20. PubMed.

71. Ling Z, Kong J, Jia P, Wei C, Wang Y, Pan Z, et al. Analysis of oral microbiota in children with dental caries by PCR-DGGE and barcoded pyrosequencing. Microb Ecol. 2010;60(3):677–90. PubMed.

72. Foxman B, Srinivasan U, Wen A, Zhang L, Marrs CF, Goldberg D, et al. Exploring the effect of dentition, dental decay and familiality on oral health using metabolomics. Infect Genet Evol. 2014;22:201–7. PubMed Pubmed Central PMCID: 3943654.

73. Takahashi N, Washio J, Mayanagi G. Metabolomics of supragingival plaque and oral bacteria. J Dent Res. 2010;89(12):1383–8. PubMed.

# Personalized Medicine Approaches to the Prevention, Diagnosis, and Treatment of Chronic Periodontitis

8

Carlos Garaicoa-Pazmino, Ann M. Decker, and Peter J. Polverini

**Abstract**
Over the years, the multifactorial and interactive nature of periodontal disease challenged clinicians in an attempt to delineate a pattern for its destructive progression. Periodontal disease is caused by persistent inflammation of the periodontium in response to the colonization of microbes upon the tooth surface near the gingival margin and a subsequent biofilm formation resulting in irreversible attachment loss of marginal alveolar bone and associated periodontal ligament and migration of the junctional epithelium. In spite of the infectious nature of periodontal disease, identification of the oral microbiome and a complete understanding of its pathogenic pathway seem the most logical step toward the development of newer and effective approaches for periodontal therapy.

## Introduction

Periodontitis is a multifactorial inflammatory disease that disrupts the periodontium, which collectively includes the gingiva, alveolar bone, periodontal ligament, and cementum. This disease is pervasive throughout human history and remains a public health concern today, affecting individuals on a global scale [1, 2]. Defining features of this disease include the spread of inflammatory infiltrate progressively deeper into the periodontal tissue, resulting in irreversible attachment loss of marginal alveolar bone and associated periodontal ligament and migration of the junctional epithelium [3].

Clinical presentation of periodontitis involves bone loss, periodontal pocket formation, and

C. Garaicoa-Pazmino, DDS (✉)
A.M. Decker, DMD • P.J. Polverini, DDS, DMSc
Department of Periodontics and Oral Medicine, University of Michigan School of Dentistry, Ann Arbor, MI, USA
e-mail: garaicoa@umich.edu; andecker@umich.edu; neovas@umich.edu



P.J. Polverini (ed.), *Personalized Oral Health Care: From Concept Design to Clinical Practice*, DOI 10.1007/978-3-319-23297-3_8 possibly gingival recession; however, patterns of bone loss can be more variable between patients [4]. Periodontitis can be broadly categorized as either chronic or aggressive and further characterized by the extent of bone loss and severity of the disease [5]. Slowly progressing chronic periodontitis characteristically displays generalized horizontal bone loss, which affects most teeth and occurs over an extended period of time [6, 7]. Alternatively, in rapidly advancing aggressive periodontitis, bone loss can be highly irregular at specific sites, creating deeper pockets and infrabony defects in a short period of time [8]. In addition to local effects, recent studies have shown systemic effects of periodontal diseases through increased risk of atherosclerosis, rheumatoid arthritis, respiratory infections, adverse pregnancy outcomes, and cancer [9–15].

## Risk Factors of Periodontal Disease Initiation and Progression

Periodontal disease is caused by persistent inflammation of the periodontium in response to the colonization of microbes on the tooth surface near the gingival margin and subsequent biofilm formation [16]. Bacterial colonization is an unavoidable event; salivary glycoproteins form a pellicle upon the tooth surface shortly following a professional cleaning [17]. Within minutes, primary colonizing bacteria (primarily gram-positive streptococci) adhere to the pellicle and begin proliferating [18]. Following the primary colonizers, a diverse group of microorganisms colonize, forming a unique microenvironment that increases in diversity as time passes [19].

Biofilm diversity and maturation depend on retention features and environmental factors, such as nutrients and oral hygiene practices [20, 21]. Plaque is physically retained by calculus deposits, anatomical features such as crowded dentition, and iatrogenic features such as overhanging restorations [22]. Though onset of periodontal disease is determined by presence of bacterial plaque biofilm, many studies have shown that plaque biofilm is necessary but insufficient to initiate the disease process, suggesting that there are other patient-specific factors involved [23].

To this end, susceptibility of the patient to disease onset and progression is guided by a number of different factors, as the host is ultimately responsible for periodontal tissue destruction in response to the plaque biofilm formation [24]. Host response and susceptibility are further guided by genetic, environmental, and lifestyle factors, which directly affect the progression of an existing disease process [25]. These patient-specific risk factors for progressive periodontal disease include smoking, genetic factors, epigenetic modifications, diabetes, and stress. Understanding the mechanisms by which these components function in the context of health and disease can help clinicians elucidate personalized preventative strategies for at-risk patients.

## Smoking

Smoking has been well established as a risk factor for periodontal disease. It has been reported to increase the risk of periodontal disease two- to eightfold [26]. Furthermore, there is a dose-response relationship between the number of cigarettes smoked per day and the odds ratio of periodontal disease, whereby there was an increased risk of periodontal disease in patients who smoked a higher number of cigarettes [27]. Furthermore, the study by Tomar and Asma [27], with the use of epidemiologic formulas, calculated that 41.9 % of periodontitis cases in the United States' adult population were attributed to current smoking. Several clinical studies demonstrate further that smokers have both increased susceptibility and severity of disease and disease progression [28–31]. Despite exacerbated periodontal disease progression, smokers present clinically with decreased inflammation, including decreased gingival bleeding, erythema, and gingival exudate [32–34].

Smoking may affect periodontal tissue breakdown in a number of different ways, including disruption of periodontal cell migration and/or function, diminished microcirculation, and dysregulated inflammatory response [35]. Ryder et al. demonstrated that smoke exposure to primary peripheral neutrophils impaired migration through upregulation of adhesion integrins, downregulation of L-selectin, and alterations in F-actin kinetics [36, 37]. Gingival fibroblasts and osteoblasts exposed to cigarette smoke increased production of matrix metalloproteinases (MMPs) and decreased production of tissue inhibitors of MMPs (TIMPs) [38–40]. In addition, epithelial cells and periodontal ligament cells showed decreased survival and proliferation in the presence of cigarette smoke [41, 42]. Furthermore, animal studies confirmed these in vitro data demonstrating smoking and tobacco-associated particulate increased alveolar bone loss, increased MMP levels, decreased fibroblast-like cell proliferation, and reduced periodontal tissue repair [43–46].

In humans, however, the mechanism of periodontal breakdown observed in response to tobacco use has not been fully elucidated. Consensus of literature is present on the deleterious effects of typical periodontal treatment therapy, scaling, and root planning in smokers [47–49]. The use of adjuncts such as antimicrobials and anti-inflammatory agents has been utilized in the treatment of smokers. However, inconsistencies in clinical reports have yielded meta-analyses with inconclusive results [50]. Taken together, these results highlight the complex nature of the host response within the tobacco-periodontal disease relationship and variant response among sampled patients.

## Diabetes

Diabetes is characterized by chronic hyperglycemia as a result of defects in insulin secretion, insulin action, or both. In addition, diabetic patients have disturbances in carbohydrate, protein, and fat metabolism [51]. These combined metabolic disturbances can result in long-term damage to many vital organs and increase risk of other diseases, including periodontal disease [52–54].

Diabetes affects periodontal disease by increasing its prevalence, severity, extent, and progression [55]. The relationship between diabetes and periodontal disease was suspected with the observation that the severity of periodontitis was statistically worse in individuals with diabetes compared to those individuals without diabetes [56, 57]. Longitudinal studies have demonstrated that poor glycemic control is associated with increased rate of attachment loss and alveolar bone loss for both males and females [58–60].

The relationship between diabetes and periodontal disease has been expressed as bidirectional (1) due to the associations reported of periodontal disease severity and glycemic control and (2) through the biological mechanism that inflammation can dysregulate glycemia [61]. To this point, patients with worsened glycemic control showed increased risk of periodontal disease [62]. Likewise, periodontal disease adversely affected glycemic control in diabetic patients [63, 64]. This relationship is corroborated evidence that treatment of periodontitis can decrease elevated levels of glycated hemoglobin [65–67].

Treatment of periodontal disease associated with diabetes is not without complications. Diabetic patients generally have delayed wound healing and a diminished response to periodontal treatment [68]. Mechanisms for these outcomes include a hyperreactive inflammatory response, increased cellular apoptosis, increased levels of pro-inflammatory mediators such as advanced glycation end-products (AGEs), and altered immune response such as impaired phagocytosis and neutrophil chemotaxis [69–71].

Due to rising global incidence of diabetes mellitus, clinicians must be able to identify this disease in both diagnosed and undiagnosed patients. Additionally, dental clinicians must work with both the individual patient and comprehensive medical team to manage both local and systemic effects of diabetes mellitus.

## Genetic Factors

Periodontal disease is initiated by colonization of microorganisms and subsequent biofilm formation; however, genetic factors may also modify the susceptibility of the host. Genetic factors that may influence the onset of periodontal disease include specific genes, gene-gene interactions, and gene-environmental interactions [55].

Strong evidence that genetic factors influence the risk of periodontitis is rooted in studies between adult twins [72]. Specifically, Michalowicz et al. demonstrated that monozygotic twins were more similar than dizygotic twins [73]. Additionally, this work showed that chronic periodontitis was estimated to have an approximately 50 % heritability, thus signifying that about half of the variance in periodontal disease is attributed to genetic factors. The authors further pointed out that there was no evidence for the heritability for gingivitis.

In addition to twin studies, familial aggregation studies have demonstrated that aggressive periodontitis is an inherited autosomal dominant trait in black families [74]. Other familial aggregate studies have demonstrated that aggressive periodontitis is very high among specific families, affecting siblings up to 40–50 % [75]. In the case of aggressive periodontitis, studies often concomitantly report an underlying cause of leukocyte dysfunction, which may also be genetic.

Familial aggregation studies have also reported a basis for shared environmental factors in addition to shared genetic factors, which in many cases cannot be distinguished. Shearer et al. demonstrated that parents with poor oral hygiene tend to have children with poor oral hygiene; however, they were unable to distinguish between genetic and environmental factors [76].

Association studies have also been conducted to determine to the relationship of genetic polymorphisms and chronic periodontitis [77, 78]. Karimbux et al. [79] identified two interleukin (IL) gene variations that increased the risk of chronic periodontitis in adult whites: IL-1A (odds ratio = 1.48) and IL-1B (odds ratio = 1.54). In addition, other genetic polymorphisms have been identified to potentially influence the onset of periodontal disease, including IL-6 and Toll-like receptors (TLRs) [80–82].

Furthermore, genome-wide association studies have also been conducted and provide a larger analysis of the entire genome for more than a million polymorphisms [83]. While polymorphisms have not been statistically significantly associated with chronic periodontitis, one study reported an associated genetic polymorphism with aggressive periodontitis [84, 85]. Schaefer et al. demonstrated a single nucleotide polymorphism associated with intron 2 of glucosyltransferase 6 domain containing 1 (GLT6D1) correlated with generalized aggressive periodontitis [85]. This finding was recently replicated in the study of aggressive periodontitis in a Sudanese population [86].

The potential of genome-wide association studies provides a means to more clearly identify the mechanisms involved in the onset and progression of periodontal disease. Precisely identifying the etiology of a patient's disease will support personalized treatment and improve patient care.

## Epigenetics

Changes in the gene expression that are not related to alterations in the DNA sequence serve as the basis for epigenetics. Such modifications are associated with chemical alterations of the DNA and packing proteins responsible for the shape and structure of the chromatin, leading to activation or inactivation of genes [87]. DNA methylation and histone modifications represent two of the major epigenetic modifications as result of the exposure to environmental factors. While different possible mechanisms of DNA methylation in periodontal disease have been suggested [88, 89], studies emphasizing histone modification mechanisms remain scarce and limited [90].

Epigenetic modifications have been identified among carcinogenesis and autoimmune and chronic inflammatory diseases, such as periodontitis. As discussed earlier, the multifactorial nature of periodontal disease and its destructive progression can be impacted by several risk factors [91]. In such instances, it has been hypothesized that the constant exposure of these environmental factors to the gingival tissues is capable of modifying gene expression and thus increasing the susceptibility for disease activity or explains the presence of unresponsive sites despite receiving periodontal therapy.

The epigenetic patterns of environmental factors associated with periodontal disease have not been fully elucidated. Identification of these DNA modifications may represent a viable approach for patient stratification, adjustments in recalls for dental care, and more personalized treatment according to the patient's disease susceptibility.

## Stress

Stress was first identified to negatively impact the periodontal tissues in necrotizing periodontal diseases [92]. However, there might be connections between stress and chronic diseases, including periodontitis [93, 94]. Several studies have reported that stress increased the odds of periodontal disease more than twofold [95, 96]. Furthermore, Genco et al. [95] reported that individuals who were under stress, such as financial strain, but who had developed effective coping methods had no increased risk of periodontal disease relative to individuals without stress.

The mechanisms by which stress affects a patient's susceptibility to periodontal diseases include both immune modulation and behavior modification. Stress modulates immune response via neurons located in the hypothalamic-pituitary-adrenal axis that produce biological mediators that modulate immune cell activity [97]. When activated through stress, the hypothalamic-pituitary-adrenal axis stimulates secretion of corticotropin-releasing hormone and glucocorticoid hormones [98]. Immune cells have receptors for these biological mediators, and stimulation of these receptors may lead to immune dysregulation [97]. Immune dysfunction as a result of stress is expressed in a number of ways, including decreased natural killer cells, decreased antibody production to vaccination, increased susceptibility to infectious diseases, and latent virus activation [99]. Immune suppression caused through the hypothalamic-pituitary-adrenal axis increases susceptibility to periodontal infections [100].

Additionally, the autonomic nervous system may be activated by stress. Stimulation of the autonomic nervous system induces catecholamine release [101]. In turn, catecholamines promote release of proteases and prostaglandins [102]. Increased proteases and prostaglandins in the periodontal tissues can amplify periodontal tissue destruction [101, 103]. As such, there are multiple biological mechanisms by which stress influences the onset and progression of periodontal disease.

In addition to the biological mechanisms involved in stress-mediated susceptibility to periodontal disease, stress also modifies behaviors that can promote periodontal disease [103]. These behaviors include increased smoking, decreased oral hygiene, and/or fewer dental visits [95]. Combining the biological mechanisms and behavior modifications induced by stress, the effects of stress can be harmful to both the periodontal health and systemic health of patients. Identifying patients at risk for periodontal disease who have poor stress-coping skills may be important in the development of a personalized treatment strategy for those patients.

## Pathogenesis of Periodontal Disease

Over the years, the multifactorial and interactive nature of periodontal disease challenged clinicians in an attempt to delineate a pattern for its destructive progression. A series of cross-sectional studies by Löe and colleagues initiated a new era in understanding periodontitis by using an untreated population of Sri Lankan tea workers to evaluate the natural progression of periodontal disease [104–107]. Their findings reported different rates of progression patterns, with a small part of the population in whom gingivitis never progressed to periodontal disease [108]. Later studies revealed a dynamic condition with random and asynchronous periods of disease exacerbation and remission, as well as periods of inactivity, suggesting linear and nonlinear destructive patterns [109, 110].

Despite its natural progression, the main finding focused on the impact of biofilm upon the gingival tissues as a true etiology for the development of periodontal disease. The following section will discuss the ecological community of the periodontium and the host immunological and adaptive responses against the periodontopathic microorganisms.

## Microbiome

In spite of the infectious nature of periodontal disease, identification of the healthy and pathogenic microorganism seems the most logical step toward the development of an effective periodontal therapy. Limited by technological advances, early studies used DNA probes; polymerase chain reactions (PCRs) and immunoessays were molecular diagnostic tests meant to fulfill this purpose. Cross-sectional studies in combination with culture techniques allowed a clear identification of early and late colonizers within the biofilm [111]. Interestingly, the short-term transition from a nonmotile gram-positive bacteria (i.e., cocci and *Actinomyces* sp.) to a motile, anaerobic gram-negative bacteria (*Veillonella* and *Bacteroides* sp.) was commonly observed as the natural recolonization pattern after providing periodontal treatment [112].

Socransky and colleagues divided the microbial populations in complexes according to their association with disease activity [110]. Members of the red complex (i.e., *Porphyromonas gingivalis*, *Treponema denticola*, *Tannerella forsythia*) and orange complex (*Fusobacterium*, *Prevotella*, and *Campylobacter* spp.) are considered meaningful in the periodontal diagnosis due to their high correlation with deep probing depths and bleeding on probing in patients affected with chronic periodontitis. On the contrary, *Aggregatibacter actinomycetemcomitans* was associated as the main etiological microorganism of aggressive periodontitis. These findings suggested a more appropriate and effective approach by targeting specific bacteria with the use of systemic or locally delivered antibiotics [112, 113].

Recently, newer molecular approaches made possible the ability to identify unrecognized species in the etiology of periodontal diseases and thus expanded our knowledge of the diversity of these oral microbiomes [114, 115]. As a matter of fact, microorganisms of the Archaea and Eukarya domains, in addition to new bacterial candidates (i.e., *Filifactor alocis*), revealed moderate association in periodontitis-affected patients [116].

To a certain point, the understanding of the composition of the subgingival biofilm extends beyond the limits of the oral cavity. A collection of 16S ribosomal RNA gene sequencing has been used by the Human Microbiome Project to establish the dynamic association of microbial communities across different sites across the human body. Patients' interactions between their surrounding environments can shape the structure of the human microbiome. Aside from its complexity, the oral microbiome reflects unstable patterns from an intra- and interpersonal perspective when compared to other ecosystems [117].

## Host Response

In a pristine periodontium, the epithelium turnover and the attachment apparatus serve as an effective barrier against the microbiological invasion and associated endotoxins in their attempt to penetrate into the underlying tissues. Saliva and gingival crevicular fluid (GCF) secretion act as defense mechanisms by removing or preventing further microbial aggregation upon the tooth surface. Furthermore, the homeostasis of the oral cavity is enhanced by humoral immune response through complement proteins and specific antibodies contained among these oral fluids.

Diffusion of bacterial endotoxins through the junctional epithelium will trigger an increased production of inflammatory mediators, including a variety of interleukins, prostaglandin E2 (PG2), histamine, and MMPs from keratinocytes, fibroblasts, macrophages, and endothelial or mast cells. Activation of these mediators leads to a hyperemic effect of the surrounding blood vessels by altering the vascular permeability. Opening of the endothelial cell junctions facilitates the extravasation of the vessel content in the extracellular matrix and the migration of leukocytes to the sulcus area in response to the chemotactic stimuli elicited by IL-8 and intercellular attachment molecule-1.

Underneath the subgingival biofilm, a cell barricade is formed following the expression of cell adhesion molecules and pro-inflammatory agents for leukocyte recruitment to prevent its further apical advancement. In early stages of inflammation, neutrophils represent the most abundant cell population within this inflammatory infiltrate, which might also include monocytes, lymphocytes, Langerhans cells, and other antigen-presenting cells. Nevertheless, the predominance of specific leukocytes will eventually shift over time from a polymorphonuclear toward a mononuclear concentrate.

Macrophages are crucial players in the transition of early to advanced lesion. Several cytokines from lipopolysaccharide-activated macrophages, such as tumor necrosis factor-α (TNF-α), IL-1B, PG2, and MMPs (such as MMP-1, MMP-3, MMP-8, MMP-9, and MMP-13), function as chemoattractant signals for mononuclear recruitment and are capable of inducing collagen degradation [118]. Macrophage-mediated expression of TIMPs has the ability to suppress collagenase activity and primarily acts as adaptive mediators. For such reason, the sole presence of macrophages, monocytes, T and B lymphocytes, and plasma cells provides evidence for the chronic nature of periodontal disease and potential risk for further disease progression [119, 120].

Receptor activator of nuclear factor kappa-B ligand (RANKL) is a cell-surface protein critical, which binds to its specific receptor RANK on hematopoietic cells for osteoclastic differentiation and activation [121]. Conversely, osteoprotegerin (OPG) binds to RANKL to inhibit the differentiation process [122, 123]. Bone resorption is regulated by the RANK/RANKL/OPG interaction. Once the balance of these bone mediators is disrupted as a result of the plaque-induced collagen degradation, an advanced lesion is established. GCF increased levels of RANKL and reduced levels of OPG have been reported during periodontal disease.

As previously discussed, the progression of the disease might differ between individuals in response to several risk factors. Eventually, tooth loss will occur if the disease remains untreated.

## Management Strategies

Proper management of all systemic and local factors affecting the periodontal condition is essential to achieve or maintain a state of health, comfort, and function [124]. Adequate home care, patient education, and motivation for compliance of dental care play significant key roles in preventing plaque accumulation and future disease progression before and after providing initial periodontal therapy.

Removal of bacterial biofilm through mechanical debridement represents the foundation of periodontal therapy. Nonsurgical therapy consists of a closed-flap approach using site-specific and ultrasonic instrumentation under local and regional anesthesia. Scaling and root planning are the most widely used methods to create a viable environment to promote the formation of new attachment upon the denuded root surface. If managed properly, significant pocket reduction and limited clinical attachment gain are among the expected treatment outcomes.

Despite efforts to obtain a complete calculus removal, surgical approaches have been proposed to overcome limitations of nonsurgical therapy [125, 126]. Periodontal surgery aims to improve the access to the affected sites and create pockets accessible for regular home care. Elimination of pockets and reduction of inflammation represent the ultimate treatment goals of periodontal surgery.

A careful assessment of the defect morphology is crucial when selecting between resective and regenerative procedures. Osseous surgery involves removal of the bony supporting tissues to correct deformities resulting from periodontal disease and increase better tissue adaptation. However, aesthetic concerns may arise from these procedures due to increased gingival recession being most critical in the anterior zone. On the other hand, modern dentistry promotes the use of bone grafting, soft tissue grafts, biological agents, and barrier membranes to restore lost periodontal structures without compromising aesthetics.

Ultimately, the use of locally delivered antibiotics is advocated to be as effective as mechanical debridement for unresponsive sites; however, these agents are limited to controlling disease activity, rather than calculus chemical dissolution [127–130]. Regardless of the approach, pocket elimination, defect correction, and reduction of inflammation reflect the successful treatment outcomes of periodontal therapy [131–133].

Periodontal maintenance is considered an extension of active periodontal therapy and consists of procedures to maintain periodontal stability. Longitudinal studies have shown the importance of periodontal maintenance following active periodontal therapy. Recurrence of periodontal disease can be observed in surgically and nonsurgically treated patients without regular or erratic maintenance recalls [134, 135]. On the contrary, long-term results of periodontal therapy can be sustained with periodic intervals [136–138].

In order to minimize risk for recurrence of periodontal disease or arrest disease progression in a timely manner, recall programs ranging between 3 and 6 months have been considered acceptable [139, 140]. Nowadays, oral hygiene and rate of microbial pocket recolonization remain as the key components to determine regular maintenance intervals; however, a personalized risk assessment of contributing factors might represent a more valid approach to establish adjustments in dental care visits [141].

## Conclusions

Current clinical periodontal diagnostic criteria used in the practice setting have limited utility to predict future disease progression [142]. The potential role of host-response biomarkers and microbial profile obtained from oral fluids has been investigated as complementary diagnostic tools for periodontal disease (see Fig. 5.3). Concentrations of host-response molecules and total percentage of bacterial DNA may represent a more accurate, real-time disease activity than conventional clinical measurements [143, 144].

Identifying a single predictive biomarker for periodontal diseases would be of great significance [142, 145]. Oral health professionals are in need of diagnostic and prognostic tools to obtain fast and valuable information in order to enhance the decision-making for periodontal therapy [146, 147]. Nevertheless, present diagnostic tests require training, major resources, and increased cost-effective healthcare delivery [148]. For that reason, biomarkers and microbial assessment with portable and simpler microfluidic screening devices might lead to acceptance from the dental community and a more efficient therapy (Fig. 8.1) [149, 150].

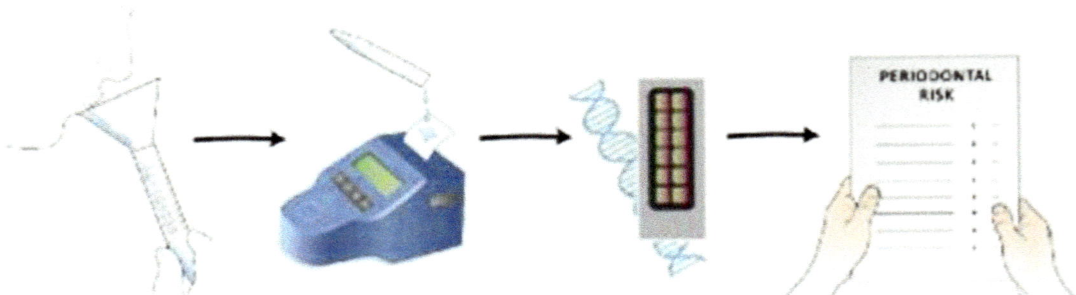


**Fig. 8.1** Application of salivary diagnostics to the periodontal practice of the future. A point-of-care diagnostic may be available in which a patient provides an oral sample that is delivered to the chairside or to a laboratory device. The result is interpreted by the oral healthcare provider, who then educates the patient about the findings from the biomarker report. The diagnostic test may reveal a patient's susceptibility to disease (e.g., a genetic test) or provide a real-time assessment of the patient's disease status via the use of microbiological or protein markers of periodontal infection, destruction, or both (Reprinted from Giannobile [148]. Copyright © 2012 with permission from Elsevier)

Despite significant advances in oral fluid diagnostics, the role of DNA testing has shown promising results and represents the key component of personalized approaches. Gene polymorphisms were initially proposed as potential indicators for disease susceptibility. Kornman and collaborators demonstrated an association of IL-1B and periodontal disease in a specific population [78]. Nowadays, the assessment of cell molecular signaling from gingival tissues has been used in an attempt to develop newer alternatives of periodontal classification systems based on genome transcriptomic profiles of chronic and aggressive periodontitis [151]. Drug-assisted therapies targeting epigenetic modifications could be considered to control disease activity as observed in cancer research [152]. Pharmacoepigenetic biomarkers may potentially be used to assess the drug effectiveness and predict their response. Epigenetic inhibitors (i.e., histone deacetylase inhibitors, DNA methyltransferase inhibitors) could represent a novel approach to repair any cellular damage caused by periodontal disease or oral inflammation [87].

There should be considerable benefits to all key stakeholders as new technologies are deployed to improve the diagnosis, prognosis, and treatment of patients. The complexity of biological systems means that not all genetic lesions may manifest as important phenotypic changes and disease patterns, making the identification of potential biomarkers and new targeted treatments more difficult. This may explain in part why the promise of personalized oral healthcare has been slow to translate scientific findings directly into improvements for patient care and why only a limited number of targeted treatments are currently available. Nowadays, for some of the more common dental diseases such as periodontitis, there is insufficient evidence to support the routine use of biomarkers in either diagnosis or targeted therapies. As such, increased support for research in areas of personalized medicine could potentially have a tremendous impact in the future of patient care, especially within the context of dentistry.

Personalized oral healthcare offers the potential to revolutionize the practice of dentistry. It also provides a unique window into the relationship between new medical technologies and new models for healthcare delivery. Using personalized medicine as a test of disruptive innovation in healthcare, it will be necessary to take a different approach to technology development. Achieving this, however, is fraught with difficulty, as innovations are deemed truly disruptive only in hindsight. A robust framework for continuing assessment, close scrutiny, and oversight of developing technologies might help protect the integrity of this process while enabling the rapid deployment of scientific discovery into the patient care environment. While there is unquestioned risk in this largely untested approach to healthcare, the benefits of investing in disruptive innovations that will truly revolutionize our approach to disease diagnosis and treatment are worth the risk.

## References


1. Albandar JM, Tinoco E. Global epidemiology of periodontal diseases in children and young persons. Periodontol 2000. 2002;29(1):153–76.
2. Eke P, Dye B, Wei L, Thornton-Evans G, Genco R. Prevalence of periodontitis in adults in the United States: 2009 and 2010. J Dent Res. 2012;91(10):914–20.
3. Kinane D, Bouchard P. Periodontal diseases and health: consensus report of the sixth European workshop on periodontology. J Clin Periodontol. 2008;35(s8):333–7.
4. Schei O, Waerhaug J, Lovdal A, Arno A. Alveolar bone loss as related to oral hygiene and age. J Periodontol. 1959;30(1):7–16.
5. Armitage GC. Development of a classification system for periodontal diseases and conditions. Ann Periodontol. 1999;4(1):1–6.
6. Mombelli A, Meier C. On the symmetry of periodontal disease. J Clin Periodontol. 2001;28(8):741–5.
7. Armitage GC, Cullinan MP. Comparison of the clinical features of chronic and aggressive periodontitis. Periodontol 2000. 2010;53(1):12–27.

8. Lang N, Bartold PM, Cullinan M, Jeffcoat M, Mombelli A, Murakami S, et al. Consensus report: aggressive periodontitis. Ann Periodontol. 1999; 4(1):53.
9. Leech MT, Bartold P. The association between rheumatoid arthritis and periodontitis. Best Pract Res Clin Rheumatol. 2015;29:189–201.
10. Seymour G, Ford P, Cullinan M, Leishman S, Yamazaki K. Relationship between periodontal infections and systemic disease. Clin Microbiol Infect. 2007;13(s4):3–10.
11. Tonetti MS, Dyke TE. Periodontitis and atherosclerotic cardiovascular disease: consensus report of the Joint EFP/AAP Workshop on Periodontitis and Systemic Diseases. J Clin Periodontol. 2013;40(s14): S24–9.
12. Krüger M, Hansen T, Kasaj A, Moergel M. The correlation between chronic periodontitis and oral cancer. Case Rep Dent. 2013;2013:262410.
13. Usher AK, Stockley RA. The link between chronic periodontitis and COPD: a common role for the neutrophil? BMC Med. 2013;11(1):241.
14. Han Y, Houcken W, Loos B, Schenkein H, Tezal M. Periodontal disease, atherosclerosis, adverse pregnancy outcomes, and head-and-neck cancer. Adv Dent Res. 2014;26(1):47–55.
15. Ide M, Papapanou PN. Epidemiology of association between maternal periodontal disease and adverse pregnancy outcomes–systematic review. J Clin Periodontol. 2013;40(s14):S181–94.
16. Socransky SS, Haffajee AD. The bacterial etiology of destructive periodontal disease: current concepts. J Periodontol. 1992;63(4s):322–31.
17. Lendenmann U, Grogan J, Oppenheim F. Saliva and dental pellicle-a review. Adv Dent Res. 2000;14(1): 22–8.
18. Saxton C. Scanning electron microscope study of the formation of dental plaque. Caries Res. 1973;7(2): 102–19.
19. Listgarten M. Formation of dental plaque and other oral biofilms. Dental plaque revisited: oral biofilms in health and disease. Cardiff: Bioline. 1999:187–210.
20. Finke M, Parker DM, Jandt KD. Influence of soft drinks on the thickness and morphology of in situ acquired pellicle layer on enamel. J Colloid Interface Sci. 2002;251(2):263–70.
21. Lie T. Early dental plaque morphogenesis. J Periodontal Res. 1977;12(2):73–89.
22. Desanctis M, Murphy KG. The role of resective periodontal surgery in the treatment of furcation defects. Periodontol 2000. 2000;22(1):154–68.
23. Bartold PM, Van Dyke TE. Periodontitis: a host-mediated disruption of microbial homeostasis. Unlearning learned concepts. Periodontol 2000. 2013;62(1):203–17.
24. Laine ML, Crielaard W, Loos BG. Genetic susceptibility to periodontitis. Periodontol 2000. 2012;58(1): 37–68.
25. Offenbacher S, Barros SP, Beck JD. Rethinking periodontal inflammation. J Periodontol. 2008;79(8S): 1577–84.
26. Johnson GK, Guthmiller JM. The impact of cigarette smoking on periodontal disease and treatment. Periodontol 2000. 2007;44(1):178–94.
27. Tomar SL, Asma S. Smoking-attributable periodontitis in the United States: findings from NHANES III. J Periodontol. 2000;71(5):743–51.
28. Phipps KR, Chan BK, Jennings-Holt M, Geurs NC, Reddy MS, Lewis CE, et al. Periodontal health of older men: the MrOS dental study. Gerodontology. 2009;26(2):122–9.
29. Kibayashi M, Tanaka M, Nishida N, Kuboniwa M, Kataoka K, Nagata H, et al. Longitudinal study of the association between smoking as a periodontitis risk and salivary biomarkers related to periodontitis. J Periodontol. 2007;78(5):859–67.
30. Rosa GM, Lucas GQ, Lucas ON. Cigarette smoking and alveolar bone in young adults: a study using digitized radiographs. J Periodontol. 2008;79(2): 232–44.
31. Hugoson A, Rolandsson M. Periodontal disease in relation to smoking and the use of Swedish snus: epidemiological studies covering 20 years (1983–2003). J Clin Periodontol. 2011;38(9):809–16.
32. Preber H, Bergström J. Occurrence of gingival bleeding in smoker and non-smoker patients. Acta Odontol. 1985;43(5):315–20.
33. Apatzidou D, Riggio M, Kinane D. Impact of smoking on the clinical, microbiological and immunological parameters of adult patients with periodontitis. J Clin Periodontol. 2005;32(9):973–83.
34. Vouros I, Kalpidis C, Chadjipantelis T, Konstantinidis A. Cigarette smoking associated with advanced periodontal destruction in a Greek sample population of patients with periodontal disease. J Int Acad Periodontol. 2009;11(4):250–7.
35. Nociti FH, Casati MZ, Duarte PM. Current perspective of the impact of smoking on the progression and treatment of periodontitis. Periodontol 2000. 2015;67(1):187–210.
36. Ryder MI, Fujitaki R, Lebus S, Mahboub M, Faia B, Muhaimin D, et al. Alterations of neutrophil L-selection and CD18 expression by tobacco smoke: implications for periodontal diseases. J Periodontal Res. 1998;33(6):359–68.
37. Ryder MI, Wu TC, Kallaos SS, Hyun W. Alterations of neutrophil f-actin kinetics by tobacco smoke: implications for periodontal diseases. J Periodontal Res. 2002;37(4):286–92.
38. Zhang W, Song F, Windsor L. Cigarette smoke condensate affects the collagen-degrading ability of human gingival fibroblasts. J Periodontal Res. 2009;44(6):704–13.
39. Zhang W, Fang M, Song F, Windsor LJ. Effects of cigarette smoke condensate and nicotine on human gingival fibroblast-mediated collagen degradation. J Periodontol. 2011;82(7):1071–9.

40. Katono T, Kawato T, Tanabe N, Tanaka H, Suzuki N, Kitami S, et al. Effects of nicotine and lipopolysaccharide on the expression of matrix metalloproteinases, plasminogen activators, and their inhibitors in human osteoblasts. Arch Oral Biol. 2009;54(2):146–55.
41. Semlali A, Chakir J, Goulet JP, Chmielewski W, Rouabhia M. Whole cigarette smoke promotes human gingival epithelial cell apoptosis and inhibits cell repair processes. J Periodontal Res. 2011;46(5):533–41.
42. Bulmanski Z, Brady M, Stoute D, Lallier TE. Cigarette smoke extract induces select matrix metalloproteinases and integrin expression in periodontal ligament fibroblasts. J Periodontol. 2012;83(6):787–96.
43. Nociti Jr FH, Nogueira-Filho GR, Primo MT, Machado MA, Tramontina VA, Barros SP, et al. The influence of nicotine on the bone loss rate in ligature-induced periodontitis. A histometric study in rats. J Periodontol. 2000;71(9):1460–4.
44. Neto JBC, de Souza AP, Barbieri D, Moreno Jr H, Sallum EA, Nociti Jr FH. Matrix metalloproteinase-2 may be involved with increased bone loss associated with experimental periodontitis and smoking: a study in rats. J Periodontol. 2004;75(7):995–1000.
45. Milanezi de Almeida J, Bosco AF, Bonfante S, Theodoro LH, Nagata MJH, Garcia VG. Nicotine-induced damage affects gingival fibroblasts in the gingival tissue of rats. J Periodontol. 2011;82(8):1206–11.
46. Benatti BB, César-Neto JB, Gonçalves PF, Sallum EA, Nociti FH. Smoking affects the self-healing capacity of periodontal tissues. A histological study in the rat. Eur J Oral Sci. 2005;113(5):400–3.
47. Grossi SG, Goodson JM, Gunsolley JC, Otomo-Corgel J, Bland PS, Doherty F, et al. Mechanical therapy with adjunctive minocycline microspheres reduces red-complex bacteria in smokers. J Periodontol. 2007;78(9):1741–50.
48. Heasman L, Stacey F, Preshaw P, McCracken G, Hepburn S, Heasman P. The effect of smoking on periodontal treatment response: a review of clinical evidence. J Clin Periodontol. 2006;33(4):241–53.
49. Wan CP, Leung WK, Wong M, Wong R, Wan P, Lo E, et al. Effects of smoking on healing response to non-surgical periodontal therapy: a multilevel modelling analysis. J Clin Periodontol. 2009;36(3):229–39.
50. Angaji M, Gelskey S, Nogueira-Filho G, Brothwell D. A systematic review of clinical efficacy of adjunctive antibiotics in the treatment of smokers with periodontitis. J Periodontol. 2010;81(11):1518–28.
51. Alberti K, Zimmet PF. Definition, diagnosis and classification of diabetes mellitus and its complications. Part 1: diagnosis and classification of diabetes mellitus provisional report of a WHO consultation. Diabet Med. 1998;15:539–53.
52. Nathan DM. Long-term complications of diabetes mellitus. N Engl J Med. 1993;328(23):1676–85.
53. Taylor GW. Bidirectional interrelationships between diabetes and periodontal diseases: an epidemiologic perspective. Ann Periodontol. 2001;6(1):99–112.
54. Löe H. Periodontal disease: the sixth complication of diabetes mellitus. Diabet Care. 1993;16(1):329–34.
55. Genco RJ, Borgnakke WS. Risk factors for periodontal disease. Periodontol 2000. 2013;62(1):59–94.
56. Emrich LJ, Shlossman M, Genco RJ. Periodontal disease in non-insulin-dependent diabetes mellitus. J Periodontol. 1991;62(2):123–31.
57. Shlossman M, Knowler WC, Pettitt DJ, Genco RJ. Type 2 diabetes mellitus and periodontal disease. J Am Dent Assoc. 1990;121(4):532–6.
58. Taylor GW, Burt BA, Becker MP, Genco RJ, Shlossman M. Glycemic control and alveolar bone loss progression in type 2 diabetes. Ann Periodontol. 1998;3(1):30–9.
59. Chávarry N, Vettore MV, Sansone C, Sheiham A. The relationship between diabetes mellitus and destructive periodontal disease: a meta-analysis. Oral Health Prev Dent. 2009;7(2):107–27.
60. Bandyopadhyay D, Marlow NM, Fernandes JK, Leite RS. Periodontal disease progression and glycaemic control among Gullah African Americans with type-2 diabetes. J Clin Periodontol. 2010;37(6):501–9.
61. Lalla E, Papapanou PN. Diabetes mellitus and periodontitis: a tale of two common interrelated diseases. Nat Rev Endocrinol. 2011;7(12):738–48.
62. Grossi SG, Genco RJ. Periodontal disease and diabetes mellitus: a two-way relationship. Ann Periodontol. 1998;3(1):51–61.
63. Genco RJ, Grossi SG, Ho A, Nishimura F, Murayama Y. A proposed model linking inflammation to obesity, diabetes, and periodontal infections. J Periodontol. 2005;76(11-s):2075–84.
64. Taylor GW, Borgnakke W. Periodontal disease: associations with diabetes, glycemic control and complications. Oral Dis. 2008;14(3):191–203.
65. Kiran M, Arpak N, Ünsal E, Erdoğan MF. The effect of improved periodontal health on metabolic control in type 2 diabetes mellitus. J Clin Periodontol. 2005;32(3):266–72.
66. Jones JA, Miller DR, Wehler CJ, Rich SE, Krall-Kaye EA, McCoy LC, et al. Does periodontal care improve glycemic control? The department of veterans affairs dental diabetes study. J Clin Periodontol. 2007;34(1):46–52.
67. Darré L, Vergnes J-N, Gourdy P, Sixou M. Efficacy of periodontal treatment on glycaemic control in diabetic patients: a meta-analysis of interventional studies. Diabet Metab. 2008;34(5):497–506.
68. Salvi GE, Carollo-Bittel B, Lang NP. Effects of diabetes mellitus on periodontal and peri-implant conditions: update on associations and risks. J Clin Periodontol. 2008;35(s8):398–409.

69. Darby IA, Bisucci T, Hewitson TD, MacLellan DG. Apoptosis is increased in a model of diabetes-impaired wound healing in genetically diabetic mice. Int J Biochem Cell Biol. 1997;29(1):191–200.
70. Graves DT, Liu R, Oates TW. Diabetes-enhanced inflammation and apoptosis–impact on periodontal pathosis. Periodontol 2000. 2007;45(1):128–37.
71. Liu R, Desta T, He H, Graves DT. Diabetes alters the response to bacteria by enhancing fibroblast apoptosis. Endocrinology. 2004;145(6):2997–3003.
72. Michalowicz BS, Aeppli D, Virag JG, Klump DG, Hinrichs E, Segal NL, et al. Periodontal findings in adult twins. J Periodontol. 1991;62(5):293–9.
73. Michalowicz BS, Diehl SR, Gunsolley JC, Sparks BS, Brooks CN, Koertge TE, et al. Evidence of a substantial genetic basis for risk of adult periodontitis. J Periodontol. 2000;71(11):1699–707.
74. Marazita ML, Burmeister JA, Gunsolley JC, Koertge TE, Lake K, Schenkein HA. Evidence for autosomal dominant inheritance and race-specific heterogeneity in early-onset periodontitis. J Periodontol. 1994;65(6):623–30.
75. Meng H, Ren X, Tian Y, Feng X, Xu L, Zhang L, et al. Genetic study of families affected with aggressive periodontitis. Periodontol 2000. 2011;56(1): 87–101.
76. Shearer DM, Thomson WM, Caspi A, Moffitt TE, Broadbent JM, Poulton R. Inter-generational continuity in periodontal health: findings from the Dunedin Family History Study. J Clin Periodontol. 2011;38(4):301–9.
77. Divaris K, Monda KL, North KE, Olshan AF, Reynolds LM, Hsueh W-C, et al. Exploring the genetic basis of chronic periodontitis: a genome-wide association study. Hum Mol Genet. 2013; 22(11):2312–24.
78. Kornman KS, Crane A, Wang HY, di Giovine FS, Newman MG, Pirk FW, et al. The interleukin-1 genotype as a severity factor in adult periodontal disease. J Clin Periodontol. 1997;24(1):72–7. PubMed.
79. Karimbux NY, Saraiya VM, Elangovan S, Allareddy V, Kinnunen T, Kornman KS, et al. Interleukin-1 gene polymorphisms and chronic periodontitis in adult whites: a systematic review and meta-analysis. J Periodontol. 2012;83(11):1407–19.
80. Taylor JJ, Preshaw PM, Donaldson PT. Cytokine gene polymorphism and immunoregulation in periodontal disease. Periodontol 2000. 2004;35(1): 158–82.
81. Schröder N, Meister D, Wolff V, Christan C, Kaner D, Haban V, et al. Chronic periodontal disease is associated with single-nucleotide polymorphisms of the human TLR-4 gene. Genes Immun. 2005;6(5): 448–51.
82. Zhang HY, Feng L, Wu H, Xie XD. The association of IL-6 and IL-6R gene polymorphisms with chronic periodontitis in a Chinese population. Oral Dis. 2014;20(1):69–75.
83. Vaithilingam R, Safii S, Baharuddin N, Ng C, Cheong S, Bartold P, et al. Moving into a new era of periodontal genetic studies: relevance of large case–control samples using severe phenotypes for genome-wide association studies. J Periodontal Res. 2014;49(6):683–95.
84. Schaefer AS, Bochenek G, Manke T, Nothnagel M, Graetz C, Thien A, et al. Validation of reported genetic risk factors for periodontitis in a large-scale replication study. J Clin Periodontol. 2013;40(6): 563–72.
85. Schaefer AS, Richter GM, Nothnagel M, Manke T, Dommisch H, Jacobs G, et al. A genome-wide association study identifies GLT6D1 as a susceptibility locus for periodontitis. Hum Mol Genet. 2009:ddp508.
86. Hashim NT, Linden GJ, Ibrahim ME, Gismalla BG, Lundy FT, Hughes FJ, et al. Replication of the association of GLT6D1 with aggressive periodontitis in a Sudanese population. J Clin Periodontol. 2015;42(4):319–24.
87. Larsson L, Castilho RM, Giannobile WV. Epigenetics and its role in periodontal diseases: a state-of-the-art review. J Periodontol. 2015;86(4):556–68. PubMed.
88. Zhang S, Barros SP, Moretti AJ, Yu N, Zhou J, Preisser JS, et al. Epigenetic regulation of TNFA expression in periodontal disease. J Periodontol. 2013;84(11):1606–16. PubMed Pubmed Central PMCID: 3986590.
89. Uehara O, Abiko Y, Saitoh M, Miyakawa H, Nakazawa F. Lipopolysaccharide extracted from Porphyromonas gingivalis induces DNA hypermethylation of runt-related transcription factor 2 in human periodontal fibroblasts. J Microbiol Immunol Infect. 2014;47(3):176–81. PubMed.
90. Larsson L, Thorbert-Mros S, Rymo L, Berglundh T. Influence of epigenetic modifications of the interleukin-10 promoter on IL10 gene expression. Eur J Oral Sci. 2012;120(1):14–20. PubMed.
91. Van Dyke TE, Sheilesh D. Risk factors for periodontitis. J Int Acad Periodontol. 2005;7(1):3–7. PubMed Pubmed Central PMCID: 1351013.
92. Johnson BD, Engel D. Acute necrotizing ulcerative gingivitis. A review of diagnosis, etiology and treatment. J Periodontol. 1986;57(3):141–50. PubMed.
93. Chrousos GP. Stress and disorders of the stress system. Nat Rev Endocrinol. 2009;5(7):374–81.
94. Halawany H, Abraham N, Jacob V, Al Amri M, Patil S. Is psychological stress a possible risk factor for periodontal disease. A systematic review. J Psychiatry. 2015;18(217):2.
95. Genco RJ, Ho AW, Grossi SG, Dunford R, Tedesco L. Relationship of stress, distress, and inadequate coping behaviors to periodontal disease. J Periodontol. 1999;70(7):711–23.
96. Moss ME, Beck JD, Kaplan BH, Offenbacher S, Weintraub JA, Koch GG, et al. Exploratory case-control

analysis of psychosocial factors and adult periodontitis. J Periodontol. 1996;67(10s):1060–9.
97. Padgett DA, Glaser R. How stress influences the immune response. Trends Immunol. 2003;24(8):444–8.
98. Glaser R, Kiecolt-Glaser JK. Stress-induced immune dysfunction: implications for health. Nat Rev Immunol. 2005;5(3):243–51.
99. Guo S, DiPietro LA. Factors affecting wound healing. J Dent Res. 2010;89(3):219–29.
100. Hilgert J, Hugo F, Bandeira D, Bozzetti M. Stress, cortisol, and periodontitis in a population aged 50 years and over. J Dent Res. 2006;85(4):324–8.
101. Boyapati L, Wang HL. The role of stress in periodontal disease and wound healing. Periodontol 2000. 2007;44(1):195–210.
102. Dimsdale JE, Moss J. Plasma catecholamines in stress and exercise. JAMA. 1980;243(4):340–2.
103. Peruzzo DC, Benatti BB, Ambrosano GM, Nogueira-Filho GR, Sallum EA, Casati MZ, et al. A systematic review of stress and psychological factors as possible risk factors for periodontal disease. J Periodontol. 2007;78(8):1491–504.
104. Anerud A, Loe H, Boysen H, Smith M. The natural history of periodontal disease in man. Changes in gingival health and oral hygiene before 40 years of age. J Periodontal Res. 1979;14(6):526–40. PubMed.
105. Loe H, Anerud A, Boysen H, Smith M. The natural history of periodontal disease in man. Study design and baseline data. J Periodontal Res. 1978;13(6):550–62. PubMed.
106. Loe H, Anerud A, Boysen H, Smith M. The natural history of periodontal disease in man. The rate of periodontal destruction before 40 years of age. J Periodontol. 1978;49(12):607–20. PubMed.
107. Loe H, Anerud A, Boysen H, Smith M. The natural history of periodontal disease in man. Tooth mortality rates before 40 years of age. J Periodontal Res. 1978;13(6):563–72. PubMed.
108. Loe H, Anerud A, Boysen H, Morrison E. Natural history of periodontal disease in man. Rapid, moderate and no loss of attachment in Sri Lankan laborers 14 to 46 years of age. J Clin Periodontol. 1986;13(5):431–45. PubMed.
109. Goodson JM, Tanner AC, Haffajee AD, Sornberger GC, Socransky SS. Patterns of progression and regression of advanced destructive periodontal disease. J Clin Periodontol. 1982;9(6):472–81. PubMed.
110. Socransky SS, Haffajee AD, Cugini MA, Smith C, Kent Jr RL. Microbial complexes in subgingival plaque. J Clin Periodontol. 1998;25(2):134–44. PubMed.
111. Kolenbrander PE, London J. Adhere today, here tomorrow: oral bacterial adherence. J Bacteriol. 1993;175(11):3247–52. PubMed Pubmed Central PMCID: 204720.
112. Slots J, Mashimo P, Levine MJ, Genco RJ. Periodontal therapy in humans. I. Microbiological and clinical effects of a single course of periodontal scaling and root planing, and of adjunctive tetracycline therapy. J Periodontol. 1979;50(10):495–509. PubMed.
113. Loesche WJ, Giordano JR, Hujoel P, Schwarcz J, Smith BA. Metronidazole in periodontitis: reduced need for surgery. J Clin Periodontol. 1992;19(2):103–12. PubMed.
114. Kumar PS, Mason MR, Brooker MR, O'Brien K. Pyrosequencing reveals unique microbial signatures associated with healthy and failing dental implants. J Clin Periodontol. 2012;39(5):425–33. PubMed Pubmed Central PMCID: 3323747.
115. Dabdoub SM, Tsigarida AA, Kumar PS. Patient-specific analysis of periodontal and peri-implant microbiomes. J Dent Res. 2013;92(12 Suppl):168S–75. PubMed Pubmed Central PMCID: 3827621.
116. Perez-Chaparro PJ, Goncalves C, Figueiredo LC, Faveri M, Lobao E, Tamashiro N, et al. Newly identified pathogens associated with periodontitis: a systematic review. J Dent Res. 2014;93(9):846–58. PubMed.
117. Ding T, Schloss PD. Dynamics and associations of microbial community types across the human body. Nature. 2014;509(7500):357–60. PubMed Pubmed Central PMCID: 4139711.
118. Yu X, Graves DT. Fibroblasts, mononuclear phagocytes, and endothelial cells express monocyte chemoattractant protein-1 (MCP-1) in inflamed human gingiva. J Periodontol. 1995;66(1):80–8. PubMed.
119. Seymour GJ, Powell RN, Aitken JF. Experimental gingivitis in humans. A clinical and histologic investigation. J Periodontol. 1983;54(9):522–8. PubMed.
120. Page RC, Schroeder HE. Pathogenesis of inflammatory periodontal disease. A summary of current work. Lab Invest. 1976;34(3):235–49. PubMed.
121. Theill LE, Boyle WJ, Penninger JM. RANK-L and RANK: T cells, bone loss, and mammalian evolution. Annu Rev Immunol. 2002;20:795–823. PubMed.
122. Ross AB, Bateman TA, Kostenuik PJ, Ferguson VL, Lacey DL, Dunstan CR, et al. The effects of osteoprotegerin on the mechanical properties of rat bone. J Mater Sci Mater Med. 2001;12(7):583–8. PubMed.
123. Kostenuik PJ, Shalhoub V. Osteoprotegerin: a physiological and pharmacological inhibitor of bone resorption. Curr Pharm Des. 2001;7(8):613–35. PubMed.
124. Parameter on periodontal maintenance. American Academy of Periodontology. J Periodontol. 2000;71(5 Suppl):849–50. PubMed.
125. Stambaugh RV, Dragoo M, Smith DM, Carasali L. The limits of subgingival scaling. Int J Periodontics Restorative Dent. 1981;1(5):30–41. PubMed.
126. Waerhaug J. The infrabony pocket and its relationship to trauma from occlusion and subgingival plaque. J Periodontol. 1979;50(7):355–65. PubMed.

127. Garrett S, Adams DF, Bogle G, Donly K, Drisko CH, Hallmon WW, et al. The effect of locally delivered controlled-release doxycycline or scaling and root planing on periodontal maintenance patients over 9 months. J Periodontol. 2000;71(1):22–30. PubMed.
128. Caton JG, Ciancio SG, Blieden TM, Bradshaw M, Crout RJ, Hefti AF, et al. Subantimicrobial dose doxycycline as an adjunct to scaling and root planing: post-treatment effects. J Clin Periodontol. 2001;28(8):782–9. PubMed.
129. Heasman PA, Heasman L, Stacey F, McCracken GI. Local delivery of chlorhexidine gluconate (PerioChip) in periodontal maintenance patients. J Clin Periodontol. 2001;28(1):90–5. PubMed.
130. Leiknes T, Leknes KN, Boe OE, Skavland RJ, Lie T. Topical use of a metronidazole gel in the treatment of sites with symptoms of recurring chronic inflammation. J Periodontol. 2007;78(8):1538–44. PubMed.
131. Ochsenbein C. A primer for osseous surgery. Int J Periodontics Restorative Dent. 1986;6(1):8–47. PubMed.
132. Tibbetts Jr LS, Ochsenbein C, Loughlin DM. Rationale for the lingual approach to mandibular osseous surgery. Dent Clin North Am. 1976;20(1):61–78. PubMed.
133. Cortellini P, Tonetti MS. Focus on intrabony defects: guided tissue regeneration. Periodontol 2000. 2000;22:104–32. PubMed.
134. Nyman S, Lindhe J, Rosling B. Periodontal surgery in plaque-infected dentitions. J Clin Periodontol. 1977;4(4):240–9. PubMed.
135. DeVore CH, Duckworth JE, Beck FM, Hicks MJ, Brumfield FW, Horton JE. Bone loss following periodontal therapy in subjects without frequent periodontal maintenance. J Periodontol. 1986;57(6):354–9. PubMed.
136. Knowles JW, Burgett FG, Nissle RR, Shick RA, Morrison EC, Ramfjord SP. Results of periodontal treatment related to pocket depth and attachment level. Eight years. J Periodontol. 1979;50(5):225–33. PubMed.
137. Lindhe J, Nyman S. Long-term maintenance of patients treated for advanced periodontal disease. J Clin Periodontol. 1984;11(8):504–14. PubMed.
138. Rosling B, Serino G, Hellstrom MK, Socransky SS, Lindhe J. Longitudinal periodontal tissue alterations during supportive therapy. Findings from subjects with normal and high susceptibility to periodontal disease. J Clin Periodontol. 2001;28(3):241–9. PubMed.
139. Ramfjord SP, Morrison EC, Burgett FG, Nissle RR, Shick RA, Zann GJ, et al. Oral hygiene and maintenance of periodontal support. J Periodontol. 1982;53(1):26–30. PubMed.
140. Rosen B, Olavi G, Badersten A, Ronstrom A, Soderholm G, Egelberg J. Effect of different frequencies of preventive maintenance treatment on periodontal conditions. 5-Year observations in general dentistry patients. J Clin Periodontol. 1999;26(4):225–33. PubMed.
141. Giannobile WV, Braun TM, Caplis AK, Doucette-Stamm L, Duff GW, Kornman KS. Patient stratification for preventive care in dentistry. J Dent Res. 2013;92(8):694–701. PubMed Pubmed Central PMCID: 3711568.
142. Ramseier CA, Kinney JS, Herr AE, Braun T, Sugai JV, Shelburne CA, et al. Identification of pathogen and host-response markers correlated with periodontal disease. J Periodontol. 2009;80(3):436–46. PubMed.
143. Syndergaard B, Al-Sabbagh M, Kryscio RJ, Xi J, Ding X, Ebersole JL, et al. Salivary biomarkers associated with gingivitis and response to therapy. J Periodontol. 2014;85(8):e295–303. PubMed.
144. Sexton WM, Lin Y, Kryscio RJ, Dawson 3rd DR, Ebersole JL, Miller CS. Salivary biomarkers of periodontal disease in response to treatment. J Clin Periodontol. 2011;38(5):434–41. PubMed Pubmed Central PMCID: 3095429.
145. Kinney JS, Morelli T, Oh M, Braun TM, Ramseier CA, Sugai JV, et al. Crevicular fluid biomarkers and periodontal disease progression. J Clin Periodontol. 2014;41(2):113–20. PubMed.
146. Giannobile WV, Beikler T, Kinney JS, Ramseier CA, Morelli T, Wong DT. Saliva as a diagnostic tool for periodontal disease: current state and future directions. Periodontol 2000. 2009;50:52–64. PubMed.
147. Agrawal P, Sanikop S, Patil S. New developments in tools for periodontal diagnosis. Int Dent J. 2012;62(2):57–64. PubMed.
148. Giannobile WV. Salivary diagnostics for periodontal diseases. J Am Dent Assoc. 2012;143(10 Suppl):6S–11. PubMed.
149. Yager P, Edwards T, Fu E, Helton K, Nelson K, Tam MR, et al. Microfluidic diagnostic technologies for global public health. Nature. 2006;442(7101):412–8. PubMed.
150. Giannobile WV, McDevitt JT, Niedbala RS, Malamud D. Translational and clinical applications of salivary diagnostics. Adv Dent Res. 2011;23(4):375–80. PubMed Pubmed Central PMCID: 3172998.
151. Kebschull M, Demmer RT, Grun B, Guarnieri P, Pavlidis P, Papapanou PN. Gingival tissue transcriptomes identify distinct periodontitis phenotypes. J Dent Res. 2014;93(5):459–68. PubMed Pubmed Central PMCID: 3988627.
152. Ivanov M, Barragan I, Ingelman-Sundberg M. Epigenetic mechanisms of importance for drug treatment. Trends Pharmacol Sci. 2014;35(8):384–96. PubMed.

# The Brain as a Therapeutic Target in TMD and Orofacial Pain: The Next Frontier in Personalized Pain Medicine and Health Technology

9

Alexandre F. DaSilva

**Abstract**

There is growing evidence that the cause for the chronicity in many TMD and orofacial pain patients may lie in the brain, instead of the peripheral areas where the symptoms reside. Accumulating data, stemming primarily from the area of neuroimaging, show that the transition from acute to chronic pain appears to be due to an alteration of specific neural systems as a maladaptation to the prolonged suffering, a phenomenon called neuroplasticity. As described by William James, a pioneering American psychologist, in his book *The Principles of Psychology* (1890): "*Plasticity* [...] *means the possession of a structure weak enough to yield to an influence, but strong enough not to yield all at once*." He attributed this inherent ability of adaptive changes to any organic matter, especially the nervous system, granting it a special degree of plasticity. Based on this principle, prolonged pain may induce ingrained alterations in the brain, which could explain the resilience of TMD and orofacial pain to conventional treatments in countless patients.

This chapter will describe new technologies that represent a change of paradigm in personalized treatment of pain patients: They objectively evaluate and modulate in vivo neuromechanisms in the brain depending on the patient's symptoms, even in the clinical environment, reaching far beyond the traditional clinical translational models.

## Introduction

Temporomandibular disorders (TMD) and orofacial pain are chronic conditions that highly affect patients' quality of life and productivity in our society. For example, TMD prevalence ranges from 8 to 15 % for women and 3 to 10 % for men [1]. A sizable number of TMD patients have a tendency

A.F. DaSilva, DDS, DMedSc
Biologic and Material Sciences Department, University of Michigan School of Dentistry, Ann Arbor, MI, USA
e-mail: adasilva@umich.edu





P.J. Polverini (ed.), *Personalized Oral Health Care: From Concept Design to Clinical Practice*, DOI 10.1007/978-3-319-23297-3_9 for chronicity and aggravation of their symptoms. In a study of 45,711 US households, nearly 11 % described TMD symptoms that persisted over a 6-month period [2]. In another large population-based study, 10 % of participants who reported TMD had severe pain upon jaw function [3]. Patients suffering from chronic TMD are frequently followed by multiple healthcare professionals and are subjected to various treatment modalities, including medications (e.g., tricyclic antidepressants, muscle relaxants), occlusal adjustment and appliances, trigger point (TP) injections, physical therapy, behavioral therapy, and surgeries [4, 5]. Approximately 10 % of TMD patients will not experience an improvement of their symptoms [6], and around 75 % of patients who fail to respond to conservative treatments are not suitable for TMJ surgery [7]. Unfortunately, it is not known which patients will benefit from the treatments described above at the acute stages and which will be at risk to experience perpetuation and/or worsening of the TMD symptoms even when the peripheral trigger or etiologic factor is eliminated.

Other orofacial pain conditions that contribute to patient distress are trigeminal neuropathic pain (TNP) disorders, such as post-herpetic and classical trigeminal neuralgias. They are debilitating chronic conditions that usually affect older adults, and their excruciating symptoms can be either spontaneous or intensely evoked by a light touch to the skin. However, one of the most common pain conditions in the dental office is dentin hypersensitivity, which is characterized by pain evoked by normally non-noxious thermal stimuli. This pain is often caused by unprotected dentinal tubules of the tooth caused by erosion, corrosion, abrasion, or periodontal recession. When affected by this condition, patients have to change their daily drinking and feeding habits.

The frustration that conventional treatments fail to relieve symptoms in a large number of TMD and orofacial pain patients [6] demonstrates that chronic pain and dysfunction must, in part, be sustained by more than peripheral-dependent mechanisms. It is believed that chronic pain may be induced by maladaptive changes that result in hyperexcitability of cortical and subcortical systems, rather than by the initial peripheral trigger (e.g., trauma), and may be influenced by other comorbidities, such as depression and anxiety, depending on the cortical area studied. This is reinforced by the fact that TMD and orofacial pain patients exhibit greater temporal summation on pain and unpleasantness and more frequent and stronger aftersensations than healthy subjects [8]. This increased sensitivity to sensory stimuli may be the result of peripheral and central sensitization and abnormal facilitation and disinhibition of afferent and/or efferent pathways. Previous studies show that the trigeminal sensorimotor cortex is susceptible to lasting neuroplastic changes following manipulation of afferent sensory and motor inputs [9].

In this chapter we will discuss novel neuroimaging and neuromodulatory techniques that have provided new tailored approaches into some brain mechanisms of chronic TMD and orofacial pain disorders. Many insights regarding the future of personalized diagnosis and treatment in those patients will be covered. First, how can brain mechanisms, even at the molecular level, in TMD and orofacial pain patients be assessed in vivo? Second, how can we apply these technologies in the clinical environment? Third, how can multiple cortical systems be directly and safely modulated for therapeutic and research purposes in pain patients? The understanding of these processes is crucial to determining the neuromechanisms involved in the persistence and, most importantly, the alleviation of symptoms based on the patients' condition and pain disorder.

## Neuroimaging of TMD and Orofacial Pain

The cortical mantle is a highly specialized, folded structure composed of a thin layer of gray matter. Abnormal variations in the thickness of the cortical mantle might reflect pathophysiological changes of intrinsic structure and integrity of the cortical laminae. Recently, some studies have shown this correlation in chronic pain diseases such as back pain [10], migraine [11, 12], and trigeminal neuropathic pain [13].. The implications of an alteration in these diseases are neuroplastic-associated mechanisms for each pain patient. Apkarian and colleagues [10] found reduction in the gray matter of the dorsolateral prefrontal cortex (DLPFC) of chronic back pain patients when compared to healthy controls using a volumetric-based approach. Similar results were found using highly sensitive and reliable neuroimaging tools [14] in trigeminal pain patients: Cortical thickness changes were spatially co-localized with functional allodynic (brush-induced pain) activation [13]. It seems that the pattern of concurrent structural and functional changes in the TNP patients was influenced by somatotopic localization (sensorimotor cortex), known functionality of the specific region (sensory-discriminative and affective-motivational), underlying activation/deactivation following allodynic stimulation, and the duration of the disorder. This suggests that overstimulation of the sensory-discriminative and affective-motivational neuronal systems in chronic pain induces structural alterations in the cortex that is co-localized with inefficient pain modulation by the opioid system. Recently, it was reported that cortical thickness in M1 and the anterior mid-cingulate cortices (aMCC) were negatively correlated to pain intensity in TMD patients [15]. The authors also reported that the gray matter volume in the sensory thalamus positively correlated to TMD duration.

## Molecular Assessment of the Brains of TMD and Orofacial Pain Patients

Endogenous opioid systems have long been implicated in regulating pain (nociceptive) signals, with μ-opioid receptors (μORs) being the primary mediators of opiate analgesia [16]. Both elements, endogenous opioid release and μOR concentrations, are therefore important components for the understanding of chronification and alleviation of pain in TMD patients. Our center was one of the first to publish direct evidence of endogenous μ-opioid activation during sustained trigeminal pain in healthy humans using PET, measured with external imaging as reductions in the in vivo availability of μOR binding potential ($BP_{ND}$) quantified with [$^{11}$C]carfentanil [17]. Immediate decreases in μOR $BP_{ND}$ were observed in several pain-related regions including the thalamus, periaqueductal gray matter, and nucleus accumbens, which correlated with reductions of sensory-emotional qualities of the pain task.

Comparable findings were observed with [$^{11}$C]diprenorphine in central poststroke and infarction pain patients [18, 19], which indicated neuroplasticity of receptor-mediated opioid mechanisms at rest in response to chronic pain. Using the selective μOR radiotracer [$^{11}$C]carfentanil, reductions in μOR $BP_{ND}$ localized in the ACC, nucleus accumbens, and amygdala were also observed in patients diagnosed with fibromyalgia syndrome [20]. In this sample, lower receptor concentrations were in fact associated with higher ratings of clinical pain.

We examined the regional μOR availability in vivo of TNP patients who were non-opiate users [21]. The clinical pain profile of the TNP patients recruited for this study was accessed using an in-house and free mobile application developed by the lab (PainTrek®, University of Michigan). This application provides a 3D map of orofacial pain that facilitates data entry and visualization by pain patients, including the elderly, as well as its tracking and analysis. Four TNP patients and eight age- and gender-matched healthy controls were scanned with PET. TNP patients had reduced μOR $BP_{ND}$ in the nucleus accumbens, an area associated with pain modulation and reward/aversive behaviors. Furthermore, the μOR $BP_{ND}$ in the NAc was negatively correlated with the McGill sensory and total pain ratings in the TNP patients.

The information above indicates that opioid mechanisms are highly influenced by the type of chronic pain disorder, therapeutic method, and cortical area studied. This technology can be used at the individual level in an extremely interactive way for research, clinical, and educational purposes. For instance, we investigated for the first time the brain of a migraine patient using fully immersive virtual 3D reality in vivo, which included unrestricted navigation through the neuroimaging data regarding availability of μ-opioid receptors (μOR $BP_{ND}$) [22]. The personalized and interactive approach demonstrated a

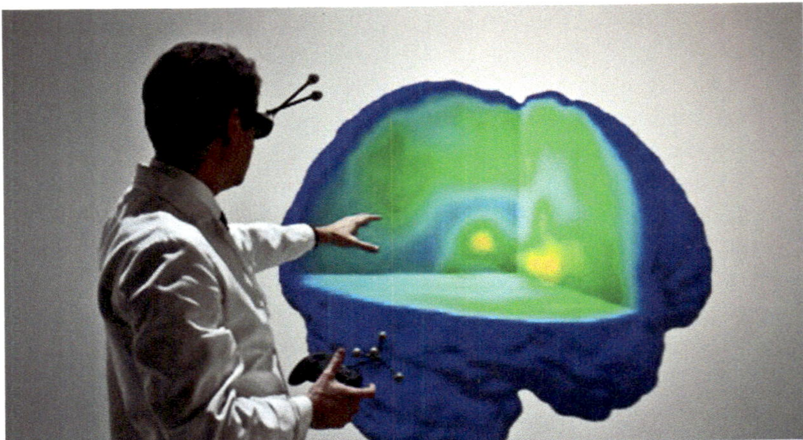

**Fig. 9.1** Full virtual reality 3D data navigation in a migrainous brain. We investigated for the first time actual migraine neuroimaging data in a fully immersive virtual 3D reality (3D-IIN), which includes unrestricted navigation through the data (by students, clinicians, and researchers) regarding availability of μ-opioid receptors (μOR $BP_{ND}$) in the brain during the migraine attack in vivo. We have been using it for data analysis and as a novel educational tool for our residents (From DaSilva et al. [22], used with permission from JoVE)

decrease in μ-opioid receptor availability (μOR $BP_{ND}$) in the brain of the patient during clinical pain. Reductions in μOR $BP_{ND}$ imply that there was a higher occupancy and/or a loss of μ-opioid receptors in the central nervous system. Acute reductions in μOR $BP_{ND}$ in pain-matrix regions during the ictal scan (headache phase) as compared to the interictal scan (non-headache phase) are expected to occur as a consequence of the release of endogenous opioids interacting with μORs as a modulatory response to the ongoing pain, making less μORs available to the radiotracer. We have been using this emerging 3D technology for data analysis and as a novel educational tool for our residents (Fig. 9.1).

## Assessment of the Brain Activity of Orofacial Pain Patients in a Dental Chair

The advancements in neuroimaging above have allowed for the study of many different neuroplastic mechanisms in TMD and orofacial pain patients. However, the use of those technologies in the clinic is often restricted due to their financial and functional characteristics. For instance, the patient has to be secluded and immobile in the scanner during the evaluation, and the costs of the neuroimaging scanners are too expensive for a clinical environment. Furthermore, MRI and PET scanners look at brain activation in a delayed temporal resolution, leading to possible artifacts in the data analysis.

Recently, a novel neuroimaging technology that enables real-time measurement of brain activity noninvasively has become available with several advantages over MRI and PET imaging; it is called functional near-infrared spectroscopy (fNIRS). fNIRS measures deoxyhemoglobin and oxyhemoglobin concentrations by using the specific absorption of near-infrared light to monitor their attenuation changes [23–25], allowing for the prompt measure of brain response during pain. fNIRS also requires short sessions, has relatively low cost, and is movable and safe to use (e.g., no radiation). These unique qualities are highly suitable to clinical and surgical environments for the evaluation of the cortical activity of TMD and orofacial pain patients in a personalized manner.

We have recently studied patients with hypersensitive teeth by using painful and non-painful stimuli in a clinical setting. While in a dental chair, subjects were tested using fNIRS to measure cortical activity during thermal stimulation of their affected tooth. In the somatosensory

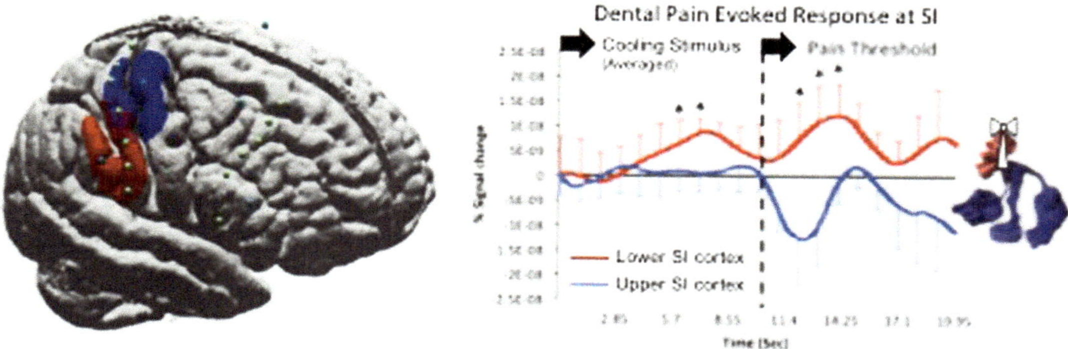


**Fig. 9.2** Dental pain evoked response at the somatosensory cortex. The *red/blue line* separately indicates the averaged responses at the lower/upper sensory cortex. The *vertical lines* indicate start of painful cooling stimulus and pain perception/threshold. The *blue and green dots* indicate the location of fNIRS probes (*blue*: light emitter, *green*: light detector) (From: Racek et al. [49]. Used with permission from SAGE Publications)

cortex contralateral to the stimulus, there were well-defined double hemodynamic peaks in the homuncular orofacial cortical region: an early peak during the cold, but non-painful phase and a late peak when the cold pain thresholds were trespassed. Furthermore, in the prefrontal cortices there were activations only in the non-painful phase, before the pain level was reached [26]. Interestingly, the prefrontal cortical areas deactivated during the actual dental pain experience. Then, we further investigated with fNIRS the immediate changes in resting-state functional connectivity (RSFC) between those two cortical regions, the primary somatosensory and bilateral prefrontal cortices, following the dental pain in the clinical environment. Increases in RSFC were found between the primary somatosensory cortex contralateral to the pain and the bilateral prefrontal cortices, as well as the prefrontal cortices. However, we noticed a decrease in RSFC between the bilateral inferior prefrontal cortices, with negative correlation with the level of pain intensity.

These findings indicate that clinical dental pain and experience have an immediate effect on the patients' brains not only during the expectation and experience of pain in the dental chair but also immediately after its occurrence by changing the sensory and cognitive function and connectivity in the patient's brain. Hence, these studies demonstrated for the first time that the individual global dental pain experience in the clinical setting elicits multiple hemodynamic cortical responses and may induce an ingrained aftereffect on the patients' brains (Fig. 9.2).

## Neuromodulation of the Brain Activity of Orofacial Pain Patients

Therapies that directly modulate brain activity might be implemented in the future to relieve chronic pain in individuals with TMD and orofacial pain when other conventional options fail. Amid the methods of brain neurostimulation, transcranial magnetic stimulation (TMS) and transcranial direct current stimulation (tDCS) are attractive as they can change brain activity in a noninvasive and safe manner. TMS was developed in 1985 [27] and is based on a time-varying magnetic field that creates an electric current and targets brain areas using appropriate stimulation coils [28]. It induces cortical modulation that can persist beyond the time of stimulation when applied frequently [29]. Although tDCS has dissimilar mechanisms of action, animal studies have consistently shown that it reliably modulates brain activity [30–32].

tDCS has potential advantages for the research of acute and chronic TMD and orofacial pain in comparison to TMS, including small portable size and non-expensive cost, and, most important, it can provide a more reliable placebo condition [33]. Several studies have shown the efficacy of tDCS in pain alleviation [34]. DCS is based on the application of a weak direct current to the scalp that flows between two electrodes, the anode and cathode. Its effects depend on polarity of stimulation, such that cathodal stimulation tends to induce a decrease in cortical excitability and anodal stimulation an increase in cortical excitability. In fact, application of tDCS for 13 min to the motor cortex can modulate cortical excitability for hours [35, 36]. Nonetheless, the efficacy of tDCS depends on the electrode montage and the duration and strength of the session [37, 38]. For example, M1 is a reliable target to modulate the sensory and motor subthalamic activity associated with chronic pain, independent of the type of stimulation applied [39–42], which also affects other pain-matrix structures. This occurs directly and indirectly because of the multiple connections between the corticospinal tract and thalamus. In fact, we were able to significantly decrease pain in chronic migraine patients following 10 M1-tDCS sessions. In our initial investigation, the immediate effect of M1-tDCS application induced great thalamic activation of the μ-opioid system in trigeminal neuropathic pain, even when controlling for placebo effect.

Using a finite element (FE) program (Simpleware Ltd., Exeter, UK), we analyzed the effect of our M1 cortex electrode montage, described above, on the current flow in the brain, taking into consideration the electrical properties of cortical and subcortical structures [43]. The human head model was based on a single high-spatial-resolution 3T MRI-derived FE from a healthy subject. The spatial focality of the analysis was restricted to our montage: the anode electrode over the motor cortex and the cathode electrode at the forehead above the contralateral supraorbital area (SO). Afterward, the head was segmented into compartments representing the brain tissues, cerebrospinal fluid, skull, muscle, fatty tissue, eyes, blood vessels, and scalp. One good analogy of our forward-tDCS analysis is the prediction of earthquake diffusion, taking into consideration a particular seismic strength and the terrain's geography and geology. Here, instead, it is the current strength, size/location of electrodes, head/brain anatomy, and white/gray matter constitution that dictate the flow of electricity. Our results show for the first time that significant electric fields are generated, not only in target cortical regions (M1) as previously reported but also in the posterior thalamus (e.g., VPM) and other pain-matrix regions: insula, ACC, and even the brain stem. Using this tDCS montage, we were able to decrease pain levels in patients with chronic migraine. Therefore, derived from our forward-tDCS analysis, this direct modulation of the pain matrix, especially the thalamus, may explain the therapeutic effects associated with our protocol.

Subsequently, we developed a unique protocol where the tDCS stimulation (20 min) is performed during the actual PET session without creating artifacts on the μOR $BP_{ND}$ or posing risks to the patient (e.g., controlling amount of resistance). To the best of our knowledge, this was the first time we are able to demonstrate that there is an immediate reduction in μ-opioid receptor binding in response to an acute motor cortex neuromodulation. During a single tDCS application, levels of μOR $BP_{ND}$ in a chronic trigeminal pain patient (post-herpetic neuralgia) were significantly reduced in the thalamus and other pain-matrix structures, including the nucleus accumbens, ACC, and insula, as predicted in our forward-tDCS model. Hence, the analgesic effect of tDCS is possibly due to an acute increase of endogenous opioid release, by direct and indirect effect of M1 stimulation on the thalamus and pain matrix [44].

M1 neuromodulation induces immediate changes in sensory perception in healthy subjects [45]. Acute tDCS modulates functional connectivity depending on its polarity [46], as anodal M1 and cathodal SO stimulation immediately increases functional coupling between the ipsilateral motor cortex and thalamus. In contrast, cathodal M1 modulation with tDCS decreases functional coupling between ipsilateral M1 and contralateral putamen.

We conducted further analysis to demonstrate that tDCS can significantly modulate μ-opioid mechanisms and trigeminal pain measures in vivo, even immediately [47]. This is a unique advancement in pain translation research in humans, previously only possible in animal models. We examined with PET healthy volunteers with no history of chronic pain or systemic disorders. The protocol consisted of two PET scans using [$^{11}$C]carfentanil, a selective μOR radiotracer. The first PET provided a baseline evaluation of regional μOR $BP_{ND}$. During the second PET, placebo and active (2 mA) M1(−SO) tDCS sessions were delivered sequentially for 20 min each, the same tDCS montage in our migraine study. When analyzed separately, placebo and active tDCS were both associated with an acute reduction in μOR $BP_{ND}$ in the periaqueductal gray matter, indicating activation of this neurotransmitter system. In addition, the initial placebo tDCS phase induced immediate activation of μORs in the left thalamus (Thal) and postcingulate cortex (PCC) and, subsequently, in the left prefrontal cortex (PreF) and precuneus (PreC) during the active tDCS phase. Furthermore, μOR system activation was positively correlated with improvements of hot and cold pain thresholds, measured by quantitative sensory testing. Our results suggest that immediate analgesia induced by the M1(−SO) tDCS application, placebo and active, can be related to the recruitment of shared and also dissimilar endogenous mu-opioid mechanisms.

In order to evaluate the analgesic effect of focally targeted M1 modulation, we have developed a novel M1 HD-tDCS montage with 2×2 electrode design and tested it on a cohort of patients with another chronic trigeminal pain illness, temporomandibular disorder (TMD) [48]. Our computational model simulated the montage's current flow through tissues captured with 3D imaging, accounting for the tissue type, tissue shape, tissue resistance, electrode positioning, and strength of the current. The greatest density was focused on the lower region of the precentral gyrus/sulcus, targeting the putative homuncular craniofacial M1 region, and immediately within the HD-tDCS ring electrodes. TMD patients were randomized into active and placebo

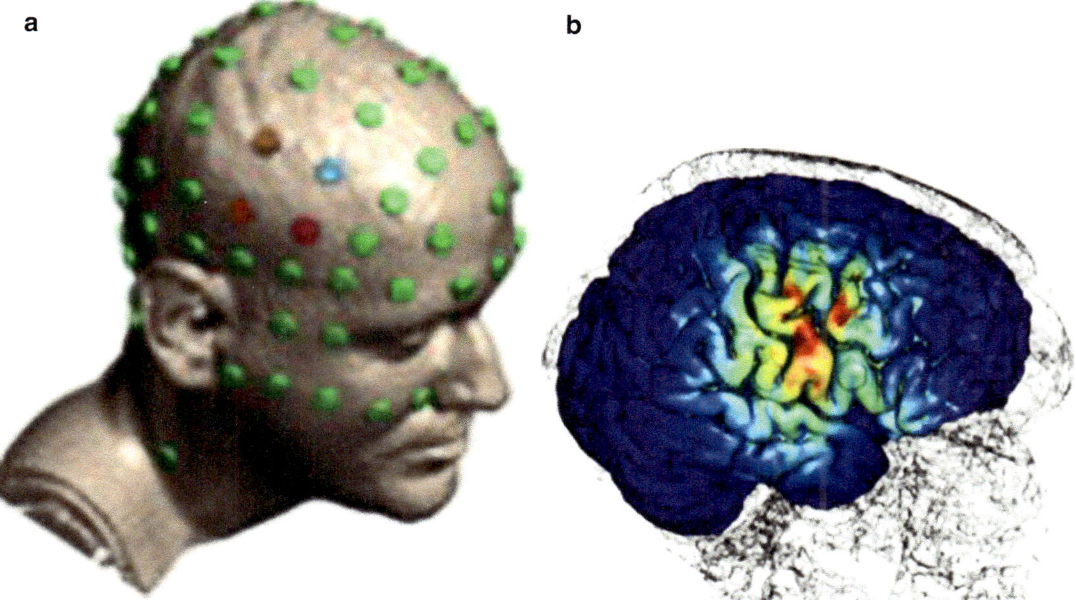


**Fig. 9.3** (**a**, **b**) M1 HD-tDCS montage: computational model of current distribution (right) showing predicted focalized peak on the lower homuncular portion of the precentral gyrus and sulcus in patients with chronic TMD during neuromodulation

groups. All patients completed the active or placebo 5-daily sessions of M1 HD-tDCS according to the protocol. There were statistically significant differences between groups for sensorimotor measurements, including VAS 50 % responders at one month follow-up, pain-free mouth opening at one week follow-up, and most important "exclusive" improvement of contralateral sensory-discriminative pain measures as collected by PainTrek (e.g., pain intensity, area, and their summation), not ipsilateral pain measures, during the treatment week (Fig. 9.3).

**Conclusions**

While understanding brain mechanisms in pain is important, equally important is applying these concepts to the clinical side of science. Novel neuroscience-driven technologies have improved immensely our ability to navigate and track brain activity related to acute and chronic pain at the individual level, even amid clinical and surgical procedures in situ, especially in patients who cannot express their suffering. In addition, we can now noninvasively modulate those dysfunctional activities in the brain of pain patients based on their own needs. Therefore, the brain is presenting itself as an objective and more reliable target for multiple emerging technologies to advance personalized treatment of chronic TMD and orofacial pain.

## References


1. LeResche L. Epidemiology of temporomandibular disorders: implications for the investigation of etiologic factors. Crit Rev Oral Biol Med. 1997;8: 291–305.
2. Lipton JA, Ship JA, Larach-Robinson D. Estimated prevalence and distribution of reported orofacial pain in the United States. J Am Dent Assoc. 1993;124: 115–21.
3. Salonen L, Hellden L, Carlsson GE. Prevalence of signs and symptoms of dysfunction in the masticatory system: an epidemiologic study in an adult Swedish population. J Craniomandib Disord. 1990;4:241–50.
4. DaSilva AF, Shaefer J, Keith DA. The temporomandibular joint: clinical and surgical aspects. Neuroimaging Clin N Am. 2003;13:573–82.
5. DaSilva AF, Acquadro MA. Orofacial pain. In: Ballantyne JC, editor. The Massachusetts General Hospital handbook of pain management. 3rd ed. Philadelphia: Lippincott Williams & Wilkins; 2005.
6. Okeson J. Management of temporomandibular disorders and occlusion. St. Louis: Mosby; 2003.
7. Dimitroulis G. The role of surgery in the management of disorders of the temporomandibular joint: a critical review of the literature. Part 2. Int J Oral Maxillofac Surg. 2005;34:231–7.
8. Sarlani E, Greenspan JD. Why look in the brain for answers to temporomandibular disorder pain? Cells Tissues Organs. 2005;180:69–75.
9. Sessle BJ, Yao D, Nishiura H, Yoshino K, Lee JC, Martin RE, et al. Properties and plasticity of the primate somatosensory and motor cortex related to orofacial sensorimotor function. Clin Exp Pharmacol Physiol. 2005;32:109–14.
10. Apkarian AV, Sosa Y, Sonty S, Levy RM, Harden RN, Parrish TB, et al. Chronic back pain is associated with decreased prefrontal and thalamic gray matter density. J Neurosci. 2004;24:10410–5.
11. Granziera C, DaSilva AF, Snyder J, Tuch DS, Hadjikhani N. Anatomical alterations of the visual motion processing network in migraine with and without aura. PLoS Med. 2006;3:e402.
12. DaSilva AF, Granziera C, Snyder J, Hadjikhani N. Thickening in the somatosensory cortex of patients with migraine. Neurology. 2007;69:1990–5.
13. DaSilva AF, Becerra L, Pendse G, Chizh B, Tully S, Borsook D. Colocalized structural and functional changes in the cortex of patients with trigeminal neuropathic pain. PLoS One. 2008;3:e3396.
14. Han X, Jovicich J, Salat D, van der Kouwe A, Quinn B, Czanner S, et al. Reliability of MRI-derived measurements of human cerebral cortical thickness: the effects of field strength, scanner upgrade and manufacturer. Neuroimage. 2006;32:180–94.
15. Moayedi M, Weissman-Fogel I, Crawley AP, Goldberg MB, Freeman BV, Tenenbaum HC, et al. Contribution of chronic pain and neuroticism to abnormal forebrain gray matter in patients with temporomandibular disorder. Neuroimage. 2011;5:277–86.
16. Sora I, Takahashi N, Funada M, Ujike H, Revay RS, Donovan DM, et al. Opiate receptor knockout mice define μ receptor roles in endogenous nociceptive responses and morphine-induced analgesia. Proc Natl Acad Sci U S A. 1997;94.
17. Zubieta JK, Smith YR, Bueller JM, Xu Y, Kilbourn MR, Meyer CR, et al. Regional mu opioid receptor regulation of sensory and affective dimensions of pain. Science. 2011;293:311–5.
18. Willoch F, Tolle TR, Wester HJ, Munz F, Petzold A, Schwaiger M, et al. Central pain after pontine infarction is associated with changes in opioid receptor binding: a PET study with 11C-diprenorphine. Am J Neuroradiol. 1999;20:686–90.
19. Willoch F, Schindler F, Wester HJ, Empl M, Straube A, Schwaiger M, et al. Central poststroke pain and reduced opioid receptor binding within pain processing circuitries: a [11C]diprenorphine PET study. Pain. 2004;108:213–20.
20. Harris RE, Clauw DJ, Scott DJ, McLean SA, Gracely RH, Zubieta JK. Decreased central mu-opioid receptor availability in fibromyalgia. J Neurosci. 2007;27: 10000–6.

21. DosSantos MF, Martikainen IK, Nascimento TD, Love TM, Deboer MD, Maslowski EC, et al. Reduced basal ganglia mu-opioid receptor availability in trigeminal neuropathic pain: a pilot study. Mol Pain. 2012;8:74.
22. DaSilva AF, Nascimento TD, Love T, DosSantos MF, Martikainen IK, Cummiford CM, et al. 3D-neuronavigation in vivo through a patient's brain during a spontaneous migraine headache. J Vis Exp. 2014;(88):e50682. doi:10.3791/50682.
23. Villringer A, Chance B. Non-invasive optical spectroscopy and imaging of human brain function. Trends Neurosci. 1997;20:435–42.
24. Chance B, Anday E, Nioka S, Zhou S, Hong L, Worden K, et al. A novel method for fast imaging of brain function, non-invasively, with light. Opt Express. 1998;2:411–23.
25. Izzetoglu M, Izzetoglu K, Bunce S, Ayaz H, Devaraj A, Onaral B, et al. Functional near-infrared neuroimaging. IEEE Trans Neural Syst Rehabil Eng. 2005;13:153–9.
26. Racek AJ, Xu XS, Nascimento TD, Bender MA, DaSilva AF. Real-time assessment of brain activity during dental pain and percussion in a clinical setting. IADR/AADR/CADR General Session, Boston; 2015.
27. Barker AT, Jalinous R, Freeston IL. Non-invasive magnetic stimulation of human motor cortex. Lancet. 1985;1:1106–7.
28. Pascual-Leone A, Tarazona F, Keenan J, Tormos JM, Hamilton R, Catala MD. Transcranial magnetic stimulation and neuroplasticity. Neuropsychologia. 1999; 37:207–17.
29. Pascual-Leone A, Bartres-Faz D, Keenan JP. Transcranial magnetic stimulation: studying the brain-behaviour relationship by induction of 'virtual lesions'. Philos Trans R Soc Lond B Biol Sci. 1999; 354:1229–38.
30. Brunoni AR, Fregni F, Pagano RL. Translational research in transcranial direct current stimulation (tDCS): a systematic review of studies in animals. Rev Neurosci. 2011;22:471–81.
31. Nitsche MA, Fricke K, Henschke U, Schlitterlau A, Liebetanz D, Lang N, et al. Pharmacological modulation of cortical excitability shifts induced by transcranial direct current stimulation in humans. J Physiol. 2003;553:293–301.
32. Nitsche MA, Liebetanz D, Antal A, Lang N, Tergau F, Paulus W. Modulation of cortical excitability by weak direct current stimulation – technical, safety and functional aspects. Suppl Clin Neurophysiol. 2003;56: 255–76.
33. Gandiga PC, Hummel FC, Cohen LG. Transcranial DC stimulation (tDCS): a tool for double-blind sham-controlled clinical studies in brain stimulation. Clin Neurophysiol. 2006;117:845–50.
34. Lima MC, Fregni F. Motor cortex stimulation for chronic pain: systematic review and meta-analysis of the literature. Neurology. 2008;70:2329–37.
35. Nitsche MA, Paulus W. Excitability changes induced in the human motor cortex by weak transcranial direct current stimulation. J Physiol. 2000;527(Pt 3):633–9.
36. Nitsche MA, Paulus W. Sustained excitability elevations induced by transcranial DC motor cortex stimulation in humans. Neurology. 2001;57:1899–901.
37. Nitsche MA, Liebetanz D, Lang N, Antal A, Tergau F, Paulus W. Safety criteria for transcranial direct current stimulation (tDCS) in humans. Clin Neurophysiol. 2003;114:2220–2; author reply 2222–3.
38. Nitsche MA, Nitsche MS, Klein CC, Tergau F, Rothwell JC, Paulus W. Level of action of cathodal DC polarisation induced inhibition of the human motor cortex. Clin Neurophysiol. 2003;114:600–4.
39. Garcia-Larrea L, Peyron R, Mertens P, Gregoire MC, Lavenne F, Bonnefoi F, et al. Positron emission tomography during motor cortex stimulation for pain control. Stereotact Funct Neurosurg. 1997;68:141–8.
40. Garcia-Larrea L, Peyron R, Mertens P, Gregoire MC, Lavenne F, Le Bars D, et al. Electrical stimulation of motor cortex for pain control: a combined PET-scan and electrophysiological study. Pain. 1999;83:259–73.
41. Strafella AP, Vanderwerf Y, Sadikot AF. Transcranial magnetic stimulation of the human motor cortex influences the neuronal activity of subthalamic nucleus. Eur J Neurosci. 2004;20:2245–9.
42. Lang N, Siebner HR, Ward NS, Lee L, Nitsche MA, Paulus W, et al. How does transcranial DC stimulation of the primary motor cortex alter regional neuronal activity in the human brain? Eur J Neurosci. 2005;22:495–504.
43. Dasilva AF, Mendonca ME, Zaghi S, Lopes M, Dossantos MF, Spierings EL, et al. tDCS-induced analgesia and electrical fields in pain-related neural networks in chronic migraine. Headache. 2012;52(8): 1283–95.
44. DosSantos MF, Love TM, Martikainen IK, Nascimento TD, Fregni F, Cummiford C, et al. Immediate effects of tDCS on the μ-opioid system of a chronic pain patient. Front Psychiatry. 2012;3:93.
45. Bachmann CG, Muschinsky S, Nitsche MA, Rolke R, Magerl W, Treede RD, et al. Transcranial direct current stimulation of the motor cortex induces distinct changes in thermal and mechanical sensory percepts. Clin Neurophysiol. 2010;121:2083–9.
46. Polania R, Paulus W, Nitsche MA. Modulating cortico-striatal and thalamo-cortical functional connectivity with transcranial direct current stimulation. Hum Brain Mapp. 2012;3:2499–508.
47. DosSantos MF, Martikainen IK, Nascimento TD, Love TM, DeBoer MD, Schambra HM, et al. Building up analgesia in humans via the endogenous mu-opioid system by combining placebo and active tDCS: a preliminary report. PLoS One. 2014;9:e102350.
48. Donnell A, Nascimento TD, Lawrence M, Gupata V, Zieba T, Truong DQ, et al. High-definition non-invasive brain modulation of sensorimotor dysfunction in chronic TMD. ADR/AADR/CADR General Session, Boston; 2015.
49. Racek AJ, Hu X, Nascimento TD, Bender MC, Khatib L, Chiego Jr D, Holland GR, Bauer P, McDonald N, Ellwood RP, DaSilva AF. Different brain responses to pain and its expectation in the dental chair. J Dent Res. 2015;94(7):998–1003.

# 10 Preparing the Next Generation of Oral Healthcare Professionals for a Personalized Oral Healthcare Environment

Peter J. Polverini

**Abstract**

A prospective healthcare system proposes shifting the focus from disease management to disease prevention and health promotion. Dentistry has a unique opportunity to embrace this model of healthcare and focus its attention on the management of oral health. To prepare future oral healthcare professionals to succeed in this new healthcare environment, dental schools will need to provide students with the scientific and technical knowledge required to understand and assess risk, employ new strategies to minimize disease progression, and place a greater emphasis on disease prevention. This will require innovative approaches to curriculum that include expanding knowledge domains such as genomic medicine and health policy and define new competencies to facilitate interprofessional education and high-value collaborative care. Dental schools must also consider developing career paths and new work force models that will accelerate the development of a prospective oral healthcare environment, increase access to care, and insure that dentistry maintains its leadership role in fostering optimal oral health.

## Introduction: Prospective Healthcare and The Emerging Personalized Healthcare Environment

A healthcare system that shifts the focus from disease management to disease prevention and health promotion defines the emerging "prospective" healthcare environment [1–7]. It is a system of care that encourages interprofessional education and high-value collaborative care [8–13]. By embracing this prospective and collab-

P.J. Polverini, DDS, DMSc
Department of Periodontics and Oral Medicine,
University of Michigan School of Dentistry,
Ann Arbor, MI, USA
e-mail: neovas@umich.edu





P.J. Polverini (ed.), *Personalized Oral Health Care: From Concept Design to Clinical Practice*,
DOI 10.1007/978-3-319-23297-3_10

orative model of care, the dental profession can focus more on the management of oral health by managing risk and developing innovative diagnostic and interventional strategies designed to minimize disease progression [3, 14]. In many settings there continues to be limited or no access to care, and when care is delivered, it is often sporadic, uncoordinated, and fragmented [8, 11–13]. Our current healthcare system focuses primarily on disease management and less so on health promotion and prevention. In many respects, dentists employ the same ineffective approach to care delivered by other healthcare professionals [3–7]. Dentists, like physicians, take a reductionist approach to disease diagnosis [5, 6]. They use scientific principles to identify the chief complaint, develop a series of differentials, and, using diagnostic aids, arrive at a diagnosis that guides treatment. While this approach has enabled health professionals to better manage, and in some cases cure, disease, it tends to oversimplify and discount the impact of culture, lifestyle choices, and environmental influences. More importantly, it tends to look at optimal health as the absence of disease rather than the result of a well-designed, personalized plan to maintain health [3]. We are a product of our genetic constitution and the environment we live in. Lifestyle choices and the availability of care will determine our risk for disease and the stage at which disease is first detected (Fig. 10.1). What is missing in today's healthcare setting is a personalized plan for disease prevention and health promotion, one that focuses more on prevention, risk assessment, and early intervention [1–8, 11, 13, 15–17].

As the prospective healthcare environment takes shape, healthcare professionals, including dentists, will be expected to place greater emphasis on assessing disease risk, focus more on prevention and personalized treatment, and enable greater involvement of patients in the decision-making process [9]. Driven largely by the rapid acceleration in the cost of providing care, a prospective approach to healthcare has the potential to address the need to improve patient care while reducing costs and increasing efficiencies [1–7, 9].

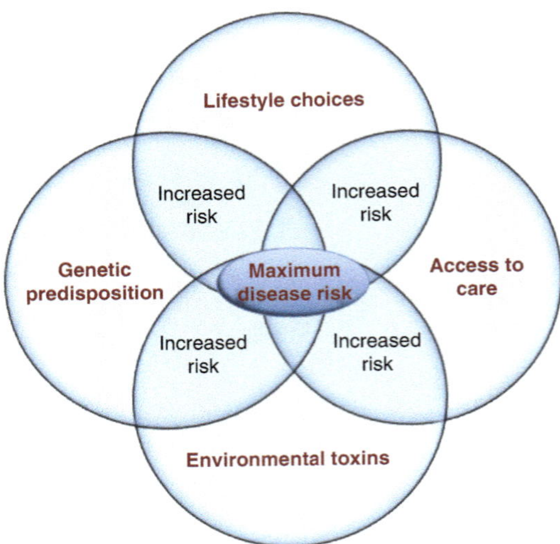


**Fig. 10.1** The impact of genetic constitution, the environment, lifestyle choices, and the availability of care on disease risk and disease onset are shown

## Personalized Oral Healthcare and the Changing Education and Practice Environment

Providing the patients with the right care at the right time that results in a measurable improvement in health outcomes at a lower cost will define personalized oral healthcare [3]. This process will require a very different approach to healthcare. Providers will be incentivized and reimbursed for preventing disease and helping patients develop a personal plan for achieving optimal oral health. Oral healthcare professionals will be expected to manage a diverse workforce and spend more time promoting health literacy and partnering with patients in the provision of care [9, 18]. They will also need to develop a deeper understanding of the complex interplay between factors that both determine health and those that lead to chronic disease. To be successful in this new healthcare environment, oral healthcare professionals will need to be conversant with the emerging sciences of genomic medicine, bio- and health-informatics and health policy, and be knowledgeable about the power and limitation of the emerging "omic" technologies [19–26].

To overcome the current fragmented and uncoordinated healthcare environment, dental professionals will be expected to function in collaborative healthcare teams working shoulder to shoulder with other healthcare providers and community leaders [13, 27–39]. Dentists will be expected to embrace their health professional colleagues in a setting that is both challenging and exciting. The IOM report "Health Professions Education, a Bridge to Quality" outlines a series of core competencies for an outcome-based education system that better prepares practitioners to meet the needs of their patients and enables them to function effectively as a member of a patient-centered healthcare team [10]. First, healthcare professionals will be expected to work with other healthcare professionals and allied healthcare providers in nonhierarchical, interdisciplinary teams. Second, healthcare professionals will be expected to routinely employ evidence-based principals in the care of their patients. Third, team members will be expected to apply quality improvement in the context of a learning healthcare environment [40, 41]. This is expected to be an iterative process whereby data from patient care and team-based experiences is translated into evidence-based practice that leads to improved outcomes and increased efficiencies. In this setting the learning healthcare system utilizes health information technology, databases, the electronic healthcare record, and a supporting research infrastructure that continues to advance and improve patient outcomes. The application of the most up-to-date evidence in all aspects of the patient care environment will continue to define and refine those processes that underpin a learning healthcare system. Most importantly, patients will be expected to participate in the decisions that affect their care. Oral health professionals must have an understanding of the values and ethics that underpin a successful collaborative care environment and understand and respect the roles and responsibilities of the provider team. To be effective in this setting, the healthcare team must develop skills in interprofessional communication and understand the goals that promote successful teamwork [13, 27, 29–34, 36–42].

Health professional schools will need to provide the foundation for a continuous learning environment that supports new interprofessional competencies and their adoption across the health professions. These competencies will serve to guide curricula development, encourage innovative approaches to learning and teaching, and advance assessment strategies to achieve productive outcomes. Competencies will be driven by individual patient needs and communities of interest. The proposed new competencies will require periodic assessment to fine-tune and shape the educational and practice setting outcomes (Fig. 10.2). Ongoing evaluation of existing knowledge domains and competencies will require the development of a creative educational research agenda that will serve to strengthen scholarship and promote innovation. Continued evaluation and refinement of competencies will be needed to ensure an optimal environment for collaborative practice that supports patient needs. It will be important to integrate core interprofessional educational content with current

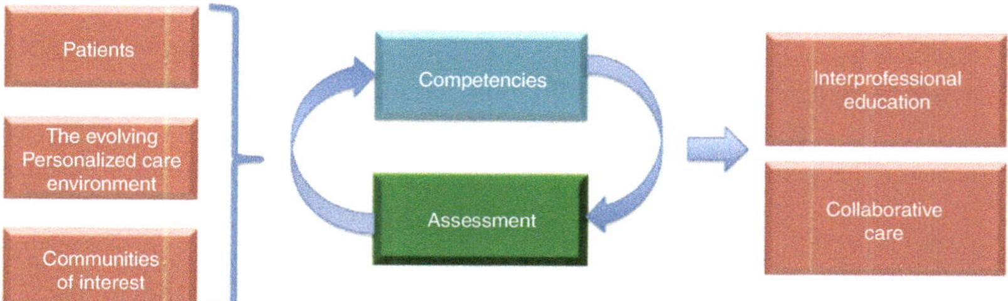


**Fig. 10.2** Dentistry has long employed a competency-based educational program to guide curricular design. All too often however, schools change their objectives to meet what the faculty want to teach so that the objectives drive the curriculum. Many of these changes lead to incremental rather than transformative curricular changes that fail to improve care or reflect what patients need and want. As healthcare becomes more patient centered, patient needs will play a key role in recalibrating patient-centered competencies and in curriculum development

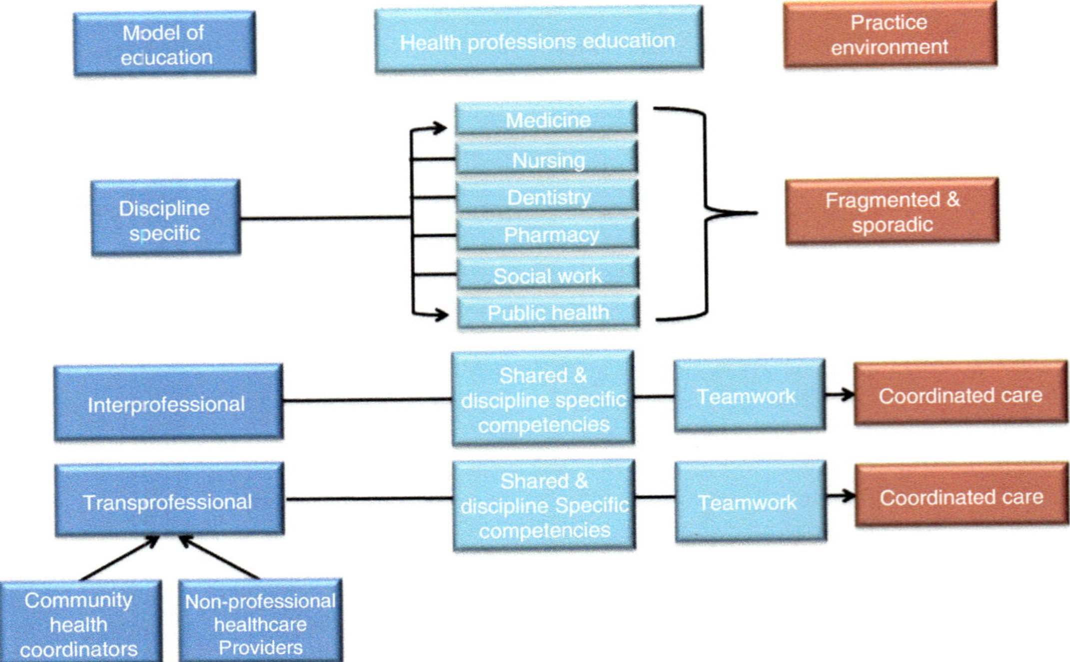


**Fig. 10.3** The health professions education models depicted here contrast the current principal model of siloed education with the emerging interprofessional and transprofessional models of education and practice. Healthcare professionals working in teams with and without nonprofessional providers will become the norm in the near future, replacing the inefficient silo-like approach to healthcare

accreditation standards for each of the health professions. Education programs and accrediting agencies will need to set common standards across the health professions that support interprofessional education and collaborative care. These new core competencies will inform professional licensing and credentialing bodies in defining appropriate content for the purpose of developing credentialing standards for collaborative practice. Figure 10.3, adapted from Frenk et al. shows how the evolving interprofessional and transprofessional education and practice environment may take shape and replace the siloed education that health professional students now experience [43].

## Essential Knowledge Domains for the New Oral Healthcare Professional

In the 1894 Gies report, it was acknowledged that dentistry should be considered an integral member of the university community and strive to attain the highest level of scholarly excellence [44]. The report stipulated that the dental professional must be a product of a continuous learning environment, one that encourages self-reflection and uses the rigorous application of scientific evidence to advance the profession and patient care. These expectations take on even greater significance in the emerging prospective healthcare environment. Dental schools must take the lead in advancing the profession by reaffirming the rigorous application of science as it educates future oral healthcare providers and by embracing research and discovery as a core value. A fundamental requirement for a successful oral healthcare environment in the future will be the creation of a more collaborative and integrated approach to overall healthcare [13, 27–41].

Advances in the "omic" technologies (i.e., genomic, proteomics, metabolomics, transcripotomics) are rapidly changing the healthcare landscape. What that change will mean in the long run, while uncertain, necessitates that oral healthcare professionals not only acquire the knowledge and skills required to understand both the power and limitations of this new technology but also understand how to apply this knowledge to develop a personalized approach to care for patients. As lifelong learners, oral healthcare professionals will be expected to keep pace with the rapidly advancing field of genomic medicine to more rationally apply this knowledge to their patients and, most importantly, to understand underlying concepts that will be required to develop an appreciation for the clinical application of this knowledge to the care of their patients [18–26, 45–52].

Greater emphasis will need to be placed on existing and new knowledge domains that better prepare oral healthcare professionals to practice in a personalized healthcare environment. As knowledge of the genetic basis of common oral disease continues to advance, healthcare providers will be expected to have a working knowledge of genomic medicine if they are to manage their patients effectively. The knowledge value of genomic medicine lies in its application to disease risk. The healthcare professionals who understand the potential impact of genomic medicine on patient care will be well prepared to effectively apply advances in genomic medicine to the care of their patients. At a minimum, oral healthcare professionals will need to use genomic data to assess risk and how best to inform and interpret the results for their patients. This is particularly true today where over-the-counter genetic testing is often used inappropriately to assess risk, leading to misinterpretation of results [53]. While there are a number of single-gene disorders that affect the orofacial structures, as genomic medicine continues to develop a genetic basis for many of the most common dental diseases, more will no doubt be revealed [45–52]. As with all health-related disciplines, educating oral healthcare professionals about genetics and genomics will be essential for clinical practice. Although medical schools continue to increase genetic content of the undergraduate curriculum, students in the dental profession in United States and Europe continue to lag behind other healthcare professionals in their knowledge of genetic and genomic medicine [54–60]. While most dentists may believe that genomic medicine is peripheral to their practice, the ability to understand the power and limitations of genetic testing will be an important part of the oral healthcare professional's toolbox in the emerging personalized healthcare environment [56].

Another knowledge domain that will be necessary to navigate in the emerging personalized oral healthcare environment is healthcare policy. A number of medical schools have developed programs to educate physicians about the impact of healthcare systems and healthcare economics on health policy [61–63]. For example, an understanding of the values and importance of comparative and cost-effective research and evidence-based practice will require that dental schools develop curricula in this domain. If the personalized oral healthcare environment is to have a meaningful impact of the oral health of patients, dental schools must embrace these new educational initiatives.

## How Interprofessional Education and Collaborative Care Will Influence the Future of Personalized Oral Healthcare

The long-term outcomes of a successful collaboration among the health professions include optimized patient care, enhanced health system efficiency, lower costs, and an increase in both patient and provider satisfaction [9, 40, 41]. The framework for a successful interprofessional education program and collaborative care environment rests on four core competencies. These are: (1) communication that enhances interprofessional collaboration and team work; (2) role clarification that defines the scope of practice for each of the collaborating health professions; (3) understanding the roles, responsibility, and value added by of each member of the team; and (4) periodic critical evaluation to assess the impact of the collaborative care team on the health outcomes of patients [9–11, 13, 43].

As interprofessional learning better prepares health professional students for an ever-changing healthcare system, collaborative care and teamwork will be key to a successful personalized healthcare environment. Workforce-ready graduates will need skills to meet increasingly complex patient needs, adapt to changing technology that will influence dental practice, and function effectively in diverse practice settings. Given the prohibitive cost of the current healthcare system and the increasing inaccessibility of high-value healthcare to a large segment of the population, there is little reason not to embrace that collaborative approach to education and patient care. Breaking down the current siloed approach to health profession education and practice care can only enhance the value of each of the health professions, while at the same time advancing a healthcare system that is more efficient, patient centered, and health management driven. In addition to making better use of existing services, the dental profession must explore new workforce models that help meet the oral healthcare needs of the growing underserved population [9–11, 13, 43].

## How a Personalized Oral Healthcare Environment Will Reshape Dental Practice

Collaboration with and integration of the health professions will significantly alter the practice landscape [13, 27–39, 64]. Dental students will be expected to share educational and patient care experiences with other healthcare providers. The scope of the dental practice will likely change as we see more routine dental procedures being performed by other health professionals, freeing the dentist to focus more on managing the care of patients as part of an integrated healthcare team. New dental graduates will be expected to serve in leadership and advisory roles in the development of oral healthcare policies. The emerging prospective healthcare environment will continue to put pressure on all health professions to personalize care and increase access to underserved populations. This will require dental schools to expand educational and professional opportunities for our graduates in support of these new opportunities. New graduates must have a working knowledge of the latest scientific advances that shape an emerging prospective oral healthcare environment. This will require a number of fundamental changes in the educational content of dental education programs and the environment in which dental students are educated [31, 32, 54–63, 65–71].

The concept of the "Health Home"—where primary care providers, families, and patients work collaboratively to improve health outcomes and quality of life for patients with chronic disabilities and disease—will only become a reality when dentistry embraces an integrated healthcare environment [9]. As the concept of prospective oral healthcare gains momentum, there will be increased pressure on the academic dentistry and the profession to focus more on risk assessment and disease prevention rather than on restorative and surgical care. This will no doubt lead to significant changes in the scope of dental practice. The successful practitioners will focus more on helping patients learn to manage their own health and less on the management of common chronic oral diseases such as dental caries and periodontal disease.

A greater focus on managing disease risk and disease prevention will be another defining feature of the personalized oral healthcare environment. New technologies will provide dentists with greater capabilities to predict early disease onset and minimize disease progression and thus initiate treatment that it is more cost-effective [3–7]. This concept of prospective healthcare will have a transformative effect on the healthcare system. If dentistry is to be part of a prospective healthcare environment, future practitioners must be able to utilize the most up-to-date technologies that will enable risk assessment and facilitate the creation of a personalized health plan for their patients.

Many of these new technologies that are designed to aid in point-of-care decisions about disease risk or early diagnoses are evolving rapidly and reflect technological and knowledge-driven advances in genomics, proteomics, and metabolomics [19–26]. It will no longer be necessary for dentists to rely solely on clinical biomarkers to assess disease risk, onset, and progression. Rather, the identification of patient-specific molecular profiles that reveal disease susceptibility or predict early disease onset will be among the principal tools used by the new practitioner. Genomic medicine will be a major catalyst in the implementation of point-of-care diagnostics and patient-specific biomarkers. These advances will rapidly accelerate the adoption of personalized oral healthcare [19–26, 45–52].

## Conclusions

Both William Gies and Abraham Flexner had a profound influence on the education of dentists and physicians, respectively [44, 66]. Their influence on the standardization of curricula, their emphasis of scientific rigor, and their insistence on academic integrity remain the cornerstone of a modern health professions curriculum. There are several opportunities to be considered when envisioning a prospective oral healthcare curriculum. If students are expected to compete successfully in this new healthcare environment and be productive members of an integrated team of health professionals, several important elements in curriculum development must be taken into consideration [31, 32]. The emerging prospective healthcare environment will provide enormous opportunities for innovation and leadership. The exploration of new academic partnerships with the other health professions will enable future dental practitioners to deliver the highest quality, patient-centered oral healthcare to an increasingly diverse patient population. Figure 10.4 envisions what an interprofessional curriculum might look like. While each of the health professions would have their discipline-specific competencies and course work, there would also be a significant investment in a shared educational environment. This would extend to collaborative practice experiences that would serve as a model for the "Health Home."

To meet these objectives, it will also be necessary to recast traditional dental educational programs and consider developing alternative career tracks that will enable students to assume important leadership roles in public health, public policy, research, leadership, and community service. This new emphasis on alternative career pathways, along with the adoption of new knowledge domains and reintegration of dental education with medicine, will produce a dental graduate more capable of managing patient health in a

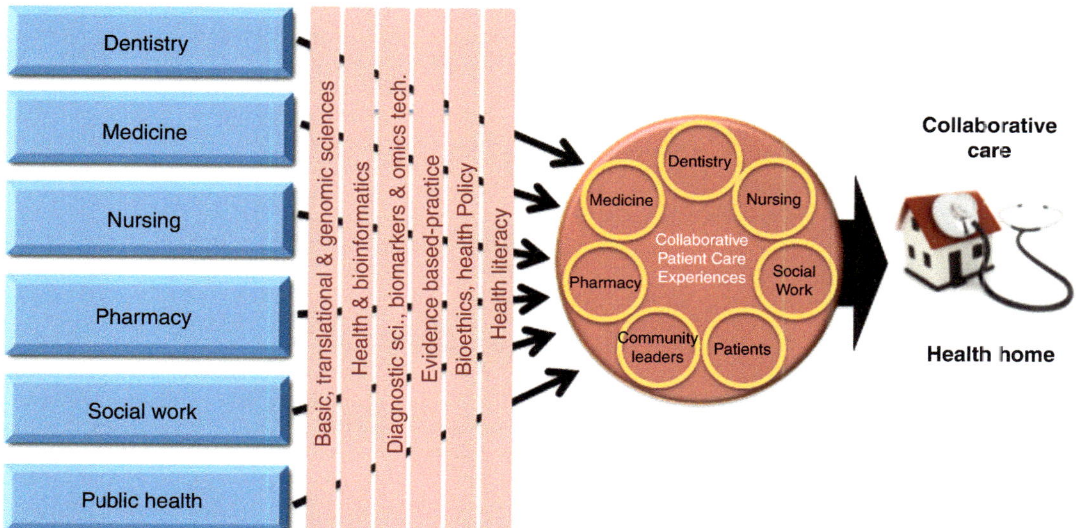


**Fig. 10.4** This depicts how discipline-specific and shared education and patient care experiences will prepare health professional students for a collaborative care environment

more collaborative setting and who will be instrumental in leading this change. A recent perspective article in the *New England Journal of Medicine* points out that the continued artificial separation of dentistry from medicine and the lack of value place on oral health has imposed significant costs on the healthcare system and society. Indeed, closer integration of oral and general health at the level of education and patient care would result in greater efficiencies, lower costs, and improved patient outcomes [72].

Success in meeting the demands of a prospective healthcare environment requires empowering graduating dentists with the ability to employ the most up-to-date scientific knowledge and evidence that informs and transforms diagnosis, therapy, and patient care. The linkages between oral and systemic health must be emphasized through the entire educational experience and practice environment will all health professional students. The next generation of dental practitioners must be prepared to influence oral healthcare policy at the regional and national levels and lead teams of healthcare providers in developing new strategies to improve oral health for local, regional, and global communities. The dental practitioner of the future will be fully integrated with the other health science disciplines and will thrive on interdisciplinary and cross-disciplinary collaboration. Creating a collaborative learning and practice environment will empower future dental practitioners to function in a more efficient healthcare environment that is focused on managing oral and general health rather than disease [42, 65, 67–72].

## References


1. Dinan MA, Simmons LA, Snyderman R. Commentary: personalized health planning and the patient protection and Affordable Care Act: an opportunity for academic medicine to lead health care reform. Acad Med. 2010;85(11):1665–8.
2. Hamburg MA, Collins FS. The path to personalized medicine. N Engl J Med. 2010;363(4):301–4.
3. Snyderman R. Personalized health care: from theory to practice. Biotechnol J. 2012;7(8):973–9.
4. Snyderman R, Dinan MA. Improving health by taking it personally. JAMA. 2010;303(4):363–4.
5. Snyderman R, Williams RS. Prospective medicine: the next health care transformation. Acad Med. 2003;78(11):1079–84.
6. Snyderman R, Yoediono Z. Prospective care: a personalized, preventative approach to medicine. Pharmacogenomics. 2006;7(1):5–9.
7. Snyderman R, Yoediono Z. Perspective: prospective health care and the role of academic medicine: lead, follow, or get out of the way. Acad Med. 2008;83(8):707–14.
8. Institute of Medicine (U.S.). Committee on an Oral Health Initiative. Advancing oral health in America. Washington, D.C: National Academies Press; 2011. p. xviii, 248.
9. Institute of Medicine (U.S.). Committee on Quality of Health Care in America. Crossing the quality chasm: a new health system for the 21st century. Washington, D.C: National Academy Press; 2001. p. xx, 337.
10. Greiner A, Knebel E, Institute of Medicine (U.S.). Board on Health Care Services, Institute of Medicine (U.S.). Committee on the Health Professions Education Summit. Health professions education: a bridge to quality. Washington, D.C: National Academies Press; 2003. p. xvi, 175.
11. United States Department of Health and Human Services. Healthy people 2010: understanding and improving health. Washington, DC: U.S. Dept. of Health and Human Services; 2000. p. 63.
12. Committee on Oral Health Access to Services (U.S.), National Research Council (U.S.). Board on Children Youth and Families, Institute of Medicine (U.S.). Board on Health Care Services. Improving access to oral health care for vulnerable and underserved populations. Washington, D.C: National Academies Press; 2011. p. xvii, 279.
13. United States Department of Health and Human Services, National Institute of Dental and Craniofacial Research (U.S.). Oral health in America: a report of the Surgeon General. Rockville: U.S. Public Health Service, Dept. of Health and Human Services; 2000. p. xxiv, 308.
14. Polverini PJ. A curriculum for the new dental practitioner: preparing dentists for a prospective oral health care environment. Am J Public Health. 2012; 102(2):e1–3.
15. Godman B, Finlayson AE, Cheema PK, Zebedin-Brandl E, Gutierrez-Ibarluzea I, Jones J, et al. Personalizing health care: feasibility and future implications. BMC Med. 2013;11:179.
16. Manolio TA. Genomewide association studies and assessment of the risk of disease. N Engl J Med. 2010;363(2):166–76.
17. Payne PR, Marsh CB. Towards a "4I" approach to personalized healthcare. Clin Transl Med. 2012; 1(1):14.

18. Syurina EV, Brankovic I, Probst-Hensch N, Brand A. Genome-based health literacy: a new challenge for public health genomics. Public Health Genomics. 2011;14(4–5):201–10.
19. Chen R, Mias GI, Li-Pook-Than J, Jiang L, Lam HY, Chen R, et al. Personal omics profiling reveals dynamic molecular and medical phenotypes. Cell. 2012;148(6):1293–307.
20. Chen R, Snyder M. Systems biology: personalized medicine for the future? Curr Opin Pharmacol. 2012;12(5):623–8.
21. Chen R, Snyder M. Promise of personalized omics to precision medicine. Wiley Interdiscip Rev Syst Biol Med. 2013;5(1):73–82.
22. Ginsburg GS, Willard HF. Genomic and personalized medicine: foundations and applications. Transl Res. 2009;154(6):277–87.
23. Langheier JM, Snyderman R. Prospective medicine: the role for genomics in personalized health planning. Pharmacogenomics. 2004;5(1):1–8.
24. Miller CS, Foley JD, Bailey AL, Campell CL, Humphries RL, Christodoulides N, et al. Current developments in salivary diagnostics. Biomark Med. 2010;4(1):171–89.
25. Tanaka H. Omics-based medicine and systems pathology. A new perspective for personalized and predictive medicine. Methods Inf Med. 2010;49(2):173–85.
26. Wong DT. Salivary diagnostics powered by nanotechnologies, proteomics and genomics. J Am Dent Assoc. 2006;137(3):313–21.
27. Accreditation CD. Accreditation standards for dental education programs. Chicago: American Dental Association; 2010.
28. Blue AV, Mitcham M, Smith T, Raymond J, Greenberg R. Changing the future of health professions: embedding interprofessional education within an academic health center. Acad Med. 2010;85(8):1290–5.
29. Crall JJ. Oral health policy development since the Surgeon General's Report on Oral Health. Acad Pediatr. 2009;9(6):476–82.
30. Crosson FJ. 21st-century health care – the case for integrated delivery systems. N Engl J Med. 2009;361(14):1324–5.
31. DePaola DP. The revitalization of U.S. dental education. J Dent Educ. 2008;72(2 Suppl):28–42.
32. DePaola DP, Slavkin HC. Reforming dental health professions education: a white paper. J Dent Educ. 2004;68(11):1139–50.
33. Formicola A, Valachovic RW, Chmar JE, Mouradian W, Bertolami CN, Tedesco L, et al. Curriculum and clinical training in oral health for physicians and dentists: report of panel 2 of the Macy study. J Dent Educ. 2008;72(2 Suppl):73–85.
34. Foundation RWJ, editor. Team based competencies: building a shared foundation for education and clinical practice. Washington, D.C.: Team Based Competencies; 2011.
35. Garcia RI, Inge RE, Niessen L, DePaola DP. Envisioning success: the future of the oral health care delivery system in the United States. J Public Health Dent. 2010;70 Suppl 1:S58–65.
36. Lavin MA, Ruebling I, Banks R, Block L, Counte M, Furman G, et al. Interdisciplinary health professional education: a historical review. Adv Health Sci Educ Theory Pract. 2001;6(1):25–47.
37. Mitchell PH, Belza B, Schaad DC, Robins LS, Gianola FJ, Odegard PS, et al. Working across the boundaries of health professions disciplines in education, research, and service: the University of Washington experience. Acad Med. 2006;81(10):891–6.
38. Interprofessional Education Collaborative Expert Panel. Core competencies for interprofessional collaborative practice: report of an expert panel. Washington, D.C: American Dental Education Association; 2011.
39. Tedesco LA. Revising accreditation processes and standards to address current challenges in dental education. J Dent Educ. 2008;72(2 Suppl):46–50.
40. Friedman CP, Wong AK, Blumenthal D. Achieving a nationwide learning health system. Sci Transl Med. 2010;2(57):57cm29.
41. Olsen L, Aisner D, McGinnis JM, Institute of Medicine (U.S.) Roundtable on Evidence-Based Medicine. The learning healthcare system: workshop summary. Washington, DC: National Academies Press; 2007. p. xx, 354.
42. Garcia I, Kuska R, Somerman MJ. Expanding the foundation for personalized medicine: implications and challenges for dentistry. J Dent Res. 2013;92(7 Suppl):3S–10.
43. Frenk J, Chen L, Bhutta ZA, Cohen J, Crisp N, Evans T, et al. Health professionals for a new century: transforming education to strengthen health systems in an interdependent world. Lancet. 2010;376(9756):1923–58.
44. Gies WJ. Dental education in the United States and Canada. A report to the Carnegie Foundation for the advancement of teaching. 1926. J Am Coll Dent. 2012;79(2):32–49.
45. Davies SM. Pharmacogenetics, pharmacogenomics and personalized medicine: are we there yet? Hematology Am Soc Hematol Educ Program. 2006:111–7.
46. Feero WG, Guttmacher AE, Collins FS. Genomic medicine – an updated primer. N Engl J Med. 2010;362(21):2001–11.
47. Issa AM. Evaluating the value of genomic diagnostics: implications for clinical practice and public policy. Adv Health Econ Health Serv Res. 2008;19: 191–206.
48. Nibali L, Donos N, Henderson B. Periodontal infectogenomics. J Med Microbiol. 2009;58(Pt 10):1269–74.
49. Tanke HJ. Genomics and proteomics: the potential role of oral diagnostics. Ann N Y Acad Sci. 2007; 1098:330–4.
50. West M, Ginsburg GS, Huang AT, Nevins JR. Embracing the complexity of genomic data for personalized medicine. Genome Res. 2006; 16(5):559–66.

51. Weston AD, Hood L. Systems biology, proteomics, and the future of health care: toward predictive, preventative, and personalized medicine. J Proteome Res. 2004;3(2):179–96.
52. Wright JT, Hart TC. The genome projects: implications for dental practice and education. J Dent Educ. 2002;66(5):659–71.
53. Annas GJ, Elias S. 23andMe and the FDA. N Engl J Med. 2014;370(23):2248–9.
54. Guttmacher AE, Porteous ME, McInerney JD. Educating health-care professionals about genetics and genomics. Nat Rev Genet. 2007;8(2):151–7.
55. Haiech J, Kilhoffer MC. Personalized medicine and education: the challenge. Croat Med J. 2012;53(4):298–300.
56. Johnson L, Genco RJ, Damsky C, Haden NK, Hart S, Hart TC, et al. Genetics and its implications for clinical dental practice and education: report of panel 3 of the Macy study. J Dent Educ. 2008;72(2 Suppl): 86–94.
57. Katsanis SH, Dungan JR, Gilliss CL, Ginsburg GA. Educating future providers of personalized medicine. N C Med J. 2013;74(6):491–2.
58. McInerney JD. Genetics education for health professionals: a context. J Genet Counsel. 2008;17(2):145–51.
59. Salari K, Karczewski KJ, Hudgins L, Ormond KE. Evidence that personal genome testing enhances student learning in a course on genomics and personalized medicine. PLoS One. 2013;8(7), e68853.
60. Skirton H, Lewis C, Kent A, Coviello DA, Members of Eurogentest Unit 6 and ESHG Education Committee. Genetic education and the challenge of genomic medicine: development of core competences to support preparation of health professionals in Europe. Eur J Hum Genet. 2010;18(9):972–7.
61. Clancy TE, Fiks AG, Gelfand JM, Grayzel DS, Marci CD, McDonough CG, et al. A call for health policy education in the medical school curriculum. JAMA. 1995;274(13):1084–5.
62. Patel MS, Davis MM, Lypson ML. Advancing medical education by teaching health policy. N Engl J Med. 2011;364(8):695–7.
63. Patel MS, Lypson ML, Miller DD, Davis MM. A framework for evaluating student perceptions of health policy training in medical school. Acad Med. 2014;89(10):1375–9.
64. Schmitt M, Blue A, Aschenbrener CA, Viggiano TR. Core competencies for interprofessional collaborative practice: reforming health care by transforming health professionals' education. Acad Med. 2011;86(11):1351.
65. Deverka PA, Doksum T, Carlson RJ. Integrating molecular medicine into the US health-care system: opportunities, barriers, and policy challenges. Clin Pharmacol Ther. 2007;82(4):427–34.
66. Flexner A. Medical education in the United States and Canada. From the Carnegie Foundation for the Advancement of Teaching, Bulletin Number Four, 1910. Bull World Health Organ. 2002;80(7): 594–602.
67. Hakim F, Kachalia PR. Implementation strategies for incorporating new technologies into the dental practice. J Calif Dent Assoc. 2010;38(5):337–41.
68. Korf BR. Genomic medicine: educational challenges. Mol Genet Genomic Med. 2013;1(3):119–22.
69. Kornman KS, Duff GW. Personalized medicine: will dentistry ride the wave or watch from the beach? J Dent Res. 2012;91(7 Suppl):8S–11.
70. Slavkin HC, Santa FG. Revising the scope of practice for oral health professionals: enter genomics. J Am Dent Assoc (1939). 2014;145(3):228–30.
71. Snead ML, Slavkin HC. Science is the fuel for the engine of technology and clinical practice. J Am Dent Assoc (1939). 2009;140 Suppl 1:17S–24.
72. Donoff B, McDonough JE, Riedy CA. Integrating oral and general health care. N Engl J Med. 2014;371(24):2247–9.

# Policy and Personalized Oral Health Care

11

Burton L. Edelstein

**Abstract**

Policy—whether promulgated by government, professions, business, providers, or others—determines priorities and establishes how things are done. When applied to personalized oral healthcare, polices established by these interests may advance or impede application of science to practice with both intended and unintended consequences. Federal science and technology policy will substantially impact how personalized medicine and dentistry are advanced through scientific discovery, how the public gains an understanding of these novel approaches, and how advances in care will be integrated into health insurance coverage. Federal health policy can be expected to accelerate an existing shift from healthcare systems to health-promoting systems with attendant cost and outcome accountability. Financial incentives inherent in such health-promoting systems are intended to engage healthcare providers in mitigating risks and addressing health determinants which can be identified through genetic and epigenetic studies.

Confidentiality concerns can be expected to remain paramount to policymakers even as tensions between privacy and utility expand with greater volumes of genetic testing. The future of policymaking can be anticipated to be as dynamic and far-reaching as the field of healthcare genomics itself. Whether policymaking, in the end, will keep up with science and whether it will facilitate or hamper the institutionalization of personalized medicine and dentistry are yet to be seen.

B.L. Edelstein, DDS, MPH
Section of Population Oral Health,
Columbia University College of Dental Medicine,
New York, NY, USA

Children's Dental Health Project,
Washington, DC, USA
e-mail: ble22@cumc.columbia.edu

## Introduction

Careful consideration of the interplay between policy and personalized dentistry first requires an appreciation of policy's definition and the roles it plays in setting priorities, implementing actions,



P.J. Polverini (ed.), *Personalized Oral Health Care: From Concept Design to Clinical Practice*,
DOI 10.1007/978-3-319-23297-3_11

and accelerating or inhibiting scientific advances in patient care. Policy can be simultaneously determinative and aspirational, both restraining and accelerating advances in personalized dentistry. Applications of genomics to oral health and dental care will, of necessity, engage federal policymakers who routinely struggle with competing interests as they apply national science and technology policy to ever more complex questions on behalf of the public's interest. Public and private policymakers may also regard scientific advances as gateways to improved healthcare, greater cost accountability, and cost savings, yet such expectations remain controversial. This chapter explores these issues and seeks to anticipate the range of relationships that hold promise to move personalized dentistry into the mainstream.

## Policy

Policy seeks to facilitate actions or resolve problems that are shared by constituents. Policy may be promulgated by government to address concerns of the populace, by professional organizations to address membership, by business and nonprofits to address customers and stakeholders, or by service providers like dentists to address their operations and care of their clients or patients. Policy promulgated by these agents influences a wide range of stakeholders who, in turn, seek to influence these agents as they develop policy. Considering only federal policymaking, the Congressional Research Service has identified 18 organizations and individuals who directly impact science and technology policy (Fig. 11.1). Similar constellations of interest groups and stakeholders impact policy decision-making in the private sectors. The larger the issue, the more people it impacts, and the more dollars that are at stake, the greater the numbers and intensities of groups and individuals who seek to influence its promulgation.

Policy sets a course of action, guides decisions, dictates operations, and advances objectives. It establishes priorities, promotes the common good, and maximizes use of available resources. Expressed as legislation, regulation, rules, and procedures, policy defines how things are done, creates options, sets limits, and dictates processes and outcomes. It determines who is authorized to take actions under specified circumstances, including where, when, and how those actions are permissible.

Applied to the advent of personalized dentistry, policy established by government, professional associations, educators, insurers, and vendors will directly influence how new technologies and procedures come to the dental marketplace, how they are distributed, who will use

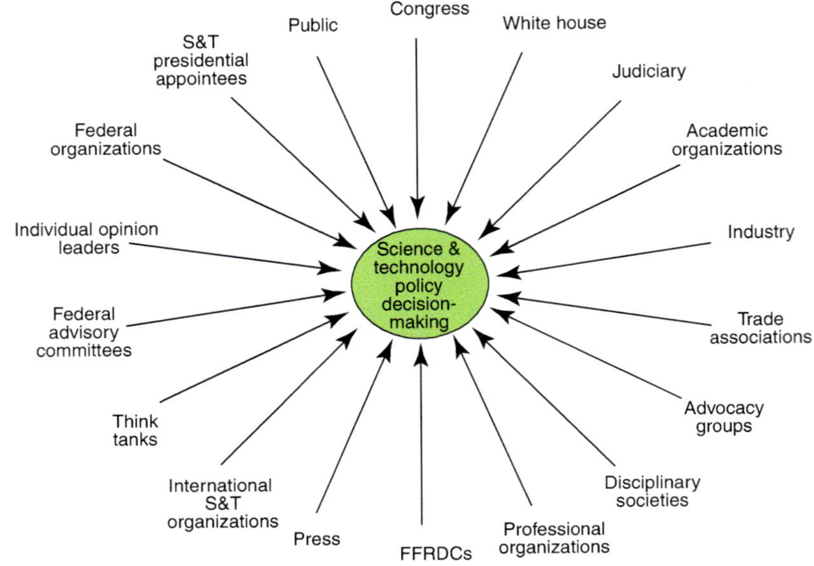


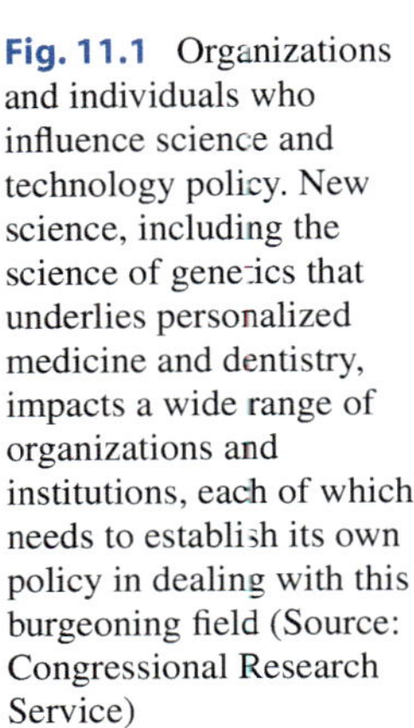
**Fig. 11.1** Organizations and individuals who influence science and technology policy. New science, including the science of genetics that underlies personalized medicine and dentistry, impacts a wide range of organizations and institutions, each of which needs to establish its own policy in dealing with this burgeoning field (Source: Congressional Research Service)

them, and who will benefit (or is placed at risk) from them. Policy will determine when genetic-based tests will be delivered and paid for, when genetic-influenced individualized medications are prescribed, and when and if genetically modified organisms—including us—are utilized to improve health.

While all policies seek to support action related to an identified need or problem, any such need or problem can be addressed through a myriad of competing policy approaches advanced by various stakeholders with divergent agendas and interests. This is especially true when the issue under consideration, like personalized medicine, is controversial, with some promoting the potential for improved health and others warning of dire consequences from "tinkering with nature." Which approach is selected—typically through a political, legislative, or administrative process which itself is governed by policies—will determine all subsequent actions while also benefiting some stakeholders and potentially harming or inhibiting others.

Policies typically yield both intended and unintended consequences [1]. That is, they both address the action or resolve the problem under consideration but also create the need for additional actions or generate new problems. Unintended consequences arise from inherent temporal and political constraints of policymaking. The Institute of Medicine (IOM) reflects on temporal disjunctions that often characterize governmental policymaking, noting that "Regulations to implement a new program are developed over time but must operate in different health policy environments that include dynamics not present when the legislation was passed." Unintended consequences also arise from the political process itself as "Political realities often deter policy modification and refinement to correct unintended consequences arising from imperfect legislation." Political considerations, including demands of reelection, can result in legislation that is either incomplete or inflexible as compromises are made to secure legislation's passage. The IOM also notes that frequently "politics trumps science" with one observer stating, "Conversations of politically correct versus scientifically accurate policy proposals are independent monologues that fail to converge through the entire policy debate."

These policy attributes are reflected in the Merriam-Webster Dictionary's pragmatic definition of policy as "a definite course or method of action selected from among alternatives and in light of given conditions to guide and determine present and future decisions." The dictionary, however, goes further by additionally defining policy as "prudence or wisdom in the management of affairs" [2]. This aspirational definition highlights the wide-ranging impacts of policymaking by suggesting that policies function best when they are holistic in approach, visionary in anticipating the future, appreciative of the social and political environment, and accountable in ways that maximize outcomes. In contrast, narrowly defined policies tend to inhibit creativity while failing to keep up with changes in the environment like the creation of new science.

Policymaking, both public and private, is particularly challenging when action must be taken in environments of uncertainty, as when policymakers seek to address issues related to cutting-edge science and technology, as is the case with personalized medicine and dentistry. Policymaking is similarly challenging when addressing large and far-reaching economic sectors such as healthcare because the consequences of action are so significant to the economy, the delivery system, and to individual providers, beneficiaries, and patients/constituents. When governmental policymakers seek to guide decisions in such cutting-edge environments (Webster definition #1), they must also seek to demonstrate "prudence and wisdom" (Webster definition #2), by taking actions that protect the public, promote fairness, and advance the collective good while also avoiding unintended consequences that inhibit progress or backfire. An example of these tensions is reflected in controversial state and federal policymaking over the appropriate labeling of genetically modified food, for example, whether they can be called "natural." Often these tensions are referred to the judicial branch of government for resolution—resolution that is effective only until the issue at hand evolves and is again addressed by the legislative and executive branches.

## Federal Science and Technology Policy

Public policymakers often struggle when addressing issues related to science and technology, for example, when addressing climate change, embryonic research, nanotechnology, or applied genetics. When confronted with issues like these, policymakers are often ill-equipped to assess the scientific evidence and arguments, may be frustrated by varying interpretations of the same evidence by competing interests, and may be uncomfortable with sciences' inherent ambiguities and frequent revisions.

Yet science and technology policymaking is critical both for government to support the development of new science and for government to be informed by new science in its roles of protecting the public and advancing the common good. In its primer on science and technology policy for members of congress, the Congressional Research Service captures the tremendous range of issues regarding new scientific and technologic knowledge creation and the utility and application of that knowledge for the betterment of society, stating, "Science and technology policy is concerned with (1) the allocation of resources for and encouragement of scientific and engineering research and development; (2) the use of scientific and technical knowledge to enhance the nation's response to societal challenges; and (3) the education of Americans…" [3].

Government policy plays a leading role in the "allocation of resources" for the advancement of genomic medicine. Through a wide variety of agencies—the National Institutes of Health (NIH), Patient-Centered Outcomes Research Institute (PCORI), Center for Medicare and Medicaid Innovation (CMMI), National Science Foundation, Department of Defense, and other sponsoring units—congress authorizes and appropriates funding for research and development. In so doing, it establishes priorities that are translated into specific research opportunities. Examples of government's role in advancing genomic medicine include:

- NIH's sponsorship of "genomic medicine pilot demonstration grants" that seek to "develop methods for, and evaluate the feasibility of, incorporating an individual patient's genomic findings into his or her clinical care." This research priority seeks to "expand and link existing genomic medicine efforts, and develop new collaborative projects and methods, in diverse settings and populations; contribute to the evidence base regarding outcomes of incorporating genomic information into clinical care; and define and share the processes of genomic medicine implementation, diffusion, and sustainability in diverse settings" [4].
- PCORI's research approach to individualized care extends beyond genetics to include an active role for patients in their care as well as care that is enhanced by "personalized information about a patient's profile … that could affect their outcomes including but not limited to biology, demography, culture, socioeconomic status, comorbidity, and geography" [5]. This framing mirrors the field of epigenetics by placing biology, with its genetic components, within the broader contexts of individual characteristics relative to family, community, and society.
- CMMI's support for "initiatives to speed the adoption of best practices." Noting that "it takes nearly 17 years on average before best practices—backed by research—are incorporated into widespread clinical practice," CMMI has called for studies of new delivery and payment models for "disseminating evidence-based best practices" like genomic medicine and dentistry and "significantly increasing speed of adoption" [6]. The Personalized Medicine Coalition, a trade group, recognizes that new payment mechanisms could incentivize personalized medicine but that these mechanisms need to reflect new approaches to care and new advances in medicine rather than build on current standards of care that may discourage advances in medicine [7].

Federal allocation of resources to basic and applied health-related genomics extends across a wide range of additional agencies that apply new science to personalized healthcare [8]. The Centers for Disease Control and Prevention "integrates human genetics into public health research, policies, and programs." The National Science Foundation has since 1998 led a Plant Genome Research Program that seeks to "understand the structure, organization and function of plant genomes important to agriculture, the environment, energy, and health," and the Department of Agriculture supports plant and animal genomic databases that inform human genomics research. Even the Department of Energy contributes to health-related genomic research by developing "bioinformatics tools to ultimately predict and design biological function" [9]. All of these efforts are coordinated through a Department of Health and Human Services Secretary's Advisory Committee on Genetics, Health, and Society that attends to "use and potential misuse of genetic technologies."

Another of government's roles is the "use of scientific and technical knowledge to enhance the nation's response to societal challenges" through translation of science to practice. Depending upon how policies are developed and programs deployed, personalized medicine and dentistry may help resolve or may exacerbate societal challenges that include reining in the high cost of a healthcare system that fails to produce commensurately favorable health outcomes compared to other advanced countries; addressing the rapidly escalating costs of publicly financed healthcare through Medicare, Medicaid, and CHIP; and addressing inequities in health and healthcare across subpopulations as low-income and minority populations continue to experience worse oral and general health outcomes. Governmental approaches to reducing the rate of healthcare cost escalations while simultaneously improving outcomes include incentives to develop accountable care organizations (ACOs) and patient-centered medical homes (PCMHs). These emerging delivery systems seek to demonstrate better health outcomes at lower costs through more efficient and effective quality care of defined populations. Among key strategies are targeted prevention and disease management, such as may result from personalized medicine and dentistry.

In an era of rapidly developing new health technologies, medications, and treatments, a critical societal challenge is ensuring both patient and public safety of new drugs and devices. People in need of new interventions seek their facilitated approval and availability, while others ask government to exercise extreme prudence and caution while awaiting results of thorough testing. It falls on the Food and Drug Administration (FDA) to balance these competing societal needs in meeting its responsibility to "monitor and regulate these new therapies to protect consumers" [8]. FDA's purview, however, does not extend to advertising of genetic-based disease risk tests that are made direct to the consumer through print and electronic media. In reviewing direct-to-consumer advertising of genetic testing, the agency has noted that "advertisements increased consumers' awareness about diseases, but failed to accurately convey risk information," with many advertisements promoting tests that are not valid [10].

A third governmental role is the "education of Americans" to better participate in their own care, particularly for the management of chronic conditions like the four oral diseases addressed in this book. Effective chronic care management anticipates a therapeutic dyad that engages a "prepared proactive practice team" with an "informed activated patient" in "productive interactions" that result in "improved health outcomes" [11]. Doing so requires that patients be educated about their own unique health risks and conditions—the essence of personalized medical and dental care. Federal agencies engage in policy and programs to enhance the genomic education of the populace. Examples include NIH's role in informing the public through its patient portal, for example, its posting on "Personalized Medicine: Matching Treatments to your Genes" [12]; the CDC Office of Public Health Genomics' blogs, tweets, reports, and consumer guides [13]; and the FDA's efforts to update the public about pharmacogenomics [14]. Government is also actively engaged in policies related to the education of health professionals to learn and apply genomic-based care. Through its Bureau of Health Professions, the Health Resources and

Services Administration is funded to support health professional education in "developing and expanding [trainees'] genetic and genomic knowledge base related to specific disease processes encountered in the clinical setting" [8].

Taken together, the three roles of government in advancing science and technology defined by the Congressional Research Service work synergistically to create new science, prepare the population and providers for its use, and attempt to leverage its potential for the improvement of the public good.

## Policy and Emerging Health Systems

US healthcare, including dental care, is engaged in a metamorphosis from a past orientation on repair and remediation to a future orientation on prevention and disease management. This reorientation is propelled by new financing systems that reward healthcare providers on the value of care they deliver, expressed as health outcomes per unit cost, rather than the volume of services they deliver, expressed as the aggregate and associated costs of individual clinical services delivered regardless of outcome. These payment mechanisms include global payments, bundled payments, pay-for-performance incentives, and shared savings strategies. They are being implemented modestly short term in the traditionally disaggregated delivery system comprised of solo and small-group delivery units (including private dental practices), while larger, more integrated, systems that are designed to handle global payments continue to evolve. These include ACOs and PCMHs, both of which seek to integrate multilevel care around the holistic needs of individual patients while measuring their impact at the level of populations served.

Changes in orientation and payment are forcing a merger of clinical care and public health into the unique domain of "population health." Population health concerns itself with health determinants and resulting aggregate health status of a defined population, typically characterized by geography (e.g., a county) or group (e.g., large employer group). While definitions of population health continuously evolve, they commonly encompass two essential components: (1) inclusion of health determinants—environmental, social, and behavioral—that expands and integrates concepts of both public health and clinical care; and (2) goals of fairness expressed as reduced disparities and inequities within a defined population [15]. Subsequent to its establishment by the Affordable Care Act, the federal Center for Medicare and Medicaid Innovation seeks to animate and promote population health through demonstrations focused on health determinants that "encourage better health for entire populations by addressing underlying causes of poor health, such as physical inactivity, behavioral risk factors, lack of preventive care and poor nutrition" [16]. The focus on fairness is evident in the Institute for Healthcare Improvement's schema (Fig. 11.2) which seeks "equity" through both health promotion and disease prevention, the traditional domain of public health, and healthcare, the traditional domain of the clinician.

Population health anticipates that a comprehensive healthcare system, ideally including oral health services, is financed at least in part based on risk-adjusted health outcomes of the covered population over time. This shift from "healthcare systems" to "health-promoting systems" presages a variety of tactics that are informed by personalized medicine and dentistry. Proponents argue, for example, that "The concept of personalized medicine not only promises to enhance the life of patients and increase the quality of clinical practice and targeted care pathways, but also to lower overall healthcare costs through early detection, prevention, accurate risk assessments, and efficiencies in care delivery" [17]. Detractors, however, note that new technologies bring new expenses and argue that personalized medicine will further exacerbate costs of care and drive even greater social inequities because drug and device companies are motivated to recover development costs and generate profits.

When health financing policies that reward providers based on a defined populations' health outcomes are instituted, there is inherent incentive for providers to identify and rigorously manage those individuals within the group who

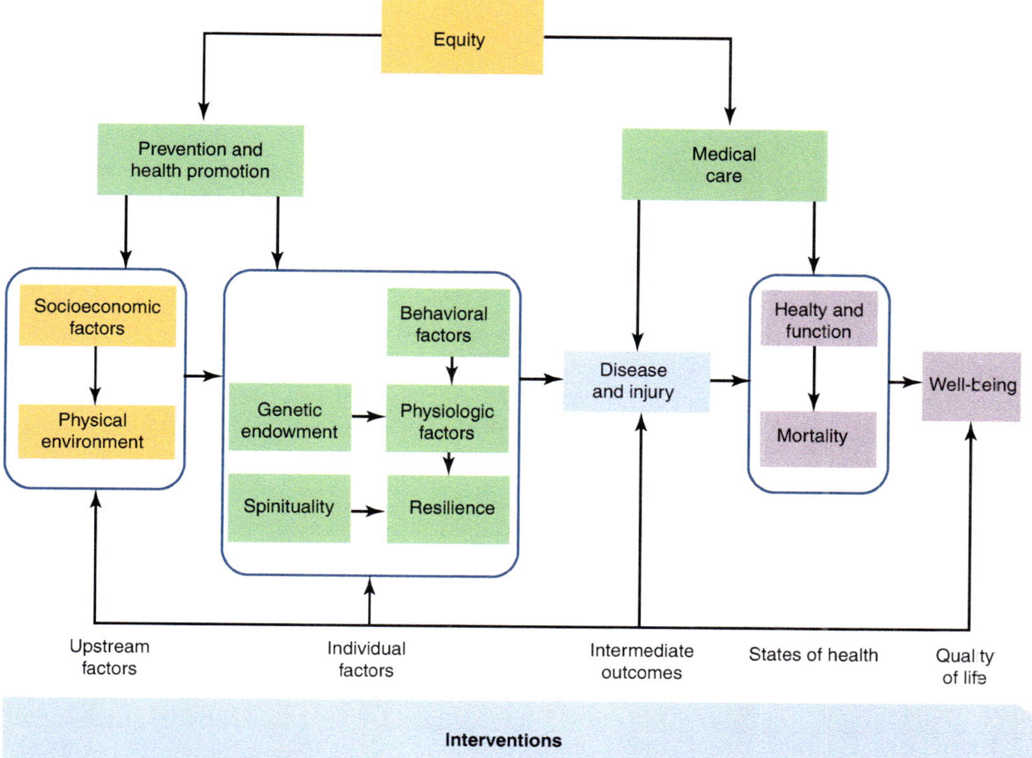


**Fig. 11.2** Components of health systems that are replacing healthcare systems. Evolving health systems consider both the populations they serve and the individuals who comprise those populations, through a holistic approach that addresses social, biological, behavioral, and environmental disease determinants. They are designed to realize positive health outcomes that support quality of life and overall well-being. Genomic medicine and dentistry are essential components of these evolving systems, as genetic endowment is a critical element of risk and susceptibility for disease, as well as response to treatment (Source: Adapted from Stiefel and Nolan [28] (Available on www.IHI.org))

are at greatest risk of and experience the most severe and costly diseases. Identifying these individuals—a process dubbed "hot spotting"—and addressing their risks of disease expression and exacerbation are potentially cost saving [18]. Doing so is facilitated by epigenetics.

Epigenetics—the modification of gene expression by exposure triggers and interactions—suggests that successful health-promoting systems will, of necessity, extend their scope of care to include management of social, environmental, and behavioral health determinants while retaining support for remedial healthcare services when needed. To control costs under a global budget and effectuate efficiencies, such systems will operate on sound management principles that promote accountability at controlled costs including delegation, best use of informatics, management through care coordination and continuous quality improvement, and application of systems science. Systems that are concerned with health determinants as well as health status will build on knowledge gleaned from studies of social determinants, life-course determinants, and common risk factors. They will actively engage in interprofessional practice not only among health professionals but between health professionals and helping professions (e.g., social workers, health educators, dieticians, public health professionals) and lay health workers (e.g., community health workers, *promotores*, care coordinators, case managers). Keys to such advances in population health are the identification, management, and monitoring of highest-risk patients who can be identified in part through genetic testing and the control of triggering exposures that activate genetic predispositions by addressing environmental, social, and behavioral risk factors. Knowing that a person has a genetic susceptibility or predisposition to an oral condition when social, environmental, and/or behavioral determinants are present demands that health-promoting systems become as involved in managing the triggers of disease in individuals as public health professionals have traditionally done for triggers of disease in populations. Thus, the advent of "omics" science accelerates clinical movement from repair and remediation to prevention and disease management.

## Privacy, Confidentiality, and Race

A significant healthcare policy issue of direct relevance to genomic dentistry is the privacy and security of personal health information. At issue is whether current HIPAA requirements will be sufficient to protect genomic data. Alzu'bi et al. detailed this issue in a 2014 journal for health information management professionals, stating: "Personal genomic data are highly sensitive and need to be protected properly because each record contains not just the health information about one particular patient, but potentially information about a large group of people who have a blood relation with the person who takes the genetic test. This impact can last for generations because the genomic information will be passed to these people's descendants."

Reflecting on long-term consequences of revealing genomic information, they add, "The privacy of the individual and his or her relatives may be threatened, and the confidentiality of the personal genomic data is lost. The threat to the individual's offspring could be even more serious because research in genomics will likely enable the discovery of more information from a human genome in the future. Therefore, a stronger and more sophisticated security measure may be needed for personal genomic data protection, and this system should be set up before the wide application of genomic information in clinical practice" [19].

According to the National Human Genome Research Institute, a branch of the National Institutes of Health, HIPAA prohibits insurers from excluding an individual from group coverage or charging a higher premium to an individual than to the group based on genetic information, but it does not prohibit the use of genetic information in setting group premiums or limit the disclosure of genetic information by insurers [20]. Thus, the cost of dental insurance may become predicated upon the genomically identified risk factors in an employer or demographic group seeking coverage.

Recognizing that release of personal genetic information could also lead to employment discrimination because of employers' concerns over both risk of disease and potential impact on health insurance premiums, the congress enacted the Genetic Information Nondiscrimination Act of 2008 [21] "to prohibit discrimination on the basis of genetic information with respect to health insurance and employment." The law seeks to establish a national standard for genetic nondiscrimination that supersedes a patchwork of state policies and assures that the public can uniformly benefit from genetic testing and new treatments as they become available.

The law's preamble explicates a series of findings to justify the need for the protections it offers. It first acknowledges that "advances in genetics open new opportunities for medical progress" in diagnosis and treatment while also acknowledging "the potential misuse of genetic information to discriminate in health insurance and employment." It then delves into significant past misuses of early genetic science in American history, noting that a majority of states enacted sterilization laws "to correct apparent genetic traits or tendencies" without constitutional protections and that these laws led to discrimination and stigmatization of racial and ethnic subgroups. The law notes that many genetic conditions and disorders are associated with particular racial and ethnic groups, as some genetic traits are more prevalent in particular population subgroups. Depending upon how this biological fact is interpreted and addressed, it may lead to positive outcomes of better targeted preventive and remedial care or to negative outcomes of discrimination and racism.

### More Challenging Policy Questions

Beyond issues of privacy, discrimination, test and drug regulation, and advertising to consumers are a range of policy issues that need to be resolved for personalized medicine and dentistry to evolve into day-to-day healthcare practice. The National Human Genome Research Institute (NHGRI) at NIH has outlined many of these issues and their potential consequences as policymakers grapple with new science [22]:

- Intellectual property protections and commercial interests: NHGRI's Policy and Program Branch describes a "thicket of patents" that may slow the capacity of US biotechnology companies to bring tests and treatments to market, putting the nation at a competitive commercial disadvantage. How can policy balance intellectual property interests against commercialization and improvements in healthcare?
- Therapeutic lag: Healthcare providers' capacity to interpret and utilize genetic information is expected to lag behind the availability of accurate and affordable genomic testing. How can policy support healthcare providers, particularly those already in practice, in gaining knowledge and skills in interpreting genomic information and factoring such information into diagnoses and treatments?
- Iterative development of science: Genetic-based risk estimates for various diseases will become increasingly refined as research progresses. How can governmental regulatory policies stay current? How can providers stay up to date?
- Ethical concerns: Genetic testing typically yields more information than sought by the prescribing practitioner. What policies should govern the use of such information?

## Genomic Policy and the Future of Dentistry

Personalized oral healthcare needs to be considered within policies, like the Affordable Care Act, that promote value in terms of accountability, efficiency, effectiveness, and quality. Nongovernmental agencies are actively contributing to these advances in health promotion. Of direct interest to dentistry, the DentaQuest Institute has sponsored a National Oral Health Quality Improvement Committee to develop and guide a "vision for the US oral health system for 2023" [23]. Personalized dentistry directly supports visionary elements of a future dental delivery system. The vision of "improved population health coupled with enhanced value" is supported by personalized dentistry when genetic testing identifies high-risk patients needing the most intensive care. Similarly, the vision of "prioritizing prevention and disease management" can be most effective when highest-risk patients are targeted.

The Affordable Care Act facilitates the adoption of personalized dentistry as a component of health-promoting systems by replacing the long-held paradigm of the "iron triangle" with the refreshed notion of the "Triple Aim." Healthcare policymaking, like all policymaking, starts with needs or problems that require resolution within constraints of the best available information. Healthcare policymaking addresses problems that relate both to the multiple concerns inherent in the provision of health services—financing, workforce, and care delivery systems (topics we will return to later)—and to the consequences of such services on cost, quality, access, utilization, and equity.

For many years, these consequences were understood to be inherently competitive and contradictory. Better access, utilization, and fairness were believed to be obtainable only through offsets in cost or quality. Lower costs were believed to be attainable only through tradeoffs in access or quality. Better quality was believed to be attainable only through lesser access or higher cost. Called the "iron triangle" by physician-policymaker William Kissick in his 1994 book, *Medicine's Dilemmas: Infinite Needs versus Finite Resources*, this belief influenced policymakers' actions even as the costs of US healthcare climbed precipitously, while objective measures of population health failed to improve. Kissick's critics note evidence that "other nations provide more, better, and cheaper care" stating that "reducing administration, the profits of health maintenance organizations, unneeded care, or seven-figure incomes need not compromise quality or access" [24].

Supplanting the "iron triangle" is the Triple Aim, "a framework for optimizing health system performance by simultaneously focusing on the health of a population, the experience of care for individuals within that population, and the per capita cost of providing that care" [25]. The Triple Aim suggests that it is possible to deliver quality healthcare to members of a group at lower costs in ways that improve the population's health and well-being, thereby allowing quality, access, and cost to coexist and become synergistic and mutually supportive. Working smarter rather than harder to realize all three aims simultaneously is possible by reducing inefficiencies, redundancies, and errors; by targeting care more precisely so that limited healthcare resources are allocated relative to individual need; and by moving care upstream to a focus on individualized, targeted prevention and health promotion. Personalized medicine and dentistry facilitate each of these strategies.

The Triple Aim is thoroughly embedded in the hallmark health policy legislation of our times, the Patient Protection and Affordable Care Act of 2010, aka "ObamaCare" or "the ACA." The law authorizes programs in population health through community needs assessments, community transformation grants, public education campaigns, and enhanced nutrition labeling. Although the law is best known for its endeavor to reform health insurance, it also seeks to fundamentally reform the US healthcare system's capacity, delivery, and financing. Both components—insurance reform and health systems reform—reflect the advent of genomic medicine. Insurance reform expands the availability of coverage through online purchasing marketplaces, standardizes benefits, controls costs, and ensures consumer protections [26]. Consumer protections "limit insurers' ability to deny, limit, or cancel coverage; end annual and lifetime spending caps; and ensure that more premium dollars are spent on delivering and improving care." They also assure guaranteed issue insurance coverage to people with preexisting conditions [27]. These protections are increasingly necessary as genomic medicine identifies people at risk for serious and costly diseases and allows previously unattainable risk stratification in coverage. Unfortunately, the list of essential health benefits which all insurers must provide does not extend specifically to genomic medicine or to adult dental coverage. As a result, dental insurers may deny or drop coverage for adults deemed high risk for oral conditions, including those identified through genomic testing.

**Conclusions**

Policies by government, industry, and the professions themselves will continue to evolve as the science and practice of genomic medicine and dentistry becomes increasingly established. Government will maintain its substantive effort to ensure public safety while expanding access to personalized healthcare that is effective, equitable, and cost-effective while also continuing to fund research that holds promise to fulfill the Triple Aim. Industry will seek policies that facilitate commercialization while protecting intellectual property. The professions can be expected to adopt continuing education policies and clinical protocols that guide their members' realization of genomic-based practice. The future of policymaking can be anticipated to be as dynamic and far-reaching as the field of healthcare genomics itself. Whether policymaking, in the end, will keep up with science and whether it will facilitate or hamper the institutionalization of personalized medicine and dentistry are yet to be seen.

## References

1. The Robert Wood Johnson Health Policy Fellowship Program. Unintended consequences of health policy programs and policies: workshop summary. Institute of Medicine; 2001. Available at http://www.nap.edu/catalog/10192/unintended-consequences-of-health-policy-programs-and-policies-workshop-summary. doi:10.17226/10192. Accessed 18 Nov 2015.

2. Miriam Webster Online Dictionary. "Definition of policy". Merriam-Webster. Undated. Available at http://www.merriam-webster.com/dictionary/policy. Accessed 18 Nov 2015.
3. Stine DD. Science and Technology Policymaking: a Primer. Congressional Research Services of the Library of Congress, 1997. http://fas.org/sgp/crs/misc/RL34454.pdf.
4. National Institutes of Health. Funding opportunity announcement HG-13-004. Genomic medicine pilot demonstration projects (U01). National Human Genome Research Institute; 2013. Available at http://grants.nih.gov/grants/guide/rfa-files/RFA-HG-13-004.html. Accessed 18 Nov 2015.
5. Patient Centered Outcomes Research Institute. National priorities for research and research agenda 2012. Patient Centered Outcomes Research Institute. Available at http://www.pcori.org/sites/default/files/PCORI-National-Priorities-and-Research-Agenda-2012-05-21-FINAL1.pdf. Accessed 18 Nov 2015.
6. Centers for Medicare and Medicaid Services. Innovation models. US Department of Health and Human Services. Available at https://innovation.cms.gov/initiatives/#views=models. Accessed 18 Nov 2015.
7. Shin A. Paying for personalized medicine: How alternative payment models could help or hinder the field. Personalized Medicine Coalition, Washington, DC; Undated. p. 40. Available at http://www.personalizedmedicinecoalition.org/Userfiles/PMCCorporate/file/paying_for_personalized_medicine.pdf. Accessed 20 Nov 2015.
8. National Human Genome Research Institute. Other federal agencies involved in genomics. National Institutes of Health, US Department of Health and Human Services; 2015. Available at http://www.genome.gov/10003899. Accessed 20 Nov 2015.
9. Genomic Science Program. About the DOE Systems Biology Knowledgebase (KBase). U.S. Department of Energy Office of Science; 2015. Available at http://genomicscience.energy.gov/compbio/kbaseindex.shtml. Accessed 20 Nov 15.
10. National Human Genome Research Institute. Direct to consumer marketing of genetic tests (archived). National Institutes of Health, US Department of Health and Human Services; 2004. Available at http://www.genome.gov/12010659. Accessed 20 Nov 2015.
11. Wagner EH. Chronic disease management: what will it take to improve care for chronic illness? Eff Clin Pract. 1998;1:2–4. http://www.improvingchroniccare.org/index.php?p=The_Chronic_CareModel&s=2.
12. NIH News in Health. Personalized medicine: matching treatments to your genes. National Institutes of Health, US Department of Health and Human Services; 2013. Available at http://newsinhealth.nih.gov/issue/dec2013/feature1. Accessed 20 Nov 2015.
13. Centers for Disease Control and Prevention. Public health genomics, precision medicine: implementation science and public health. Centers for Disease Control and Prevention, US Department of Health and Human Services; 2015. Available at http://www.cdc.gov/genomics. Accessed 20 Nov 2015.
14. Food and Drug Administration. Genomics. Food and Drug Administration, US Department of Health and Human Services; 2015. Available at http://www.fda.gov/Drugs/ScienceResearch/ResearchAreas/Pharmacogenetics/. Accessed 20 Nov 2015.
15. Soto MA. Population health in the Affordable Care Act era. Washington, DC: Academy Health; 2013. Available at http://www.academyhealth.org/files/AH2013pophealth.pdf.
16. Center for Medicare and Medicaid Innovation. Our mission. Centers for Medicare and Medicaid, US Department of Health and Human Services. Available at https://innovation.cms.gov/about/Our-Mission/index.html. Accessed 18 July 2015.
17. Jakka S, Rossbach M. An economic perspective on personalized medicine. Hum Genome Org J. 2013;7:1. doi:10.1186/1877-6566-7-1.
18. Gawande A. Medical report: the hot spotters – can we lower medical costs by giving the neediest patients better care? The New Yorker Magazine. January 24, 2011. Available at http://www.newyorker.com/magazine/2011/01/24/the-hot-spotters.
19. Alzu'bi A, Zhou L, Watzlaf V. Personal genomic information management and personalized medicine: challenges, current solutions, and roles of HIM professionals. Perspect Health Inf Manag. 2014;11:1c. Available at http://www.ncbi.nlm.nih.gov/pmc/articles/PMC3995490/.
20. National Human Genome Research Institute. Federal policy recommendations including HIPAA. National Institutes of Health, US Department of Health and Human Services; 2012. Available at http://www.genome.gov/11510216. Accessed 20 Nov 2015.
21. US Equal Employment Opportunity Commission. The Genetic Information Nondiscrimination Act of 2008. US Equal Employment Opportunity Commission; 2008. Available at http://www.eeoc.gov/laws/statutes/gina.cfm. Accessed 20 Nov 2015.
22. National Human Genome Research Institute. NHGRI policy roundtable summary, the future of genomic medicine: policy implications for research and medicine (archived). Bethesda; 2005. Available at http://www.genome.gov/17516574. Accessed 20 Nov 2015.
23. DentaQuest Institute. Report of the National Oral Health Quality Improvement Committee: a vision for the US oral health system for 2023. Westborough: DentaQuest Institute; 2014.
24. Woolhandler S, Himmelstein DU. Book review: understanding health care reform, medicine's dilemmas: infinite needs versus finite resources. N Engl J Med. 1994;331:1779. doi:10.1056/NEJM199412293312619.

25. Institute for Healthcare Improvement. About US, History. Institute for Healthcare Improvement; Undated. Available at http://www.ihi.org/about/pages/history.aspx. Accessed 20 Nov 2015.
26. American Public Health Association. Affordable Care Act overview selected provisions. 2012. Available at http://www.apha.org/~/media/files/pdf/topics/aca/aca_overview_aug2012.ashx. Accessed 20 Nov 2015.
27. Robert Wood Johnson Foundation. What Consumer Protections are Embedded in the Affordable Care Act? Health policy snapshot series. Robert Wood Johnson Foundation; 2011. Available at http://www.rwjf.org/en/research-publications/find-rwjf-research/2011/08/what-consumer-protections-are-embedded-in-the-affordable-care-ac.html. Accessed 20 Nov 2015.
28. Stiefel M, Nolan K. A guide to measuring the triple aim: population health, experience of care, and per capita cost. IHI innovation series white paper. Cambridge, MA: Institute for Healthcare Improvement; 2012.

# Opportunities and Challenges for the Future of Personalized Oral Healthcare

12

Peter J. Polverini

**Abstract**

A prospective, personalized approach to oral healthcare is gaining momentum among healthcare providers. The adoption of a personalized oral healthcare environment will be dependent upon the successful implementation of an educational program that better prepares the next generation of providers with knowledge in genomic and molecular medicine. Disruptive innovations will drive the adoption of a personalized healthcare environment through the implementation of new models of collaborative care and new workforce models. Ultimately the long-term success of personalized oral healthcare will depend on it becoming integrated within a learning healthcare system. As the predictive biomarkers that assist in the diagnosis of and treatment of common diseases are discovered and deployed chairside, the dental profession will transition to one that is more focused on disease prevention, risk assessment, and early diagnosis.

## Introduction

The traditional reactive, one-size-fits-all approach to healthcare is rapidly transitioning to one that this is proactive, with a greater focus on prevention, early intervention, and risk assessment [1–6]. The goal of this prospective approach to healthcare is designed to meet specific, individual needs of patients by incorporating patient's genomic data, cultural values, environmental challenges, and health and behavioral history to predict disease onset and the patient's response to tailored therapy [2, 7–15]. While personalized healthcare is not a new concept, only recently has this approach to care gained traction in dentistry [7, 9, 10, 13, 14].

The rapid development of patient information and communication systems is major driving forces behind the emerging personalized healthcare environment [1–6, 11, 12, 15]. With the development of new chairside technologies

P.J. Polverini, DDS, DMSc
Department of Periodontics and Oral Medicine, University of Michigan School of Dentistry, Ann Arbor, MI, USA

Department of Pathology, University of Michigan Medical School, Ann Arbor, MI, USA
e-mail: neovas@umich.edu


P.J. Polverini (ed.), *Personalized Oral Health Care: From Concept Design to Clinical Practice*,
DOI 10.1007/978-3-319-23297-3_12

designed to provide point-of-care diagnosis, the potential of personalized oral healthcare is just now being realized. For example, highly detailed information through genomic analysis and other noninvasive diagnostic technologies are enabling patient stratification to better manage patient care and achieve the best possible outcomes [7, 16]. Despite these advances, the dental profession still faces many challenges in the comprehensive implementation of personalized oral healthcare. We are at a pivotal point in time where we can transform our current disease management approach to healthcare by focusing more on a patient's unique biological, social determinants and placing greater emphasis on the management of health rather than disease. This approach to patient care has important implications not only for improving the quality of life for individual patients but also for promoting a healthy society [1].

## Factors Driving the Personalized Oral Healthcare Environment

As the personalized oral healthcare environment takes foothold, the deployment of point-of-care services and personal monitoring devises will likely become more widely available, providing both patients and healthcare providers with the ability to monitor a patient's health status and response to therapy in real time [8, 15, 17]. The increased use of information technologies in oral healthcare will accelerate the development of large-scale data sets. With system biology serving as backbone to integrate the biological and genetic information, our understanding of disease onset and progression will rapidly advance and provide guidance in the development of new prevention strategies [1, 7, 8, 10, 17, 18].

One of the most important features of the emerging personalized oral healthcare environment is the role of patients in the decision-making process [1–6]. The patient of today wants to participate and be actively involved in the decision about treatment options. The healthcare provider is no longer seen as the sole "decider" about what is best for the patient. Patients have an increasingly stronger voice as their knowledge and understanding of what is required to maintain a healthy lifestyle. Partnership and empowerment are key elements in the successful provision of care in a personalized oral healthcare environment [1]. Currently, for many (general) practitioners, personalized oral healthcare is a concept that is perceived to have little or no practical value in their practice. For this to change, it will be necessary to establish an infrastructure that makes use of our current information technologies to facilitate the communication across disciplines and between health professionals. Personalized oral healthcare will have a huge impact on reimbursement [11, 19, 20]. Assuming appropriate analytical and clinical validation, new diagnostic technologies and precision therapies will take presidence over more traditional approaches that define our reactive care environment. While no one expects the practice of dentistry to change dramatically any time soon, there will no doubt be increased pressure from patients and insurers for oral healthcare providers to place greater emphasis on risk assessment and more investment in prevention and early diagnosis and disease intervention [2, 7, 10, 13, 14, 16].

One can argue that taking responsibility for one's health is an economically and ethically sound approach to advancing personalized healthcare. The four "Ps" (prevention, predictive, personalized, and participatory) that represent the cornerstone of personalized healthcare perhaps should include a fifth P, personal responsibility. While this certainly makes sense from the standpoint of social responsibility and empowerment, there is an equally important need to provide patients with the skills to manage the deluge of information that will shape the personalized healthcare environment [1, 2, 6, 21, 22]. A diverse body of research has established the role of education as a predictor of improved health outcomes [23–26]. Our understanding of this complex relationship between patients and providers has important implications in driving continued progress in healthcare reform and even bigger implications in lifestyle reform. A broad-based dialogue among different constituencies in society is needed to discuss risks and opportunities and define an ethical framework for implementing this new personalized approach to healthcare [23–27].

## Disruptive Innovations Will Shape the Personalized Oral Healthcare Environment

Innovations that will fundamentally accelerate the adoption of a personalized oral healthcare environment have yet to be realized. While there have been rapid advances in the development of home health monitoring devices, point-of-care diagnostic systems, and precision therapies, our healthcare system continues to assume a reactive posture. If disruptive innovations are to have a meaningful impact and accelerate personalized oral healthcare, new predictive biomarkers will need to be validated analytically and clinically, and new knowledge domains must evolve to better prepare providers to succeed in a personalized oral healthcare environment [28, 29]. Changes in practice models, workforce expansion, communication strategies, and adoption of value-based reimbursement must be addressed if the current healthcare environment is to have transition to one that is personalized, preventive, predictive, and participatory.

One of the biggest challenges affecting the adoption of a personalized approach to oral healthcare by current providers is the educational deficit in genomic medicine and a broad understanding of the molecular basis of disease [30–34]. As knowledge of the genetic basis of common oral disease continues to advance and if healthcare providers are expected to manage their patients effectively, it will be essential they have a working knowledge of genetics. A major challenge for providers in the emerging personalized oral healthcare environment is communicating disease risk to patients so they can make informed decisions. An understanding of genetic principles is vital to meet this challenge. At a minimum, oral healthcare professionals will need to know how to use genetic information to assess risk and guide treatment and how best to inform and interpret the results for their patients. This is particularly true today, where over-the-counter genetic testing is often used inappropriately to assess risk, leading to misinterpretation of results [35]. While there are a number of single gene disorders that affect the orofacial structures, as genomic medicine continues to develop, many more common dental diseases that are multifactorial in nature will be reveled to a have a genetic basis [36–43]. As with all health-related disciplines, educating oral healthcare professionals about genetics and genomics will be essential for clinical practice. Although medical schools continue to increase genetic content of the undergraduate curriculum, dental students in the United States and in Europe continue to lag behind other healthcare professionals in their knowledge of genetic and genomic medicine [30–34, 44, 45], While most dentists may believe that genomic medicine is peripheral to their practice, the ability to understand the power and limitations of genetic testing will no doubt be an important part of the oral healthcare professional's toolbox in the emerging personalized healthcare environment [30–34, 44, 45].

Another discipline that will be necessary for oral healthcare providers to navigate is healthcare policy [46–48]. For example, successful implementation of a personalized healthcare environment that evolves from comparative effectiveness research and evidence-based practice will require that dental schools develop curricula to provide oral healthcare providers with the knowledge and skills necessary to work in an evolving personalized oral healthcare environment. If the personalized oral healthcare environment is to have a meaningful impact of the oral health of patients, dental schools must embrace these new educational initiatives in health policy.

The potential long-term outcomes of a successful collaboration among the health professions include an optimal patient care environment, improved health system efficiency, lower costs, and an increase in both patient and provider satisfaction [1, 49–52].

Collaborative learning enables health profession students to be better prepared to adapt to an ever-changing healthcare environment. Collaborative care and teamwork will be an essential feature of a successful personalized oral healthcare environment. Workforce-ready graduates will need skills to meet increasingly complex patient needs, adapt to changing technology that will influence dental practice, and function effectively in collaborative practice settings. Given the increasingly prohibitive cost of the current healthcare system and the increasing inaccessibility of high-value healthcare to a large segment of the population, there is little reason not to embrace that collaborative approach to education and care. Breaking down the current siloed approach to education and patient care can only enhance the value of each of the health professions, while at the same time advancing a healthcare system that is more efficient, patient centered, and health management driven. In addition to making better use of existing services, the dental profession must explore new workforce models that help meet the oral healthcare needs of the growing underserved population [1, 53–60].

What will qualify for reimbursement and how value for preventive care and risk assessment will be determined will be dependent in large part on the data generated through omics technology [21, 22, 34, 36–38, 41, 42, 45]. Revisions to current payment systems to incorporate genomic and molecular data for diagnosis and clinical management of patients will, to a great extent, determine the pace at which personalized oral healthcare is incorporated into clinical practice [9, 15, 20, 38]. A recent example of this is reported in a publication by Giannobile et al. which explores the value of IL-1 genotyping in determining the risk of severe periodontal disease [16]. Their data suggests that IL-1 genotyping may serve as a predictive measure of the potential severity of periodontal disease and thus may be used to make evidence-based decisions regarding the frequency of dental visits for "routine periodontal evaluation." Given the potential significance of this work, further corroboration is necessary [16]. Conflicting viewpoints on this matter point to the need for additional research in assessing the validity of predictive biomarkers in determining disease risk [61, 62].

## Predictive Biomarkers Will Advance Personalized Oral Healthcare

Predictive biomarkers have been effectively employed for some time in cancer diagnosis and therapy, where they have been shown to have value in disease prognosis and in targeted cancer therapy [9, 13, 14, 63–65]. Biomarkers have been detected in blood, other body fluids, and tissues and have been shown to play a key role in drug development and pharmacotherapy [66–68]. Some of the most successful examples where biomarkers have had a significant impact in both predictive diagnosis and precision therapy is in cancer. Targeted therapies for the treatment of oral and head and neck squamous cell carcinoma (OHNSCC) fall into several categories of unique and overlapping targets. These include oncogenes, biomarkers associated with metastasis, gene amplifications, mutations and translocations, epigenetic alterations including DNA methylation, and alterations in histone proteins [66, 67, 69, 70]. Some of the more promising targets include receptors for epidermal growth factor (EGFR); vascular endothelial growth factor (VEGFR) that disrupt or block signaling pathways and networks that govern cell growth, cell motility, and survival; angiogenesis inhibitors that block tumor neovascularization and accelerate vascular normalization; and activation of immune response to tumor-associated antigens and unique biomarkers that identify less aggressive forms of OHNSCC, i.e., human papillomavirus associated, and more recently microRNAs [71–89]. A number of these agents are now in clinical trials, with other more promising targets soon to be forthcoming [71, 73–76, 81, 82, 84, 88, 89]. Patient management is clearly being improved with the use of biomarkers with existing drugs. This, along with increasing knowledge of gene expression and aberrant signaling pathways, should increase the number of drugs that can be more rationally prescribed and dosed using biomarkers and also broaden the use of established drugs [72, 77, 79, 80, 83, 85, 86, 90–92]. Although biomarkers have been reported to have value in assessing the risk of developing common dental diseases, until validated, their value in predicting risk or in early diagnosis and therapy remains to be determined [9, 16, 18, 61, 62].

## Personalized Oral Healthcare and the Learning Healthcare System

Much of the impetus driving the personalized healthcare environment is the recognition that the current system of fragmented care is inherently inefficient and costly [1–6, 15]. By focusing more on prevention and early intervention, the inherent value of personalized healthcare lies in its implementation in the setting of a learning healthcare system. As outlined in two Institute of Medicine (IOM) reports, a learning healthcare system is "one in which progress in science, informatics, and care culture align to generate new knowledge as an ongoing, natural by-product of the care experience, and seamlessly refine and deliver best practices for continuous improvement in health and health care" [51, 93–96].

Learning healthcare systems emphasize a collaborative approach to care and place great value on sharing information and insights across tradition practice boundaries to deliver better, more efficient patient care. Key to this vision is the creation of systems linked by a common electronic health record and shared databases. This interconnected system is informed by new evidence-based practice through clinical research, data analysis, modern information technology, and bioinformatics. Managing and communicating information guides the decisions made by health systems, providers, patients, and communities of interest. The learning health system creates a continuous cycle or feedback loop in which scientific evidence informs clinical practice, which in turn informs scientific investigation [51, 52, 93–97]. A learning healthcare system is one that is designed to generate and apply the best evidence for determining healthcare choices of each patient and provider, drives the process of discovery as a natural outgrowth of patient care, and ensures continued innovation, improved quality and safety, and value in healthcare. The key attributes of a learning healthcare system are adaptation to the pace of change, stronger synchrony of efforts, a culture of shared responsibility, support for clinical decision support systems, universal electronic health records that link databases for the public good, and trusted scientific leadership [51]. All of these initiatives—large-scale research networks, risk assessment and clinical support tools, point-of-care trials, and living guidelines—require a "paradigm shift" in healthcare, one that redefines the relationship between research and practice as a continuous feedback loop, with the application of evidence and a continuous learning environment complementing each other and flowing in both directions. As the personalized oral healthcare environment continues to evolve, it will become more complex, and providers will be increasingly judged according to the value they provide their patients through the rapid adoption and implementation of best practices [51, 52, 97]. When dentistry makes this shift to a learning healthcare system, we should see dramatic improvement in the quality of care, increased efficiencies, and better cost containment.

## Barriers to Adopting Personalized Oral Healthcare

Advances in prevention strategies, greater use of risk assessment, and the potential of biomarkers are likely to have a major effect on both clinical practice and the development of new drugs and diagnostics [9, 15, 27, 65]. Clinical biomarkers will be used to match specific therapies to specific patient characteristics. Addressing the salient ethical and legal issues facing personalized medicine underpins the regulatory framework and markets that drive its development and adoption. To make personalized oral healthcare more readily available to patients will require the rapid transition of basic, translational, and clinical research into marketable pharmaceuticals and devices. Additionally, regulatory oversight must facilitate the deployment of discovery efforts in the clinical setting while ensuring that ethical, legal, and social obligations are met. Strategic partnerships with researchers, clinicians, policy makers, and pharmaceutical and insurance companies will need to be developed. Only interdisciplinary discovery efforts and patient care alliances will enable breakthrough of scientific discoveries to lead to the development of new products and thereby contribute to strengthening the capacity for innovation while simultaneously reforming the healthcare system. Personalized oral healthcare should not be a promise for the future but one that embraces the rapid advancement of scientific and technological effort that offer patients and healthcare practitioners up-to-date diagnostics and therapeutics.

The most important challenges to implementation of personalized oral healthcare is the perceived lack of clinical utility, the reimbursement for clinically validated diagnostic biomarkers, regulatory uncertainty, protection of genetic information, and the preparedness of providers to incorporate genomic-based technologies into clinical practice. Still other challenges include existing structures and frameworks in our healthcare system, its inherent complexity, and the current inability to fast-track discovery science into the practice environment.

**Conclusions**

The deployment of new technologies designed to improve early diagnosis, prognosis, and treatment of chronic oral diseases should significantly benefit not only patients but also the medical device and pharmaceutical industry. Because of the complex nature of most chronic diseases, not all genetic loci may prove to be reliable predictors of disease onset or prognosis. As a consequence, the predictive potential of biomarkers and their usefulness as guides for the development of new targeted therapies will require more research. This may explain in part why the promise of personalized oral healthcare has been slow to translate into improvements in patient care and why only a limited number of targeted treatments are currently available. For some of the more common dental diseases, there is insufficient evident to support the routine use of genetic biomarkers in diagnosis, as reliable measures of disease risk, or as targeted therapies. As new technologies are developed and brought to market, there needs to be improved coordination and improved partnerships between public and private funding agencies while enabling fast-tracking on potential new therapies by regulatory agencies [27].

A personalized approach to oral healthcare has the potential to revolutionize dental practice. It also provides a unique opportunity to establish a mutually beneficial relationship between emerging medical technologies and new delivery systems in healthcare. If disruptive innovation is to drive personalized medicine, it will be necessary to take a more aggressive approach to innovation and discovery. A robust framework for continuing assessment and improved oversight of developing technologies will enhance the integrity of this process while enabling the rapid deployment of discovery science into the patient care environment. While there is unquestioned risk in this largely untested approach to healthcare, one has to ask if the benefits of investing in disruptive innovations to advance personalized healthcare is a risk worth taking. When one looks at the potential of a personalized approach in oral healthcare in advancing the future healthcare environment, the investment potential seems obvious.

## References

1. Institute of Medicine (U.S.). Committee on Quality of Health Care in America. Crossing the quality chasm: a new health system for the 21st century. Washington, DC: National Academy Press; 2001. p. xx, 337.
2. Snyderman R. Personalized health care: from theory to practice. Biotechnol J. 2012;7(8):973–9.
3. Snyderman R, Dinan MA. Improving health by taking it personally. JAMA. 2010;303(4):363–4.
4. Snyderman R, Williams RS. Prospective medicine: the next health care transformation. Acad Med. 2003; 78(11):1079–84.
5. Snyderman R, Yoediono Z. Prospective care: a personalized, preventative approach to medicine. Pharmacogenomics. 2006;7(1):5–9.
6. Snyderman R, Yoediono Z. Perspective: prospective health care and the role of academic medicine: lead, follow, or get out of the way. Acad Med. 2008;83(8): 707–14.

7. Garcia I, Kuska R, Somerman MJ. Expanding the foundation for personalized medicine: implications and challenges for dentistry. J Dent Res. 2013;92 (7 Suppl):3S–10.
8. Ginsburg GS, Willard HF. Genomic and personalized medicine: foundations and applications. Transl Res. 2009;154(6):277–87.
9. Godman B, Finlayson AE, Cheema PK, Zebedin-Brandl E, Gutierrez-Ibarluzea I, Jones J, et al. Personalizing health care: feasibility and future implications. BMC Med. 2013;11:179.
10. Kornman KS, Duff GW. Personalized medicine: will dentistry ride the wave or watch from the beach? J Dent Res. 2012;91(7 Suppl):8S–11.
11. Lehrach H, Consortium IFM. A revolution in healthcare: challenges and opportunities for personalized medicine. Pers Med. 2012;9(2):105–8.
12. Regierer B, Zazzu V, Sudbrak R, Kuhn A, Lehrach H. Future of medicine: models in predictive diagnostics and personalized medicine. Adv Biochem Eng Biotechnol. 2013;133:15–33.
13. Slavkin HC. From phenotype to genotype: enter genomics and transformation of primary health care around the world. J Dent Res. 2014;93(7 suppl):3S–6.
14. Slavkin HC, Santa Fe G. Revising the scope of practice for oral health professionals: enter genomics. J Am Dent Assoc (1939). 2014;145(3):228–30.
15. Teng K, Eng C, Hess CA, Holt MA, Moran RT, Sharp RR, et al. Building an innovative model for personalized healthcare. Cleve Clin J Med. 2012;79 Suppl 1:S1–9.
16. Giannobile WV, Braun TM, Caplis AK, Doucette-Stamm L, Duff GW, Kornman KS. Patient stratification for preventive care in dentistry. J Dent Res. 2013;92(8):694–701.
17. Chen R, Snyder M. Promise of personalized omics to precision medicine. Wiley Interdiscip Rev Syst Biol Med. 2013;5(1):73–82.
18. Abrahams E, Ginsburg GS, Silver M. The Personalized Medicine Coalition: goals and strategies. Am J Pharmacogenomics. 2005;5(6):345–55.
19. Crawford JM, Aspinall MG. The business value and cost-effectiveness of genomic medicine. Pers Med. 2012;9(3):265–86.
20. Annemans L, Redekop K, Payne K. Current methodological issues in the economic assessment of personalized medicine. Value Health. 2013;16(6):S20–6.
21. Hood L. Systems biology and p4 medicine: past, present, and future. Rambam Maimonides Med J. 2013; 4(2):e0012.
22. Hood L, Flores M. A personal view on systems medicine and the emergence of proactive P4 medicine: predictive, preventive, personalized and participatory. N Biotechnol. 2012;29(6):613–24.
23. Andrulis DP, Brach C. Integrating literacy, culture, and language to improve health care quality for diverse populations. Am J Health Behav. 2007;31 Suppl 1:S122–33.
24. Baker DW. The meaning and the measure of health literacy. J Gen Intern Med. 2006;21(8):878–83.
25. Baker DW, DeWalt DA, Schillinger D, Hawk V, Ruo B, Bibbins-Domingo K, et al. "Teach to goal": theory and design principles of an intervention to improve heart failure self-management skills of patients with low health literacy. J Health Commun. 2011;16 Suppl 3:73–88.
26. Hernandez LM, Institute of Medicine (U.S.). Roundtable on Health Literacy. How can health care organizations become more health literate: workshop summary. Washington, DC: National Academies Press; 2012. p. xiv, 108.
27. Rose N. Personalized medicine: promises, problems and perils of a new paradigm for healthcare. Procedia – Soc Behav Sci. 2013;77:341–52.
28. Christensen CM, Grossman JH, Hwang J. The innovator's prescription: a disruptive solution for health care. New York: McGraw-Hill; 2009. p. ii, 441.
29. Schulman KA, Vidal AV, Ackerly DC. Personalized medicine and disruptive innovation: implications for technology assessment. Genet Med. 2009;11(8): 577–81.
30. McInerney JD. Genetics education for health professionals: a context. J Genet Couns. 2008;17(2): 145–51.
31. Johnson L, Genco RJ, Damsky C, Haden NK, Hart S, Hart TC, et al. Genetics and its implications for clinical dental practice and education: report of panel 3 of the Macy study. J Dent Educ. 2008;72(2 Suppl): 86–94.
32. Skirton H, Lewis C, Kent A, Coviello DA, Members of Eurogentest U, Committee EE. Genetic education and the challenge of genomic medicine: development of core competences to support preparation of health professionals in Europe. Eur J Hum Genet. 2010; 18(9):972–7.
33. Guttmacher AE, Porteous ME, McInerney JD. Educating health-care professionals about genetics and genomics. Nat Rev Genet. 2007;8(2): 151–7.
34. Katsanis SH, Dungan JR, Gilliss CL, Ginsburg GA. Educating future providers of personalized medicine. N C Med J. 2013;74(6):491–2.
35. Annas GJ, Elias S. 23andMe and the FDA. N Engl J Med. 2014;370(23):2248–9.
36. Davies SM. Pharmacogenetics, pharmacogenomics and personalized medicine: are we there yet? Hematology. 2006:111–7.
37. Feero WG, Guttmacher AE, Collins FS. Genomic medicine–an updated primer. N Engl J Med. 2010; 362(21):2001–11.
38. Issa AM. Evaluating the value of genomic diagnostics: implications for clinical practice and public policy. Adv Health Econ Health Serv Res. 2008; 19:191–206.
39. Nibali L, Donos N, Henderson B. Periodontal infectogenomics. J Med Microbiol. 2009;58(Pt 10): 1269–74.
40. Tanke HJ. Genomics and proteomics: the potential role of oral diagnostics. Ann N Y Acad Sci. 2007; 1098:330–4.

41. West M, Ginsburg GS, Huang AT, Nevins JR. Embracing the complexity of genomic data for personalized medicine. Genome Res. 2006;16(5): 559–66.
42. Weston AD, Hood L. Systems biology, proteomics, and the future of health care: toward predictive, preventative, and personalized medicine. J Proteome Res. 2004;3(2):179–96.
43. Wright JT, Hart TC. The genome projects: implications for dental practice and education. J Dent Educ. 2002;66(5):659–71.
44. Haiech J, Kilhoffer MC. Personalized medicine and education: the challenge. Croat Med J. 2012; 53(4):298–300.
45. Salari K, Karczewski KJ, Hudgins L, Ormond KE. Evidence that personal genome testing enhances student learning in a course on genomics and personalized medicine. PLoS One. 2013;8(7):e68853.
46. Clancy TE, Fiks AG, Gelfand JM, Grayzel DS, Marci CD, McDonough CG, et al. A call for health policy education in the medical school curriculum. JAMA. 1995;274(13):1084–5.
47. Patel MS, Davis MM, Lypson ML. Advancing medical education by teaching health policy. N Engl J Med. 2011;364(8):695–7.
48. Patel MS, Lypson ML, Miller DD, Davis MM. A framework for evaluating student perceptions of health policy training in medical school. Acad Med. 2014;89(10):1375–9.
49. Freshman B, Rubino L, Chassiakos YR. Collaboration across the disciplines in health care. Sudbury: Jones and Bartlett Publishers; 2010. p. xl, 399.
50. Roberts DW. Improving care and practice through learning health systems. Nurs Manage. 2013;44(4):19–22.
51. Olsen L, Aisner D, McGinnis JM, Institute of Medicine (U.S.). Roundtable on Evidence-Based Medicine. The learning healthcare system: workshop summary. Washington, DC: National Academies Press; 2007. p. xx, 354.
52. Friedman C, Rubin J, Brown J, Buntin M, Corn M, Etheredge L, et al. Toward a science of learning systems: a research agenda for the high-functioning Learning Health System. J Am Med Inform Assoc. 2015;22(1):43–50.
53. Institute of Medicine (U.S.). Committee on an Oral Health Initiative. Advancing oral health in America. Washington, DC: National Academies Press; 2011. p. xviii, 248.
54. Greiner A, Knebel E, Institute of Medicine (U.S.). Board on Health Care Services., Institute of Medicine (U.S.). Committee on the Health Professions Education Summit. Health professions education: a bridge to quality. Washington, DC: National Academies Press; 2003. p. xvi, 175.
55. United States. Public Health Service. Healthy people 2000. Washington, DC: U.S. Department of Health and Human Services; 1991. p. vi, 154.
56. United States. Department of Health and Human Services. Healthy people 2010. Washington, DC: U.S. Department of Health and Human Services; 2000.
57. Committee on Oral Health Access to Services (U.S.), National Research Council (U.S.). Board on Children Youth and Families., Institute of Medicine (U.S.). Board on Health Care Services. Improving access to oral health care for vulnerable and underserved populations. Washington, DC: National Academies Press; 2011. p. xvii, 279.
58. Milgrom P, Garcia RI, Ismail A, Katz RV, Weintraub JA. Improving America's access to care: The National Institute of Dental and Craniofacial Research addresses oral health disparities. J Am Dent Assoc (1939). 2004;135(10):1389–96.
59. United States. Department of Health and Human Services., National Institute of Dental and Craniofacial Research (U.S.). Oral health in America: a report of the Surgeon General. Rockville: U.S. Public Health Service, Department of Health and Human Services; p. 2000. xxiv, 308.
60. Parker RM, Hernandez LM. Oral health literacy: a workshop. J Health Commun. 2012;17(10):1232–4.
61. Greenstein G, Hart TC. Clinical utility of a genetic susceptibility test for severe chronic periodontitis: a critical evaluation. J Am Dent Assoc (1939). 2002;133(4):452–9; quiz 92–3.
62. Greenstein G, Hart TC. A critical assessment of interleukin-1 (IL-1) genotyping when used in a genetic susceptibility test for severe chronic periodontitis. J Periodontol. 2002;73(2):231–47.
63. Glick M. Personalized oral health care: providing '-omic' answers to oral health care queries. J Am Dent Assoc (1939). 2012;143(2):102–4.
64. Glick M. The curious life of the biomarker. J Am Dent Assoc (1939). 2013;144(2):126–8.
65. Kalia M. Personalized oncology: recent advances and future challenges. Metabolism. 2013;62 Suppl 1: S11–4.
66. Miller AB, International Agency for Research on Cancer. Biomarkers in cancer chemoprevention. Lyon: International Agency for Research on Cancer; 2001. p. x, 294.
67. Lenz H-J. Biomarkers in oncology: prediction and prognosis. New York: Springer; 2013. p. xvi, 447.
68. Henry NL, Hayes DF. Cancer biomarkers. Mol Oncol. 2012;6(2):140–6.
69. Williams SD, Hughes TE, Adler CJ, Brook AH, Townsend GC. Epigenetics: a new frontier in dentistry. Aust Dent J. 2014;59 Suppl 1:23–33.
70. Williams MD. Integration of biomarkers including molecular targeted therapies in head and neck cancer. Head Neck Pathol. 2010;4(1):62–9.
71. National Cancer Institute Clinical Trials [updated 2014]. Available from: http://www.cancer.gov/clinicaltrials.

72. Agrawal N, Frederick MJ, Pickering CR, Bettegowda C, Chang K, Li RJ, et al. Exome sequencing of head and neck squamous cell carcinoma reveals inactivating mutations in NOTCH1. Science. 2011;333(6046):1154–7.
73. Bernier J. Drug insight: cetuximab in the treatment of recurrent and metastatic squamous cell carcinoma of the head and neck. Nat Clin Pract Oncol. 2008;5(12):705–13.
74. Bernier J. Incorporation of molecularly targeted agents in the primary treatment of squamous cell carcinomas of the head and neck. Hematol Oncol Clin North Am. 2008;22(6):1193–208, ix.
75. Dorsey K, Agulnik M. Promising new molecular targeted therapies in head and neck cancer. Drugs. 2013;73(4):315–25.
76. Erjala K, Sundvall M, Junttila TT, Zhang N, Savisalo M, Mali P, et al. Signaling via ErbB2 and ErbB3 associates with resistance and epidermal growth factor receptor (EGFR) amplification with sensitivity to EGFR inhibitor gefitinib in head and neck squamous cell carcinoma cells. Clin Cancer Res. 2006;12(13):4103–11.
77. Folkman J. What is the evidence that tumors are angiogenesis dependent? J Natl Cancer Inst. 1990;82(1):4–6.
78. Glazer CA, Chang SS, Ha PK, Califano JA. Applying the molecular biology and epigenetics of head and neck cancer in everyday clinical practice. Oral Oncol. 2009;45(4–5):440–6.
79. Jimeno A, Kulesza P, Wheelhouse J, Chan A, Zhang X, Kincaid E, et al. Dual EGFR and mTOR targeting in squamous cell carcinoma models, and development of early markers of efficacy. Br J Cancer. 2007;96(6):952–9.
80. Mineta H, Miura K, Ogino T, Takebayashi S, Misawa K, Ueda Y, et al. Prognostic value of vascular endothelial growth factor (VEGF) in head and neck squamous cell carcinomas. Br J Cancer. 2000;83(6):775–81.
81. Morgillo F, Bareschino MA, Bianco R, Tortora G, Ciardiello F. Primary and acquired resistance to anti-EGFR targeted drugs in cancer therapy. Differentiation. 2007;75(9):788–99.
82. Nathan CO, Amirghahari N, Rong X, Giordano T, Sibley D, Nordberg M, et al. Mammalian target of rapamycin inhibitors as possible adjuvant therapy for microscopic residual disease in head and neck squamous cell cancer. Cancer Res. 2007;67(5):2160–8.
83. Olsson AK, Dimberg A, Kreuger J, Claesson-Welsh L. VEGF receptor signalling – in control of vascular function. Nat Rev Mol Cell Biol. 2006;7(5):359–71.
84. Pfister DG, Su YB, Kraus DH, Wolden SL, Lis E, Aliff TB, et al. Concurrent cetuximab, cisplatin, and concomitant boost radiotherapy for locoregionally advanced, squamous cell head and neck cancer: a pilot phase II study of a new combined-modality paradigm. J Clin Oncol. 2006;24(7):1072–8.
85. Prince A, Aguirre-Ghizo J, Genden E, Posner M, Sikora A. Head and neck squamous cell carcinoma: new translational therapies. Mt Sinai J Med. 2010;77(6):684–99.
86. Scanlon CS, D'Silva NJ. Personalized medicine for cancer therapy: lessons learned from tumor-associated antigens. Oncoimmunology. 2013;2(4):e23433.
87. Shirai K, O'Brien PE. Molecular targets in squamous cell carcinoma of the head and neck. Curr Treat Options Oncol. 2007;8(3):239–51.
88. Stransky N, Egloff AM, Tward AD, Kostic AD, Cibulskis K, Sivachenko A, et al. The mutational landscape of head and neck squamous cell carcinoma. Science. 2011;333(6046):1157–60.
89. Vermorken JB, Mesia R, Rivera F, Remenar E, Kawecki A, Rottey S, et al. Platinum-based chemotherapy plus cetuximab in head and neck cancer. N Engl J Med. 2008;359(11):1116–27.
90. Scully C, Bagan JV. Recent advances in Oral Oncology 2007: imaging, treatment and treatment outcomes. Oral Oncol. 2008;44(3):211–5.
91. Sethi S, Ali S, Sethi S, Sarkar FH. MicroRNAs in personalized cancer therapy. Clin Genet. 2014;86(1):68–73.
92. Wang Y, Alam GN, Ning Y, Visioli F, Dong Z, Nor JE, et al. The unfolded protein response induces the angiogenic switch in human tumor cells through the PERK/ATF4 pathway. Cancer Res. 2012;72(20):5396–406.
93. Grossmann C, Institute of Medicine (U.S.), Roundtable on Value & Science-driven Health Care, National Academy of Engineering. Engineering a learning healthcare system: a look at the future: workshop summary. Washington, DC: National Academies Press; 2011. p. xxiii, 313.
94. Rouse WB, Cortese DA. Engineering the system of healthcare delivery. Amsterdam: IOS Press; 2010. p. viii, 481.
95. Institute of Medicine (U.S.), McClellan MB. Evidence-based medicine and the changing nature of health care: 2007 IOM annual meeting summary. Washington, DC: The National Academies Press; 2008. p. xii, 190.
96. Olsen L, Goolsby WA, McGinnis JM, Institute of Medicine (U.S.), Roundtable on Evidence-based Medicine. Leadership commitments to improve value in health care: finding common ground workshop summary. Washington, DC: National Academies Press; 2009. p. xix, 347.
97. Friedman CP, Wong AK, Blumenthal D. Achieving a nationwide learning health system. Sci Transl Med. 2010;2(57):57cm29.

# Index




P.J. Polverini (ed.), *Personalized Oral Health Care: From Concept Design to Clinical Practice*,
DOI 10.1007/978-3-319-23297-3